Nutrition Diagnosis and Intervention:

Standardized Language for the Nutrition Care Process

Nutrition Diagnosis and Intervention:
Standardized Language for the Nutrition Care Process
ISBN: 978-0-88091-366-9

10 9 8 7 6 5 4 3 2 1

Nutrition Diagnosis and Intervention:
Standardized Language for the Nutrition Care Process

Table of Contents

Nutrition Diagnosis and Intervention:
Standardized Language for the Nutrition Care Process

Table of Contents

Please check the ADA Web site (http://www.eatright.org) for additional materials. Sign in as a member and select Research from the sidebar or Practice from the sidebar and then Quality Management.

Nutrition Diagnosis and Intervention:
Standardized Language for the Nutrition Care Process

Publication Highlights

PUBLICATIONS RELATED TO THE NUTRITION CARE PROCESS

Since its development, several publications related to the Nutrition Care Process have been developed by the American Dietetic Association (ADA). In addition to this publication, there are two articles published in the *Journal of the American Dietetic Association* and one publication available regarding the Nutrition Care Process and Model. The original article published in the 2003 *Journal* described the complete nutrition care process (1). Another 2005 *Journal* article described the implementation of Nutrition Diagnosis, Step 2 in the nutrition care process (2). Similarly, the first publication, entitled *Nutrition Diagnosis: A Critical Step in the Nutrition Care Process,* examined only Nutrition Diagnosis (3).

This publication is intended to illustrate the evolution of the nutrition care process since its introduction in 2003 and provide tools for practitioners to implement the nutrition care process into their practice.

NEW IN THIS PUBLICATION

This publication addresses the first three steps in the nutrition care process: Nutrition Assessment, Nutrition Diagnosis, and Nutrition Intervention.

The **Nutrition Assessment** section is **NEW** and provides a matrix illustrating the nutrition assessment data associated with the nutrition diagnoses. It is beyond the scope of this publication to define the nutrition assessment data with a standard taxonomy, as this has been done elsewhere in the dietetics literature.

The **Nutrition Diagnosis** section reflects the **CHANGES** to the nutrition diagnoses since the publication of the book—*Nutrition Diagnosis: A Critical Step in the Nutrition Care Process*—introduced at ADA's 2005 Food and Nutrition Conference and Exhibition.

The **Nutrition Intervention** section is **NEW** and uses a standard taxonomy to describe the nutrition interventions performed by dietetics professionals. A research study is underway to assess the usability and validity in clinical settings of the terms. The taxonomy is grouped into four classes of nutrition interventions: Food and/or Nutrient Delivery, Nutrition Education, Nutrition Counseling, and Coordination of Care. The terminology used is defined and reference sheets for each specific nutrition intervention are available for use now by the profession. A practitioner will note that while some interventions are very closely related (e.g., education and counseling), the terms are intentionally separated to distinguish between them. Further, it is believed that the information necessary for medical record documentation, billing, and the description of the nutrition interventions for research are included in the terminology.

The nutrition intervention section describes the two interrelated components of nutrition intervention—planning and implementation. It also illustrates how the nutrition diagnosis statement, also called the PES (problem, etiology, signs/symptoms) statement, labels the problems and identifies where the nutrition intervention is aimed to address the problem. Specific descriptors (e.g., individuals or groups, face to face or electronically) of a nutrition intervention encounter (i.e., interactions, visits, contacts, sessions) are also provided.

NOT INCLUDED IN THIS PUBLICATION

The **Nutrition Monitoring and Evaluation** (Step 4) section was deliberately omitted from this publication since a great deal of research is underway regarding the nutrition diagnosis and nutrition intervention terminology that may impact the nutrition monitoring and evaluation component of the nutrition care process. Therefore, the research data will be examined before terms are defined and categorized for this step. Future publications will provide updates to the first three steps and examine the fourth and final step, nutrition monitoring and evaluation.

REFERENCES

1. Lacey K, Pritchett E. Nutrition care process and model: ADA adopts road map to quality care and outcomes management. *J Am Diet Assoc.* 2003;103:1061-1072.
2. Mathieu J, Foust M, Ouellette P. Implementing nutrition diagnosis, step two in the nutrition care process and model: Challenges and lesions learned in two health care facilities. *J Am Diet Assoc.* 2005;105:1636-1640.
3. American Dietetic Association. *Nutrition Diagnosis: A Critical Step in the Nutrition Care Process.* Chicago, IL: American Dietetic Association; 2006.

Nutrition Diagnosis and Intervention:
Standardized Language for the Nutrition Care Process

INTRODUCTION

Continually emerging from the American Dietetic Association's (ADA) strategic plan are priority actions that guide work groups and taskforces in creating tools to advance the dietetics profession. In 2002, to achieve the Association's strategic goals of promoting demand for dietetic professionals and help them be more competitive in the marketplace, the ADA Quality Management Committee appointed the Nutrition Care Model Workgroup. This Workgroup developed the Nutrition Care Process and Model, a systematic process describing how dietetics professionals provide care with patients/clients (1).

The nutrition care process is designed to improve the consistency and quality of individualized patient/client care and the predictability of the patient/client outcomes. It is not intended to standardize nutrition care for each patient/client but to establish a standardized process for providing care. Of note, the terms patient/client are used in association with the nutrition care process; however, the process is also intended for use with groups. In addition, family members or caregivers of patients/clients are not specified, yet they can be an essential asset to the patient/client and professional in the nutrition care process. Therefore, groups and families and caregivers of patients/clients are implied each time a reference is made to patient/client.

There are four steps in the process—Nutrition Assessment, Nutrition Diagnosis, Nutrition Intervention, and Nutrition Monitoring and Evaluation. Three of the nutrition care process steps are very familiar to dietetics professionals and nutrition textbooks skillfully cover their content— nutrition assessment, nutrition intervention, and nutrition monitoring and evaluation. However, the Workgroup identified a less well-defined aspect of nutrition care: nutrition diagnosis. Further, it recognized that a standard taxonomy for the second step in the process would greatly enhance the profession's ability to document, communicate, and research its impact.

As a result, the ADA's Standardized Language Task Force was formed to create a taxonomy for the profession's unique nutrition diagnosis language. The language was described during presentations at the 2005 Food and Nutrition Conference and Exhibition and made available in a publication at that meeting (2). This language is currently being studied in a number of research projects and future modifications will be made based on these analyses.

Because the nutrition care process and, in particular, nutrition diagnosis represent a monumental change in the approach to nutrition services, the Standardized Language Task Force has examined, to this point, two other steps in the process: nutrition assessment and nutrition intervention. Therefore, this publication illustrates the evolution of the nutrition care process and provides tools for practitioners to implement the process into their practice.

NUTRITION CARE PROCESS STEPS

Step 1. Nutrition Assessment

Nutrition assessment is the first step in the process and is a method for obtaining, verifying, and interpreting data that is needed to identify a nutrition-related problem. From the nutrition assessment data, the practitioner is able to determine whether a nutrition diagnosis/problem exists. This step, while well-known to practitioners, offers many opportunities for continued research, which will result in improved determinations of the most appropriate nutrition assessment data to use for individuals and populations.

Step 2: Nutrition Diagnosis

Nutrition diagnosis is the new component in the nutrition care process, and is a critical step between nutrition assessment and nutrition intervention. The purpose of a standardized nutrition diagnosis language is to consistently describe nutrition problems so that they are clear within and outside the profession. The standard language will enhance communication and documentation of nutrition care, and it will provide a minimum data set and common data elements for future research.

In simple terms, a nutrition diagnosis identifies and labels a specific nutrition problem that a dietetics professional is responsible for treating independently. A nutrition diagnosis is often temporary, and with nutrition intervention the nutrition diagnosis ideally resolves. This is in contrast to medical diagnosis, which is a disease or pathology of organs or body systems (e.g., diabetes), and does not change as long as the condition exists.

ADA's Standardized Language Task Force developed a framework that outlines three domains—Clinical, Intake, and Behavioral-Environmental—within which the diagnoses/problems fall. Sixty-two diagnoses/problems have been identified. A reference was developed and it describes each diagnosis/problem and incorporates expert input (2).

It is this step in the nutrition care process that results in the nutrition diagnosis statement or PES statement. This statement is composed of three distinct components: the problem (P), the etiology (E) and the signs and symptoms (S). The PES statement is derived from the synthesis of information from the nutrition assessment data.

Step 3: Nutrition Intervention

Nutrition intervention is the third step in the nutrition care process. Nutrition interventions are specific actions used to remedy a nutrition diagnosis/problem, and can be used with individuals, a group, or the community at large. These Interventions are intended to change a nutrition-related behavior, risk factor, environmental condition, or aspect of nutritional health. A dietetics professional collaborates, whenever possible, with the patient/client(s) and other health care providers during the nutrition intervention.

Nutrition intervention consists of two interrelated components—planning and implementation. Planning involves prioritizing the nutrition diagnoses; conferring with the patient, others, and practice guides and policies; jointly establishing goals; and defining the nutrition prescription and specific nutrition intervention. Implementing the nutrition intervention is the action phase, which includes carrying out and communicating the plan of care, continuing the data collection, and revising the nutrition intervention, as warranted, based on the patient/client response. This step cannot be completed unless both components are in place to support the nutrition intervention.

The nutrition intervention is, almost always, aimed at the etiology (E) of the nutrition diagnosis/problem identified in the PES statement. In very specific instances, the nutrition intervention is directed at the signs and symptoms (S) to reduce the signs and symptoms. Generally the signs and symptoms form the basis for the next step in the nutrition care process: nutrition monitoring and evaluation (Step 4).

Four main classes of nutrition intervention have been identified—Food and/or Nutrient Provision, Nutrition Education, Nutrition Counseling, and Coordination of Care. The terminology is defined and reference sheets for each specific nutrition intervention are available for use by the profession. It is believed that the information necessary for medical record documentation, billing, and the description of the nutrition interventions for research are included in the terminology.

A practitioner will note that while some interventions are closely related (e.g., education and counseling), the terms are intentionally separated to distinguish between them. Additionally, specific descriptors of a nutrition intervention encounter (i.e., interactions, visits, contacts, sessions) are provided to assist a practitioner with the details of his/her encounters with patient/client(s). Examples of descriptors include encounters with individuals or groups, face to face or electronically, and the degree to which the practitioner is responsible for the patient/client care, to name a few.

Step 4: Nutrition Monitoring and Evaluation
A great deal of progress has been made in articulating the first three nutrition care process steps. Research is underway and a deliberate decision was made to review the data emerging from the nutrition diagnosis and nutrition intervention terms before work is attempted to categorize and define terms for this step. Dietetics professionals should continue to employ nutrition monitoring and evaluation strategies and tools that are currently available until this step is further defined in the context of the nutrition care process.

NUTRITION CARE PROCESS AND MEDICAL NUTRITION THERAPY

The nutrition care process and medical nutrition therapy (MNT) are not synonymous terms. MNT is one aspect of nutrition care, whereas, the nutrition care process describes the approach to a spectrum of nutrition care. The nutrition care process defines specific steps a practitioner uses when providing MNT. Other activities, such as referral to a community program, are not MNT, but are part of the nutrition care process.

IMPLEMENTATION OF THE NUTRITION CARE PROCESS AND FUTURE DIRECTIONS

Several exciting projects are ongoing, including pilot tests of individual steps as well as multiple steps in the nutrition care process. Although it may seem practical to wait until the nutrition care process is fully articulated, practitioners and educators are encouraged to use the nutrition care process now and participate in its development and evolution.

International Information Sharing and Standardized Medical Languages

In 2005, the ADA Foundation funded an ADA hosted meeting to expand the dialogue with other international dietetic associations about ADA's standardized nutrition diagnosis language and similar efforts other associations have made. The meeting also initiated a dialogue between the foremost medical informatics organizations and the international nutrition and dietetics community.

Indeed, as the world moves fully into electronic health care records, health informatics, and common databases, the international community of nutrition and dietetics professionals have the opportunity to work in partnership with the medical informatics organizations to ensure that data elements critical to capturing nutrition care are included in databases and collected in a consistent way.

When these relationships are established, ADA will formally submit the nutrition diagnosis terms to the nationally recognized health care databases and medical informatics languages and request that the terms are added to their language databases.

SUMMARY

This publication illustrates, to date, the first three steps in the nutrition care process and provides tools for practitioners to implement the process in their practice. Future publications will provide updates to the first three steps and examine the fourth and final step: nutrition monitoring and evaluation.

From conception of the nutrition care process in 2002 through its implementation now, the Standardized Language Task Force continues to update ADA's House of Delegates, the Board of Directors, and members through reports, articles, presentations, publications, and the ADA Web site.

However, to see the strategic goals of an increased demand for dietetic professionals who are more competitive in the marketplace come to fruition, professionals need to take a historic step by implementing the nutrition care process today.

REFERENCES

1. Lacey K, Pritchett E. Nutrition care process and model: ADA adopts road map to quality care and outcomes management. *J Am Diet Assoc.* 2003;103:1061-1072.
2. American Dietetic Association. *Nutrition Diagnosis: A Critical Step in the Nutrition Care Process.* Chicago, IL: American Dietetic Association; 2006.

Nutrition Care Process and Model: ADA adopts road map to quality care and outcomes management

KAREN LACEY, MS, RD; ELLEN PRITCHETT, RD

The establishment and implementation of a standardized Nutrition Care Process (NCP) and Model were identified as priority actions for the profession for meeting goals of the ADA Strategic Plan to "Increase demand and utilization of services provided by members" and "Empower members to compete successfully in a rapidly changing environment" (1). Providing high-quality nutrition care means doing the right thing at the right time, in the right way, for the right person, and achieving the best possible results. Quality improvement literature shows that, when a standardized process is implemented, less variation and more predictability in terms of outcomes occur (2). When providers of care, no matter their location, use a process consistently, comparable outcomes data can be generated to demonstrate value. A standardized Nutrition Care Process effectively promotes the dietetics professional as the unique provider of nutrition care when it is consistently used as a systematic method to think critically and make decisions to provide safe and effective nutrition care (3).

This article describes the four steps of ADA's Nutrition Care Process and the overarching framework of the Nutrition Care Model that illustrates the context within which the Nutrition Care Process occurs. In addition, this article provides the rationale for a standardized process by which nutrition care is provided, distinguishes between the Nutrition Care Process and Medical Nutrition Therapy (MNT), and discusses future implications for the profession.

BACKGROUND

Prior to the adoption of this standardized Nutrition Care Process, a variety of nutrition care processes were utilized by practitioners and taught by dietetics educators. Other allied health

K. Lacey is lecturer and Director of Dietetic Programs at the University of Wisconsin-Green Bay, Green Bay. She is also the Chair of the Quality Management Committee. E. Pritchett is Director, Quality and Outcomes at ADA headquarters in Chicago, IL.

If you have questions regarding the Nutrition Care Process and Model, please contact Ellen Pritchett, RD, CPHQ, Director of Quality and Outcomes at ADA, eprtitchett@eatright.org

professionals, including nursing, physical therapy, and occupational therapy, utilize defined care processes specific to their profession (4-6). When asked whether ADA should develop a standardized Nutrition Care Process, dietetics professionals were overwhelmingly in favor and strongly supportive of having a standardized Nutrition Care Process for use by registered dietitians (RD) and dietetics technicians, registered (DTR).

The Quality Management Committee of the House of Delegates (HOD) appointed a Nutrition Care Model Workgroup in May 2002 to develop a nutrition care process and model. The first draft was presented to the HOD for member input and review in September 2002. Further discussion occurred during the October 2002 HOD meeting, in Philadelphia. Revisions were made accordingly, and the HOD unanimously adopted the final version of the Nutrition Care Process and Model on March 31, 2003 "for implementation and dissemination to the dietetics profession and the Association for the enhancement of the practice of dietetics."

SETTING THE STAGE

Definition of Quality/Rationale for a Standardized Process

The National Academy of Science's (NAS) Institute of Medicine (IOM) has defined quality as "The degree to which health services for individuals and populations increase the likelihood of desired health outcomes and are consistent with current professional knowledge" (7,8). The quality performance of providers can be assessed by measuring the following: (a) their patients' outcomes (end-results) or (b) the degree to which providers adhere to an accepted care process (7,8). The Committee on Quality of Health Care in America further states that it is not acceptable to have a wide quality chasm, or a gap, between *actual* and *best possible* performance (9). In an effort to ensure that dietetics professionals can meet both requirements for quality performance noted above, the American Dietetic Association (ADA) supports a standardized Nutrition Care Process for the profession.

Standardized Process versus Standardized Care

ADA's Nutrition Care Process is a standardized process for dietetics professionals and not a means to provide standardized care. A standardized process refers to a consistent structure and framework used to provide nutrition care, whereas stan-

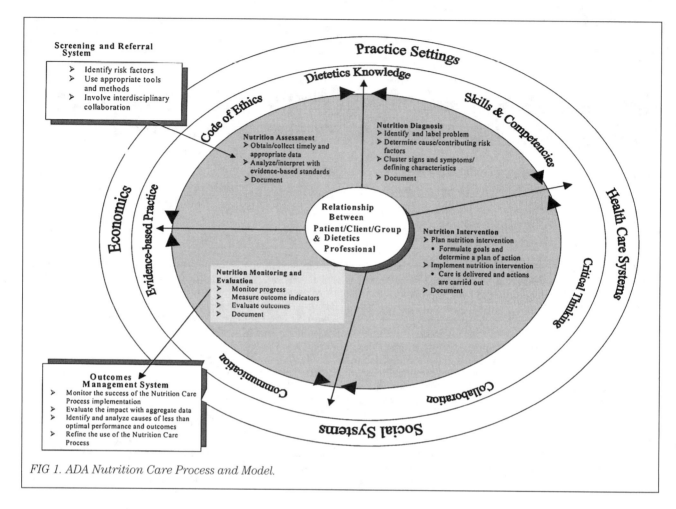

FIG 1. ADA Nutrition Care Process and Model.

dardized care infers that all patients/clients receive the same care. This process supports and promotes individualized care, not standardized care. As represented in the model (Figure 1), the relationship between the patient/client/group and dietetics professional is at the core of the nutrition care process. Therefore, nutrition care provided by qualified dietetics professionals should always reflect both the state of the science and the state of the art of dietetics practice to meet the individualized needs of each patient/client/group (10).

Using the NCP
Even though ADA's Nutrition Care Process will primarily be used to provide nutrition care to individuals in health care settings (inpatient, ambulatory, and extended care), the process also has applicability in a wide variety of community settings. It will be used by dietetics professionals to provide nutrition care to both individuals and groups in community-based agencies and programs for the purpose of health promotion and disease prevention (11,12).

Key Terms
To lay the groundwork and facilitate a clear definition of ADA's Nutrition Care Process, key terms were developed. These definitions provide a frame of reference for the specific components and their functions.

(a) Process is a series of connected steps or actions to achieve an outcome and/or any activity or set of activities that transforms inputs to outputs.

(b) Process Approach is the systematic identification and management of activities and the interactions between activities. A process approach emphasizes the importance of the following:
- understanding and meeting requirements;
- determining if the process adds value;
- determining process performance and effectiveness; and
- using objective measurement for continual improvement of the process (13).

(c) Critical Thinking integrates facts, informed opinions, active listening and observations. It is also a reasoning process in which ideas are produced and evaluated. The Commission on Accreditation of Dietetics Education (CADE) defines critical thinking as "transcending the boundaries of formal education to explore a problem and form a hypothesis and a defensible conclusion" (14). The use of critical thinking provides a unique strength that dietetics professionals bring to the Nutrition Care Process. Further characteristics of critical thinking include the ability to do the following:
- conceptualize;
- think rationally;
- think creatively;
- be inquiring; and
- think autonomously.

Edition: 2007   8

(d) Decision Making is a critical process for choosing the best action to meet a desired goal.

(e) Problem Solving is the process of the following:

- problem identification;
- solution formation;
- implementation; and
- evaluation of the results.

(f) Collaboration is a process by which several individuals or groups with shared concerns are united to address an identified problem or need, leading to the accomplishment of what each could not do separately (15).

DEFINITION OF ADA'S NCP

Using the terms and concepts described above, ADA's Nutrition Care Process is defined as "a systematic problem-solving method that dietetics professionals use to critically think and make decisions to address nutrition related problems and provide safe and effective quality nutrition care."

The Nutrition Care Process consists of four distinct, but interrelated and connected steps: (a) Nutrition Assessment, (b) Nutrition Diagnosis, (c) Nutrition Intervention, and d) Nutrition Monitoring and Evaluation. These four steps were finalized based on extensive review and evaluation of previous works describing nutrition care (16-24). Even though each step builds on the previous one, the process is not linear. Critical thinking and problem solving will frequently require that dietetics professionals revisit previous steps to reassess, add, or revise nutrition diagnoses; modify intervention strategies; and/or evaluate additional outcomes. Figure 2 describes each of these four steps in a similar format consisting of the following:

- definition and purpose;
- key components or substeps with examples as appropriate;
- critical thinking characteristics;
- documentation elements; and
- considerations for continuation, discontinuation, or discharge of care.

Providing nutrition care using ADA's Nutrition Care Process begins when a patient/client/group has been identified at nutrition risk and needs further assistance to achieve or maintain nutrition and health goals. It is also important to recognize that patients/clients who enter the health care system are more likely to have nutrition problems and therefore benefit from receiving nutrition care in this manner. The Nutrition Care Process cycles through the steps of assessment, diagnosis, intervention, and monitoring and evaluation. Nutrition care can involve one or more cycles and ends, ideally, when nutrition goals have been achieved. However, the patient/client/group may choose to end care earlier based on personal or external factors. Using professional judgment, the dietetics professional may discharge the patient/client/group when it is determined that no further progress is likely.

PURPOSE OF NCP

ADA's Nutrition Care Process, as described in Figure 2, gives dietetics professionals a consistent and systematic structure and method by which to think critically and make decisions. It also assists dietetics professionals to scientifically and holistically manage nutrition care, thus helping patients better meet their health and nutrition goals. As dietetics professionals consistently use the Nutrition Care Process, one should expect a higher probability of producing good outcomes. The Nutrition Care Process then begins to establish a link between quality

and professional autonomy. Professional autonomy results from being recognized for what we do *well*, not just for who we are. When quality can be demonstrated, as defined previously by the IOM (7,8), then dietetics professionals will stand out as the preferred providers of nutrition services. The Nutrition Care Process, when used consistently, also challenges dietetics professionals to move beyond experience-based practice to reach a higher level of evidence-based practice (9,10).

The Nutrition Care Process does not restrict practice but acknowledges the common dimensions of practice by the following:

- defining a common language that allows nutrition practice to be more measurable;
- creating a format that enables the process to generate quantitative and qualitative data that can then be analyzed and interpreted; and
- serving as the structure to validate nutrition care and showing how the nutrition care that was provided does what it intends to do.

DISTINCTION BETWEEN MNT AND THE NCP

Medical Nutrition Therapy (MNT) was first defined by ADA in the mid-1990s to promote the benefits of managing or treating a disease with nutrition. Its components included an assessment of nutritional status of patients and the provision of either diet modification, counseling, or specialized nutrition therapies. MNT soon became a widely used term to describe a wide variety of nutrition care services provided by dietetics professionals. Since MNT was first introduced, dietetics professionals have gained much credibility among legislators and other health care providers. More recently, MNT has been redefined as part of the 2001 Medicare MNT benefit legislation to be "nutritional diagnostic, therapy, and counseling services for the purpose of disease management, which are furnished by a registered dietitian or nutrition professional" (25).

The intent of the NCP is to describe accurately the spectrum of nutrition care that can be provided by dietetics professionals. Dietetics professionals are uniquely qualified by virtue of academic and supervised practice training and appropriate certification and/or licensure to provide a comprehensive array of professional services relating to the prevention or treatment of nutrition-related illness (14,26). MNT is but one specific type of nutrition care. The NCP articulates the consistent and specific steps a dietetics professional would use when delivering MNT, but it will also be used to guide nutrition education and other preventative nutrition care services. One of the key distinguishing characteristics between MNT and the other nutrition services using the NCP is that MNT always involves an in-depth, comprehensive assessment and individualized care. For example, one individual could receive MNT for diabetes and also nutrition education services or participate in a community-based weight loss program (27). Each service would use the Nutrition Care Process, but the process would be implemented differently; the components of each step of the process would be tailored to the type of service.

By articulating the steps of the Nutrition Care Process, the commonalities (the consistent, standardized, four-step process) of nutrition care are emphasized even though the process is implemented differently for different nutrition services. With a standardized Nutrition Care Process in place, MNT should not be used to describe all of the nutrition services that dietetics professionals provide. As noted above, MNT is the only application of the Nutrition Care Process (28-31). This change in

STEP 1. NUTRITION ASSESSMENT

Basic Definition & Purpose	**"Nutrition Assessment"** is the first step of the Nutrition Care Process. Its purpose is to obtain adequate information in order to identify nutrition-related problems. It is initiated by referral and/or screening of individuals or groups for nutritional risk factors. Nutrition assessment is a systematic process of obtaining, verifying, and interpreting data in order to make decisions about the nature and cause of nutrition-related problems. The specific types of data gathered in the assessment will vary depending on a) practice settings, b) individual/groups' present health status, c) how data are related to outcomes to be measured, d) recommended practices such as ADA's Evidence Based Guides for Practice and e) whether it is an initial assessment or a reassessment. Nutrition assessment requires making comparisons between the information obtained and reliable standards (ideal goals). Nutrition assessment is an on-going, dynamic process that involves not only initial data collection, but also continual reassessment and analysis of patient/client/group needs. Assessment provides the foundation for the nutrition diagnosis at the next step of the Nutrition Care Process.
Data Sources/Tools for Assessment	■ Referral information and/or interdisciplinary records ■ Patient/client interview (across the lifespan) ■ Community-based surveys and focus groups ■ Statistical reports; administrative data ■ Epidemiological studies
Types of Data Collected	■ Nutritional Adequacy (dietary history/detailed nutrient intake) ■ Health Status (anthropometric and biochemical measurements, physical & clinical conditions, physiological and disease status) ■ Functional and Behavioral Status (social and cognitive function, psychological and emotional factors, quality-of-life measures, change readiness)
Nutrition Assessment Components	■ Review dietary intake for factors that affect health conditions and nutrition risk ■ Evaluate health and disease condition for nutrition-related consequences ■ Evaluate psychosocial, functional, and behavioral factors related to food access, selection, preparation, physical activity, and understanding of health condition ■ Evaluate patient/client/group's knowledge, readiness to learn, and potential for changing behaviors ■ Identify standards by which data will be compared ■ Identify possible problem areas for making nutrition diagnoses
Critical Thinking	The following types of critical thinking skills are especially needed in the assessment step: ■ Observing for nonverbal and verbal cues that can guide and prompt effective interviewing methods; ■ Determining appropriate data to collect; ■ Selecting assessment tools and procedures (matching the assessment method to the situation); ■ Applying assessment tools in valid and reliable ways; ■ Distinguishing relevant from irrelevant data; ■ Distinguishing important from unimportant data; ■ Validating the data; ■ Organizing & categorizing the data in a meaningful framework that relates to nutrition problems; and ■ Determining when a problem requires consultation with or referral to another provider.
Documentation of Assessment	Documentation is an on-going process that supports all of the steps in the Nutrition Care Process. Quality documentation of the assessment step should be relevant, accurate, and timely. Inclusion of the following information would further describe quality assessment documentation: ■ Date and time of assessment; ■ Pertinent data collected and comparison with standards; ■ Patient/client/groups' perceptions, values, and motivation related to presenting problems; ■ Changes in patient/client/group's level of understanding, food-related behaviors, and other clinical outcomes for appropriate follow-up; and ■ Reason for discharge/discontinuation if appropriate.
Determination for Continuation of Care	If upon the completion of an initial or reassessment it is determined that the problem cannot be modified by further nutrition care, discharge or discontinuation from this episode of nutrition care may be appropriate.

FIG 2. ADA Nutrition Care Process.

Edition: 2007

10

STEP 2. NUTRITION DIAGNOSIS

Basic Definition & Purpose	**"Nutrition Diagnosis"** is the second step of the Nutrition Care Process, and is the identification and labeling that describes an actual occurrence, risk of, or potential for developing a nutritional problem that dietetics professionals are responsible for treating independently. At the end of the assessment step, data are clustered, analyzed, and synthesized. This will reveal a nutrition diagnostic category from which to formulate a specific nutrition diagnostic statement. Nutrition diagnosis should not be confused with medical diagnosis, which can be defined as a disease or pathology of specific organs or body systems that can be treated or prevented. A nutrition diagnosis changes as the patient/client/group's response changes. A medical diagnosis does not change as long as the disease or condition exists. A patient/client/group may have the medical diagnosis of "Type 2 diabetes mellitus"; however, after performing a nutrition assessment, dietetics professionals may diagnose, for example, "undesirable overweight status" or "excessive carbohydrate intake." Analyzing assessment data and naming the nutrition diagnosis(es) provide a link to setting realistic and measurable expected outcomes, selecting appropriate interventions, and tracking progress in attaining those expected outcomes.
Data Sources/Tools for Diagnosis	■ Organized and clustered assessment data ■ List(s) of nutrition diagnostic categories and nutrition diagnostic labels ■ Currently the profession does not have a standardized list of nutrition diagnoses. However ADA has appointed a Standardized Language Work Group to begin development of standardized language for nutrition diagnoses and intervention. (June 2003)
Nutrition Diagnosis Components (3 distinct parts)	**1. Problem (Diagnostic Label)** The nutrition diagnostic statement describes alterations in the patient/client/group's nutritional status. A diagnostic label (qualifier) is an adjective that describes/qualifies the human response such as: ■ Altered, impaired, ineffective, increased/decreased, risk of, acute or chronic. **2. Etiology (Cause/Contributing Risk Factors)** The related factors (etiologies) are those factors contributing to the existence of, or maintenance of pathophysiological, psychosocial, situational, developmental, cultural, and/or environmental problems. ■ Linked to the problem diagnostic label by words "related to" (RT) ■ It is important not only to state the problem, but to also identify the cause of the problem. □ This helps determine whether or not nutritional intervention will improve the condition or correct the problem. □ It will also identify who is responsible for addressing the problem. Nutrition problems are either caused directly by inadequate intake (primary) or as a result of other medical, genetic, or environmental factors (secondary). □ It is also possible that a nutrition problem can be the cause of another problem. For example, excessive caloric intake may result in unintended weight gain. Understanding the cascade of events helps to determine how to prioritize the interventions. □ It is desirable to target interventions at correcting the cause of the problem whenever possible; however, in some cases treating the signs and symptoms (consequences) of the problem may also be justified. ■ The ranking of nutrition diagnoses permits dietetics professionals to arrange the problems in order of their importance and urgency for the patient/client/group. **3. Signs/Symptoms (Defining Characteristics)** The defining characteristics are a cluster of subjective and objective signs and symptoms established for each nutrition diagnostic category. The defining characteristics, gathered during the assessment phase, provide evidence that a nutrition related problem exists and that the problem identified belongs in the selected diagnostic category. They also quantify the problem and describe its severity: ■ Linked to etiology by words "as evidenced by" (AEB); ■ The symptoms (subjective data) are changes that the patient/client/group feels and expresses verbally to dietetics professionals; and ■ The signs (objective data) are observable changes in the patient/client/group's health status.
Nutrition Diagnostic Statement (PES)	Whenever possible, a nutrition diagnostic statement is written in a PES format that states the Problem (P), the Etiology (E), and the Signs & Symptoms (S). However, if the problem is either a risk (potential) or wellness problem, the nutrition diagnostic statement may have only two elements, Problem (P), and the Etiology (E), since Signs & Symptoms (S) will not yet be exhibited in the patient. A well-written Nutrition Diagnostic Statement should be: 1. Clear and concise 2. Specific: patient/client/group-centered 3. Related to one client problem 4. Accurate: relate to one etiology 5. Based on reliable and accurate assessment data **Examples of Nutrition Diagnosis Statements (PES or PE)** ■ Excessive caloric intake (problem) "related to" frequent consumption of large portions of high fat meals (etiology) "as evidenced by" average daily intake of calories exceeding recommended amount by 500 kcal and 12-pound weight gain during the past 18 months (signs)

FIG 2 cont'd.

	■ Inappropriate infant feeding practice RT lack of knowledge AEB infant receiving bedtime juice in a bottle ■ Unintended weight loss RT inadequate provision of energy by enteral products AEB 6-pound weight loss over past month ■ Risk of weight gain RT a recent decrease in daily physical activity following sports injury
Critical Thinking	The following types of critical thinking skills are especially needed in the diagnosis step: ■ Finding patterns and relationships among the data and possible causes; ■ Making inferences ("if this continues to occur, then this is likely to happen"); ■ Stating the problem clearly and singularly; ■ Suspending judgment (be objective and factual); ■ Making interdisciplinary connections; ■ Ruling in/ruling out specific diagnoses; and ■ Prioritizing the relative importance of problems for patient/client/group safety.
Documentation of Diagnosis	Documentation is an on-going process that supports all of the steps in the Nutrition Care Process. Quality documentation of the diagnosis step should be relevant, accurate, and timely. A nutrition diagnosis is the impression of dietetics professionals at a given point in time. Therefore, as more assessment data become available, the documentation of the diagnosis may need to be revised and updated. Inclusion of the following information would further describe quality documentation of this step: ■ Date and time; and ■ Written statement of nutrition diagnosis.
Determination for Continuation of Care	Since the diagnosis step primarily involves naming and describing the problem, the determination for continuation of care seldom occurs at this step. Determination of the continuation of care is more appropriately made at an earlier or later point in the Nutrition Care Process.
STEP 3. NUTRITION INTERVENTION	
Basic Definition & Purpose	"**Nutrition Intervention**" is the third step of the Nutrition Care Process. An intervention is a specific set of activities and associated materials used to address the problem. Nutrition interventions are purposefully planned actions designed with the intent of changing a nutrition-related behavior, risk factor, environmental condition, or aspect of health status for an individual, target group, or the community at large. This step involves a) selecting, b) planning, and c) implementing appropriate actions to meet patient/client/groups' nutrition needs. The selection of nutrition interventions is driven by the nutrition diagnosis and provides the basis upon which outcomes are measured and evaluated. Dietetics professionals may actually do the interventions, or may include delegating or coordinating the nutrition care that others provide. All interventions must be based on scientific principles and rationale and, when available, grounded in a high level of quality research (evidence-based interventions). Dietetics professionals work collaboratively with the patient/client/group, family, or caregiver to create a realistic plan that has a good probability of positively influencing the diagnosis/problem. This client-driven process is a key element in the success of this step, distinguishing it from previous planning steps that may or may not have involved the patient/client/group to this degree of participation.
Data Sources/Tools for Interventions	■ Evidence-based nutrition guides for practice and protocols ■ Current research literature ■ Current consensus guidelines and recommendations from other professional organizations ■ Results of outcome management studies or Continuous Quality Index projects. ■ Current patient education materials at appropriate reading level and language ■ Behavior change theories (self-management training, motivational interviewing, behavior modification, modeling)
Nutrition Intervention Components	This step includes two distinct interrelated processes: 1. **Plan the nutrition intervention** (formulate & determine a plan of action) ■ Prioritize the nutrition diagnoses based on severity of problem; safety; patient/client/group's need; likelihood that nutrition intervention will impact problem and patient/client/groups' perception of importance. ■ Consult ADA's *MNT Evidence-Based Guides for Practice* and other practice guides. These resources can assist dietetics professionals in identifying science-based ideal goals and selecting appropriate interventions for MNT. They list appropriate value(s) for control or improvement of the disease or conditions as defined and supported in the literature. ■ Determine patient-focused expected outcomes for each nutrition diagnosis. The expected outcomes are the desired change(s) to be achieved over time as a result of nutrition intervention. They are based on nutrition diagnosis; for example, increasing or decreasing laboratory values, decreasing blood pressure, decreasing weight, increasing use of stanols/sterols, or increasing fiber. Expected outcomes should be written in observable and measurable terms that are clear and concise. They should be patient/client/group-centered and need to be tailored to what is reasonable to the patient's circumstances and appropriate expectations for treatments and outcomes.

FIG 2 cont'd.

- Confer with patient/client/group, other caregivers or policies and program standards throughout planning step.
- Define intervention plan (for example write a nutrition prescription, provide an education plan or community program, create policies that influence nutrition programs and standards).
- Select specific intervention strategies that are focused on the etiology of the problem and that are known to be effective based on best current knowledge and evidence.
- Define time and frequency of care including intensity, duration, and follow-up.
- Identify resources and/or referrals needed.

2. Implement the nutrition intervention (care is delivered and actions are carried out)
- Implementation is the action phase of the nutrition care process. During implementation, dietetics professionals:
  □ Communicate the plan of nutrition care;
  □ Carry out the plan of nutrition care; and
  □ Continue data collection and modify the plan of care as needed.
- Other characteristics that define quality implementation include:
  □ Individualize the interventions to the setting and client;
  □ Collaborate with other colleagues and health care professionals;
  □ Follow up and verify that implementation is occurring and needs are being met; and
  □ Revise strategies as changes in condition/response occurs.

Critical Thinking	Critical thinking is required to determine which intervention strategies are implemented based on analysis of the assessment data and nutrition diagnosis. The following types of critical thinking skills are especially needed in the intervention step: - Setting goals and prioritizing; - Transferring knowledge from one situation to another; - Defining the nutrition prescription or basic plan; - Making interdisciplinary connections; - Initiating behavioral and other interventions; - Matching intervention strategies with client needs, diagnoses, and values; - Choosing from among alternatives to determine a course of action; and - Specifying the time and frequency of care.
Documentation of Nutrition Interventions	Documentation is an on-going process that supports all of the steps in the Nutrition Care Process. Quality documentation of nutrition interventions should be relevant, accurate, and timely. It should also support further intervention or discharge from care. Changes in patient/client/group's level of understanding and food-related behaviors must be documented along with changes in clinical or functional outcomes to assure appropriate care/case management in the future. Inclusion of the following information would further describe quality documentation of this step: - Date and time; - Specific treatment goals and expected outcomes; - Recommended interventions, individualized for patient; - Any adjustments of plan and justifications; - Patient receptivity; - Referrals made and resources used; - Any other information relevant to providing care and monitoring progress over time; - Plans for follow-up and frequency of care; and - Rationale for discharge if appropriate.
Determination for Continuation of Care	If the patient/client/group has met intervention goals or is not at this time able/ready to make needed changes, the dietetics professional may include discharging the client from this episode of care as part of the planned intervention.

STEP 4. NUTRITION MONITORING AND EVALUATION

Basic Definition & Purpose	**"Nutrition Monitoring and Evaluation"** is the fourth step of the Nutrition Care Process. *Monitoring* specifically refers to the review and measurement of the patient/client/group's status at a scheduled (preplanned) follow-up point with regard to the nutrition diagnosis, intervention plans/goals, and outcomes, whereas *Evaluation* is the systematic comparison of current findings with previous status, intervention goals, or a reference standard. Monitoring and evaluation use selected outcome indicators (markers) that are relevant to the patient/client/group's defined needs, nutrition diagnosis, nutrition goals, and disease state. Recommended times for follow-up, along with relevant outcomes to be monitored, can be found in ADA's Evidence Based Guides for Practice and other evidence-based sources. The purpose of monitoring and evaluation is to determine the degree to which progress is being made and goals or desired outcomes of nutrition care are being met. It is more than just "watching" what is happening, it requires an active commitment to measuring and recording the appropriate outcome indicators (markers) relevant to the nutrition diagnosis and intervention strategies. Data from this step are used to create an outcomes management system. Refer to Outcomes Management System in text.

FIG 2 cont'd.

Progress should be monitored, measured, and evaluated on a planned schedule until discharge. Short inpatient stays and lack of return for ambulatory visits do not preclude monitoring, measuring, and evaluation. Innovative methods can be used to contact patients/clients to monitor progress and outcomes. Patient confidential self-report via mailings and telephone follow-up are some possibilities. Patients being followed in disease management programs can also be monitored for changes in nutritional status. Alterations in outcome indicators such as hemoglobin A1C or weight are examples that trigger reactivation of the nutrition care process.

Data Sources/Tools for Monitoring and Evaluation	■ Patient/client/group records ■ Anthropometric measurements, laboratory tests, questionnaires, surveys ■ Patient/client/group (or guardian) interviews/surveys, pretests, and posttests ■ Mail or telephone follow-up ■ ADA's *Evidence Based Guides for Practice* and other evidence-based sources ■ Data collection forms, spreadsheets, and computer programs
Types of Outcomes Collected	The outcome(s) to be measured should be directly related to the nutrition diagnosis and the goals established in the intervention plan. Examples include, but are not limited to: ■ Direct nutrition outcomes (knowledge gained, behavior change, food or nutrient intake changes, improved nutritional status); ■ Clinical and health status outcomes (laboratory values, weight, blood pressure, risk factor profile changes, signs and symptoms, clinical status, infections, complications); ■ Patient/client-centered outcomes (quality of life, satisfaction, self-efficacy, self-management, functional ability); and ■ Health care utilization and cost outcomes (medication changes, special procedures, planned/unplanned clinic visits, preventable hospitalizations, length of hospitalization, prevent or delay nursing home admission).
Nutrition Monitoring and Evaluation Components	This step includes three distinct and interrelated processes: **1. Monitor progress** ■ Check patient/client/group understanding and compliance with plan; ■ Determine if the intervention is being implemented as prescribed; ■ Provide evidence that the plan/intervention strategy is or is not changing patient/client/group behavior or status; ■ Identify other positive or negative outcomes; ■ Gather information indicating reasons for lack of progress; and ■ Support conclusions with evidence. **2. Measure outcomes** ■ Select outcome indicators that are relevant to the nutrition diagnosis or signs or symptoms, nutrition goals, medical diagnosis, and outcomes and quality management goals. ■ Use standardized indicators to: □ Increase the validity and reliability of measurements of change; and □ Facilitate electronic charting, coding, and outcomes measurement. **3. Evaluate outcomes** ■ Compare current findings with previous status, intervention goals, and/or reference standards.
Critical Thinking	The following types of critical thinking skills are especially needed in the monitoring and evaluation step: ■ Selecting appropriate indicators/measures; ■ Using appropriate reference standard for comparison; ■ Defining where patient/client/group is now in terms of expected outcomes; ■ Explaining variance from expected outcomes; ■ Determining factors that help or hinder progress; and ■ Deciding between discharge or continuation of nutrition care.
Documentation of Monitoring and Evaluation	Documentation is an on-going process that supports all of the steps in the Nutrition Care Process and is an integral part of monitoring and evaluation activities. Quality documentation of the monitoring and evaluation step should be relevant, accurate, and timely. It includes a statement of where the patient is now in terms of expected outcomes. Standardized documentation enables pooling of data for outcomes measurement and quality improvement purposes. Quality documentation should also include: ■ Date and time; ■ Specific indicators measured and results; ■ Progress toward goals (incremental small change can be significant therefore use of a Likert type scale may be more descriptive than a "met" or "not met" goal evaluation tool); ■ Factors facilitating or hampering progress; ■ Other positive or negative outcomes; and ■ Future plans for nutrition care, monitoring, and follow up or discharge.
Determination for Continuation of Care	Based on the findings, the dietetics professional makes a decision to actively continue care or discharge the patient/client/group from nutrition care (when necessary and appropriate nutrition care is completed or no further change is expected at this time). If nutrition care is to be continued, the nutrition care process cycles back as necessary to assessment, diagnosis, and/or intervention for additional assessment, refinement of the diagnosis and adjustment and/or reinforcement of the plan. If care does not continue, the patient may still be monitored for a change in status and reentry to nutrition care at a later date.

FIG 2 cont'd.

describing what dietetics professionals do is truly a paradigm shift. This new paradigm is more complete, takes in more possibilities, and explains observations better. Finally, it allows dietetics professionals to act in ways that are more likely to achieve the results that are desired and expected.

NUTRITION CARE MODEL

The Nutrition Care Model is a visual representation that reflects key concepts of each step of the Nutrition Care Process and illustrates the greater context within which the Nutrition Care Process is conducted. The model also identifies other factors that influence and impact on the quality of nutrition care provided. Refer to Figure 1 for an illustration of the model as described below:

■ Central Core: Relationship between patient/client/group and dietetics professional;
■ Nutrition Care Process: Four steps of the nutrition care process (Figure 2);
■ Outer rings:
■ Middle ring: Strengths and abilities that dietetics professionals bring to the process (dietetics knowledge, skills, and competencies; critical thinking, collaboration, and communication; evidence-based practice, and Code of Ethics) (32);
■ Outer ring: Environmental factors that influence the process (practice settings, health care systems, social systems, and economics);
■ Supporting Systems:
■ Screening and Referral System as access to Nutrition Care; and
■ Outcomes Management System as a means to provide continuous quality improvement to the process.

The model is intended to depict the relationship with which all of these components overlap, interact, and move in a dynamic manner to provide the best quality nutrition care possible.

Central to providing nutrition care is the relationship between the patient/client/group and the dietetics professional. The patient/client/groups' previous educational experiences and readiness to change influence this relationship. The education and training that dietetics professionals receive have very strong components devoted to interpersonal knowledge and skill building such as listening, empathy, coaching, and positive reinforcing.

The middle ring identifies abilities of dietetics professionals that are especially applicable to the Nutrition Care Process. These include the unique dietetics knowledge, skill, and competencies that dietetics professionals bring to the process, in addition to a well-developed capability for critical thinking, collaboration, and communication. Also in this ring is evidence-based practice that emphasizes that nutrition care must incorporate currently available scientific evidence, linking what is done (content) and how it is done (process of care). The Code of Ethics defines the ethical principles by which dietetics professionals should practice (33). Dietetics knowledge and evidence-based practice establish the Nutrition Care Process as unique to dietetics professionals; no other health care professional is qualified to provide nutrition care in this manner. However, the Nutrition Care Process is highly dependent on collaboration and integration within the health care team. As stated above, communication and participation within the health care team are critical for identification of individuals who are appropriate for nutrition care.

The outer ring identifies some of the environmental factors

such as practice settings, health care systems, social systems, and economics. These factors impact the ability of the patient/client/group to receive and benefit from the interventions of nutrition care. It is essential that dietetics professionals assess these factors and be able to evaluate the degree to which they may be either a positive or negative influence on the outcomes of care.

Screening and Referral System

Because screening may or may not be accomplished by dietetics professionals, nutrition screening is a supportive system and *not* a step within the Nutrition Care Process. Screening is extremely important; it is an identification step that is outside the actual "care" and provides access to the Nutrition Care Process.

The Nutrition Care Process depends on an effective screening and/or referral process that identifies clients who would benefit from nutrition care or MNT. Screening is defined by the US Preventive Services Task Force as "those preventive services in which a test or standardized examination procedure is used to identify patients requiring special intervention" (34). The major requirements for a screening test to be considered effective are the following:
■ Accuracy as defined by the following three components:
□ Specificity: Can it identify patients with a condition?
□ Sensitivity: Can it identify those who do not have the condition?
□ Positive and negative predictive; and
■ Effectiveness as related to likelihood of positive health outcomes if intervention is provided.

Screening parameters need to be tailored to the population and to the nutrition care services to be provided. For example, the screening parameters identified for a large tertiary acute care institution specializing in oncology would be vastly different than the screening parameters defined for an ambulatory obstetrics clinic. Depending on the setting and institutional policies, the dietetics professional may or may not be directly involved in the screening process. Regardless of whether dietetics professionals are actively involved in conducting the screening process, they are accountable for providing input into the development of appropriate screening parameters to ensure that the screening process asks the right questions. They should also evaluate how effective the screening process is in terms of correctly identifying clients who require nutrition care.

In addition to correctly identifying clients who would benefit from nutrition care, a referral process may be necessary to ensure that the client has an identifiable method of being linked to dietetics professionals who will ultimately provide the nutrition care or medical nutrition therapy. While the nutrition screening and referral is not part of the Nutrition Care Process, it is a critical antecedent step in the overall system (35).

Outcomes Management System

An outcomes management system evaluates the effectiveness and efficiency of the entire process (assessment, diagnosis, interventions, cost, and others), whereas the fourth step of the process "nutrition monitoring and evaluations" refers to the evaluation of the patient/client/group's progress in achieving outcomes.

Because outcomes management is a system's commitment to effective and efficient care, it is depicted outside of the NCP. Outcomes management links care processes and resource utilization with outcomes. Through outcomes management, relevant data are collected and analyzed in a timely manner so that performance can be adjusted and improved. Findings are compared with such things as past levels of performance; organizational, regional, or national norms; and standards or benchmarks of optimal performance. Generally, this information is reported to providers, administrators, and payors/funders and may be part of administrative databases or required reporting systems.

It requires an infrastructure in which outcomes for the population served are routinely assessed, summarized, and reported. Health care organizations use complex information management systems to manage resources and track performance. Selected information documented throughout the nutrition care process is entered into these central information management systems and structured databases. Examples of centralized data systems in which nutrition care data should be included are the following:

■ basic encounter documentation for billing and cost accounting;

■ tracking of standard indicators for quality assurance and accreditation;

■ pooling data from a large series of patients/clients/groups to determine outcomes; and

■ specially designed studies that link process and outcomes to determine effectiveness and cost effectiveness of diagnostic and intervention approaches.

The major goal of outcomes management is to utilize collected data to improve the quality of care rendered in the future. Monitoring and evaluation data from individuals are pooled/aggregated for the purposes of professional accountability, outcomes management, and systems/processes improvement. Results from a large series of patients/clients can be used to determine the effectiveness of intervention strategies and the impact of nutrition care in improving the overall health of individuals and groups. The effects of well-monitored quality improvement initiatives should be reflected in measurable improvements in outcomes.

Outcomes management comprehensively evaluates the two parts of IOM's definition of quality: outcomes and process. Measuring the relationship between the process and the outcome is essential for quality improvement. To ensure that the quality of patient care is not compromised, the focus of quality improvement efforts should always be directed at the outcome of care (36-43).

FUTURE IMPLICATIONS

Impact on Coverage for Services

Quality-related issues are gaining in importance worldwide. Even though our knowledge base is increasing, the scientific evidence for most clinical practices in all of medicine is modest. So much of what is done in health care does *not* maximize quality or minimize cost (44). A standardized Nutrition Care Process is a necessary foundation tool for gathering valid and reliable data on how quality nutrition care provided by qualified dietetics professionals improves the overall quality of health care provided. Implementing ADA's Nutrition Care Process provides a framework for demonstrating that nutrition care improves outcomes by the following: (a) enhancing the health of individuals, groups, institutions, or health systems; (b) potentially reducing health care costs by decreasing the need for medications, clinic and hospital visits, and preventing or delay-

ing nursing home admissions; and (c) serving as the basis for research, documenting the impact of nutrition care provided by dietetics professionals (45-47).

Developing Scopes and Practice Standards

The work group reviewed the questions raised by delegates regarding the role of the RD and DTR in the Nutrition Care Process. As a result of careful consideration of this important issue, it was concluded that describing the various types of tasks and responsibilities appropriate to each of these credentialed dietetics professionals was yet another professional issue beyond the intent and purpose of developing a standardized Nutrition Care Process.

A scope of practice of a profession is the range of services that the profession is authorized to provide. Scopes of practice, depending on the particular setting in which they are used, can have different applications. They can serve as a legal document for state certification/licensure laws or they might be incorporated into institutional policy and procedure guidelines or job descriptions. Professional scopes of practice should be based on the education, training, skills, and competencies of each profession (48).

As previously noted, a dietetics professional is a person who, by virtue of academic and clinical training and appropriate certification and/or licensure, is uniquely qualified to provide a comprehensive array of professional services relating to prevention and treatment of nutrition-related conditions. A Scope of Practice articulates the roles of the RD, DTR, and advanced-practice RD. Issues to be addressed for the future include the following: (a) the need for a common scope with specialized guidelines and (b) recognition of the rich diversity of practice vs exclusive domains of practice regulation.

Professional standards are "authoritative statements that describe performance common to the profession." As such, standards should encompass the following:

■ articulate the expectations the public can have of a dietetics professional in any practice setting, domain, and/or role;

■ expect and achieve levels of practice against which actual performance can be measured; and

■ serve as a legal reference to describe "reasonable and prudent" dietetics practice.

The Nutrition Care Process effectively reflects the dietetics professional as the unique provider of nutrition care when it is consistently used as a systematic method to think critically and make decisions to provide safe and effective care. ADA's Nutrition Care Process will serve as a guide to develop scopes of practice and standards of practice (49,50). Therefore, the work group recommended that further work be done to use the Nutrition Care Process to describe roles and functions that can be included in scopes of practice. In May 2003, the Board of Directors of ADA established a Practice Definitions Task Force that will identify and differentiate the terms within the profession that need clarification for members, affiliates, and DPGs related to licensure, certification, practice acts, and advanced practice. This task force is also charged to clarify the scope of practice services, clinical privileges, and accountabilities provided by RDs/DTRs based on education, training, and experience.

Education of Dietetics Students

It will be important to review the current CADE Educational Standards to ensure that the language and level of expected competencies are consistent with the entry-level practice of the Nutrition Care Process. Further work by the Commission on Dietetic Registration (CDR) may need to be done to make revisions on the RD and DTR exams to evaluate entry-level competencies needed to practice nutrition care in this way. Revision of texts and other educational materials will also need to incorporate the key principles and steps of this new process (51).

Education and Credentialing of Members

Even though dietetics professionals currently provide nutrition care, this standardized Nutrition Care Process includes some new principles, concepts, and guidelines in each of its steps. This is especially true of steps 2 and 4 (Nutrition Diagnosis and Nutrition Monitoring and Evaluation). Therefore, the implications for education of dietetics professionals and their practice are great. Because a large number of dietetics professionals still are employed in health care systems, a comprehensive educational plan will be essential. A model to be considered when planning education is the one used to educate dietetics professionals on the Professional Development Portfolio (PDP) Process (52). Materials that could be used to provide members with the necessary knowledge and skills in this process could include but not be limited to the following:

■ articles in the *Journal of the American Dietetic Association*;
■ continuing professional education lectures and presentations at affiliate and national meetings;
■ self-study materials; case studies, CD-ROM workbooks, and others;
■ hands-on workshops and training programs;
■ Web-based materials; and
■ inclusion in the learning needs assessment and codes of the Professional Development Portfolio.

Through the development of this educational strategic plan, the benefits to dietetics professionals and other stakeholders will need to be a central theme to promote the change in practice that comes with using this process to provide nutrition care.

Evidence-Based Practice

The pressure to do more with less is dramatically affecting all of health care, including dietetics professionals. This pressure is forcing the health care industry to restructure to be more efficient and cost-effective in delivering care. It will require the use of evidenced-based practice to determine what practices are critical to support outcomes (53,54). The Nutrition Care Process will be invaluable as research is completed to evaluate the services provided by dietetics professionals (55). The Nutrition Care Process will provide the structure for developing the methodology and data collection in individual settings, and the practice-based research networks ADA is in the process of initiating.

Standardized Language

As noted in Step 2 (Nutrition Diagnosis), having a standard taxonomy for nutrition diagnosis would be beneficial. Work in the area of articulating the types of interventions used by dietetics professionals has already begun by the Definitions Work Group under the direction of ADA's Research Committee. Further work to define terms that are part of the Nutrition Care Process will need to continue. Even though the work group provided a list of terms relating to the definition and key concepts of the process, there are opportunities to articulate fur-

ther terms that are consistently used in this process. The Board of Directors of ADA in May 2003 approved continuation and expansion of a task force to address a comprehensive system that includes a process for developing and validating standardized language for nutrition diagnosis, intervention, and outcomes.

SUMMARY

Just as maps are reissued when new roads are built and rivers change course, this Nutrition Care Process and Model reflects recent changes in the nutrition and health care environment. It provides dietetics professionals with the updated "road map" to follow the best path for high-quality patient/client/group-centered nutrition care.

References

1. American Dietetic Association Strategic Plan. Available at: http://eatright.org (member only section). Accessed June 2, 2003.
2. Wheeler D. *Understanding Variation: The Key to Managing Chaos.* 2nd ed. Knoxville, TN: SPC Press; 2000.
3. Shojania KG, Duncan BW, McDonald KM, Wachter RM. Making Health Care Safer: A Critical Analysis of Patient Safety Practices. Evidence Report/Technology Assessment No. 43 (Prepared by the University of California at San Francisco-Stanford Evidence-based Practice Center under Contract No. 290-97-0013). Rockville, MD: Agency for Healthcare Research and Quality; 2001. Report No.: AHRQ Publication No. 01-E058.
4. Potter, Patricia A, Perry, Anne G. *Basic Nursing Theory and Practice.* 4th ed. St Louis: C.V. Mosby; 1998.
5. American Physical Therapy Association. *Guide to Physical Therapist Practice.* 2nd ed. Alexandria, VA; 2001.
6. The Guide to Occupational Therapy Practice. *Am J Occup Ther.* 1999;53:3. Available at http://nweb.pct.edu/homepage/student/NUNJOL02/ot%20process.ppt. Accessed May 30, 2003.
7. Kohn KN, ed. *Medicare: A strategy for Quality Assurance, Volume I.* Committee to Design a Strategy for Quality Review and Assurance in Medicare. Washington, DC: Institute of Medicine. National Academy Press; 1990.
8. Kohn L, Corrigan J, Donaldson M, eds. *To Err Is Human: Building a Safer Health System.* Washington, DC: Committee on Quality of Health Care in America, Institute of Medicine. National Academy Press; 2000.
9. Institute of Medicine. *Crossing the Quality Chasm: A New Health System for the 21st Century.* Committee on Quality in Health Care in America. Rona Briere, ed. Washington, DC: National Academy Press; 2001.
10. Splett P. *Developing and Validating Evidence-Based Guides for Practice: A Tool Kit for Dietetics Professionals.* American Dietetic Association; 1999.
11. Endres JB. *Community Nutrition. Challenges and Opportunities.* Upper Saddle River, NJ: Prentice-Hall, Inc; 1999.
12. Splett P. Planning, Implementation and Evaluation of Nutrition Programs. In: Sharbaugh CO, ed. *Call to Action: Better Nutrition for Mothers, Children, and Families.* Washington, DC: National Center for Education in Maternal and Child Health (NCEMCH); 1990.
13. Batalden PB, Stoltz PA. A framework for the continual improvement of health care: Building and applying professional and improvement knowledge to test changes in daily work. *Jt Comm J Qual Improv.* 1993;19:424-452.
14. CADE Accreditation Handbook. Available at: http://www.eatright.com/cade/standards.html. Accessed March 20, 2003.
15. Alfaro-LeFevre R. Nursing process overview. *Applying Nursing Process. Promoting Collaborative Care.* 5th ed. Lippincott; 2002.
16. Grant A, DeHoog S. *Nutrition Assessment Support and Management.* Northgate Station, WA; 1999.
17. Sandrick, K. Is nutritional diagnosis a critical step in the nutrition care process? *J Am Diet Assoc.* 2002;102:427-431.
18. King LS. What is a diagnosis? *JAMA.* 1967;202:154.
19. Doenges ME. *Application of Nursing Process and Nursing Diagnosis: An Interactive Text for Diagnostic Reasoning,* 3rd ed. Philadelphia, PA: FA Davis Co; 2000.
20. Gallagher-Alred C, Voss AC, Gussler JD. *Nutrition intervention and patient outcomes: a self-study manual.* Columbus, OH: Ross Products Division, Abbott Laboratories; 1995.
21. Splett P, Myers EF. A proposed model for effective nutrition care. *J Am Diet Assoc.* 2001;101:357-363.
22. Lacey K, Cross N. A problem-based nutrition care model that is diagnostic driven and allows for monitoring and managing outcomes. *J Am Diet Assoc.* 2002;102:578-589.
23. Brylinsky C. The Nutrition Care Process. In: Mahan K, Escott-Stump S,

eds. *Krause's Food, Nutrition and Diet Therapy*, 10th ed. Philadelphia, PA: W.B. Saunders Company; 2000:431-451.

24. Hammond MI, Guthrie HA. Nutrition clinic: An integrated component of an undergraduate curriculum. *J Am Diet Assoc.* 1985;85:594.

25. Final MNT Regulations. CMS-1169-FC. Federal Register, November 1, 2001. Department of Health and Human Services. 42 CFR Parts: 405, 410, 411, 414, and 415. Available at: http://cms.hhs.gov/physicians/pfs/cms1169fc.asp. Accessed June 27, 2003.

26. Commission on Dietetic Registration CDR Certifications and State Licensure. Available at: http://www.cdrnet.org/certifications/index.htm. Accessed May 30, 2003.

27. Medicare Coverage Policy Decision: Duration and Frequency of the Medical Nutrition Therapy *(MNT) Benefit* (No. CAG-00097N). Available at: http://cms.hhs.gov/ncdr/memo.asp?id=53. Accessed June 2, 2003.

28. American Dietetic Association Medical Nutrition Therapy Evidence-Based Guides For Practice. Hyperlipidemia Medical Nutrition Therapy Protocol. CD-ROM; 2001.

29. American Dietetic Association. Medical Nutrition Therapy Evidence-Based Guides for Practice. Nutrition Practice Guidelines for Type 1 and 2 Diabetes Mellitus CD-ROM; 2001.

30. American Dietetic Association. Medical Nutrition Therapy Evidence-Based Guides for Practice. Nutrition Practice Guidelines for Gestational Diabetes Mellitus. CD-ROM; 2001.

31. American Dietetic Association Medical Nutrition Therapy Evidence-Based Guides For Practice. Chronic Kidney Disease (non-dialysis) Medical Nutrition Therapy Protocol. CD-ROM; 2002.

32. Gates G. Ethics opinion: Dietetics professionals are ethically obligated to maintain personal competence in practice. *J Am Diet Assoc.* May 2003;103: 633-635.

33. Code of Ethics for the Profession of Dietetics. *J Am Diet Assoc.* 1999;99: 109-113.

34. US Preventive Services Task Force. Guide to Clinical Preventive Services, 2nd ed. Washington, DC: US Department of Health and Human Services, Office of Disease Prevention and Health Promotion; 1996.

35. Identifying patients at risk: ADA's definitions for nutrition screening and nutrition assessment. *J Am Diet Assoc.* 1994;94:838-839.

36. Donabedian A. *Explorations in Quality Assessment and Monitoring. Volume I: The Definition of Quality and Approaches to Its Assessment.* Ann Arbor, MI: Health Administration Press; 1980.

37. Carey RG, Lloyd RC. *Measuring Quality Improvement in Health Care: A Guide to Statistical Process Control Applications.* New York, Quality Resources; 1995.

38. Eck LH, Slawson DL, Williams R, Smith K, Harmon-Clayton K, Oliver D. A model for making outcomes research standard practice in clinical dietetics. *J Am Diet Assoc.* 1998;98:451-457.

39. Ireton-Jones CS, Gottschlich MM, Bell SJ. *Practice-Oriented Nutrition Research: An Outcomes Measurement Approach.* Gaithersburg, MD: Aspen Publishers, Inc.; 1998.

40. Kaye GL. *Outcomes Management: Linking Research to Practice.* Columbus, OH: Ross Products Division, Abbott Laboratories; 1996.

41. Splett P. *Cost Outcomes of Nutrition Intervention*, a *Three Part Monograph.* Evansville, IN: Mead Johnson & Company; 1996.

42. Plsekk P. 1994. Tutorial: Planning for data collection part I: Asking the right question. *Qual Manage Health Care.* 2:76-81.

43. American Dietetic Association. Israel D, Moore S, eds. *Beyond Nutrition Counseling: Achieving Positive Outcomes Through Nutrition Therapy.* 1996.

44. Stoline AM, Weiner JP. *The New Medical Marketplace: A Physician's Guide to the Health Care System in the 1990s.* Baltimore: Johns Hopkins Press; 1993.

45. Mathematica Policy Research, Inc. Best Practices in Coordinated Care March 22, 2000. Available at: http://www.mathematica-mpr.com/PDFs/bestpractices.pdf. Accessed February 22, 2003.

46. Bisognano MA. New skills needed in medical leadership: The key to achieving business results. *Qual Prog.* 2000;33:32-41.

47. Smith R. Expanding medical nutrition therapy: An argument for evidence-based practices. *J Am Diet Assoc.* 2003;103:313-314.

48. National Council of State Boards of Nursing Model Nursing Practice Act. Available at: http://www.ncsbn.org/public/regulation/nursing_practice_model_practice_act.htm. Accessed June 27, 2003.

49. Professional policies of the American College of Medical Quality (ACMQ). Available at: http://www.acmq.org/profess/list.htm. Accessed June 27, 2003.

50. American Dietetic Association. Standards of professional practice. *J Am Diet Assoc.* 1998;98:83-85.

51. O'Neil EH and the Pew Health Professions Commission. Recreating Health Professional Practice for a New Century. The Fourth Report of the Pew Health Professions Commission. Pew Health Professions Commission; December 1998.

52. Weddle DO. The professional development portfolio process: Setting goals for credentialing. *J Am Diet Assoc.* 2002;102:1439-1444.

53. Sackett DL, Rosenberg WMC, Gray J, Haynes RB, Richardson WS. Evidence based medicine: What it is and what it isn't. *Br Med J.* 1996;312: 71-72.

54. Myers EF, Pritchett E, Johnson EQ. Evidence-based practice guides vs. protocols: What's the difference? *J Am Diet Assoc.* 2001;101:1085-1090.

55. Manore MM, Myers EF. Research and the dietetics profession: Making a bigger impact. *J Am Diet Assoc.* 2003;103:108-112.

The Quality Management Committee Work Group developed the Nutrition Care Process and Model with input from the House of Delegates dialog (October 2002 HOD meeting, in Philadelphia, PA). The work group members are the following: Karen Lacey, MS, RD, Chair; Elvira Johnson, MS, RD; Kessey Kieselhorst, MPA, RD; Mary Jane Oakland, PhD, RD, FADA; Carlene Russell, RD, FADA; Patricia Splett, PhD, RD, FADA; Suzanne Bertocchi, DTR, and Tamara Otterstein, DTR; Ellen Pritchett, RD; Esther Myers, PhD, RD, FADA; Harold Holler, RD, and Karri Looby, MS, RD. The work group would like to extend a special thank you to Marion Hammond, MS, and Naoimi Trossler, PhD, RD, for their assistance in development of the Nutrition Care Process and Model.

Nutrition Care Process Step 1. Nutrition Assessment

INTRODUCTION

Nutrition Assessment is the first of four steps in the Nutrition Care Process (1). At its simplest, it is a method of identifying and evaluating data needed to make decisions about a nutrition-related problem/diagnosis. While the types of data collected in nutrition assessments may vary among nutrition settings, the process and intention are the same. When possible, the assessment data is compared to reliable norms and standards for evaluation. Further, nutrition assessment initiates the data collection process that is continued throughout the nutrition care process and forms the foundation for reassessment and reanalysis of the data in Nutrition Monitoring and Evaluation (Step 4).

NUTRITION CARE PROCESS AND NUTRITION ASSESSMENT

Step 1, Nutrition Assessment, of the Nutrition Care Process forms the foundation for progressing through the other three steps in the process. Of initial significance, this systematic method for obtaining, verifying, and interpreting data is needed to make decisions about the significance and cause of a nutrition-related problem.

Several data sources can contribute to a nutrition assessment, such as information gained from the referring health care provider or agency, patient/client interview, medical record, patient/client rounds, community-based surveys, administrative data, and epidemiological studies. Data sources may vary among nutrition settings. Each patient/client or group presents unique aspects that may influence the approach for the nutrition assessment, and critical thinking skills are especially important at this step. The nature of the individual or group and the practice setting/environment lead to the appropriate tools to use in the assessment collection to ensure valid and reliable data. Critical thinking skills also help a practitioner distinguish relevant from irrelevant data and appropriate comparative norms and standards.

Based on the nutrition assessment, the practitioner is able to determine whether a nutrition diagnosis/problem exists. It also leads to the appropriate determination for the continuation of care, such as progression through the nutrition care process or the need for additional information/testing prior to continuing in the process. The data collection procedure persists throughout the nutrition care process and forms the foundation for reassessment and reanalysis of the data.

CATEGORIES OF NUTRITION ASSESSMENT DATA

In the development of the standardized nutrition diagnosis language, the following five categories of nutrition assessment data were identified—biochemical data, medical tests, and procedures; anthropometric measurements; physical examination findings; food/nutrition history; and client history. Because the nutrition assessment forms the basis for identifying a nutrition diagnosis, these terms are reflected on each nutrition diagnosis reference sheet (see pages 59-185) and the signs/symptoms are grouped by the categories of nutrition assessment data.

Following are some examples of data collected within each assessment category; however, these examples are not all-inclusive:

Food/Nutrition History consists of four areas: food intake, nutrition and health awareness and management, physical activity and exercise, and food availability.

Food intake may include factors such as composition and adequacy of food and nutrient intake, meal and snack patterns, environmental cues to eating, food and nutrient tolerance, and current diets and/or food modifications.

Nutrition and health awareness and management include, for example, knowledge and beliefs about nutrition recommendations, self-monitoring/management practices, and past nutrition counseling and education.

Physical activity and exercise consists of functional status, activity patterns, amount of sedentary time (e.g., TV, phone, computer), and exercise intensity, frequency, and duration.

Food availability encompasses factors such as food planning, purchasing, preparation abilities and limitations, food safety practices, food/nutrition program utilization, and food insecurity.

Biochemical Data, Medical Tests, and Procedures include laboratory data (e.g., electrolytes, glucose, lipid panel, and gastric emptying time).

Anthropometric Measurements include height, weight, body mass index (BMI), growth rate, and rate of weight change.

Physical Examination Findings include oral health, general physical appearance, muscle and subcutaneous fat wasting, and affect.

Client History consists of four areas: medication and supplement history, social history, medical/health history, and personal history.

Social history may include items such as socioeconomic status, social and medical support, cultural and religious beliefs, housing situation, and social isolation/connection.

Personal history consists of factors including age, occupation, role in family, and education level.

Medical/health history includes chief nutrition complaint, present/past illness, surgical history, chronic disease or complication risk, family medical history, mental/emotional health, and cognitive abilities.

Medication and supplement history includes, for instance, prescription and over-the-counter drugs, herbal and dietary supplements, and illegal drugs.

Standardized definitions for the nutrition assessment terms described have been published in comprehensive texts on the topic and are beyond the scope of this publication. As one example, *ADA's Pocket Guide to Nutrition Assessment*, is available and referenced at the end of this chapter (2).

In addition, for the Biochemical, Medical Tests, and Procedures category of nutrition assessment within the nutrition diagnoses, the normal test levels and ranges are provided only for guidance and professionals should be aware that values may be different depending on the laboratory performing the test. In addition, professionals are responsible for keeping abreast of national clinical guidelines that impact practice and applying them as appropriate to individual patients/clients and groups. Nutrition interventions should be individualized based on many factors, and laboratory values alone are not diagnostic. A diagnosis is assigned based on the clinical judgment of an appropriately educated, experienced individual.

NUTRITION ASSESSMENT AND DIAGNOSIS MATRIX

A nutrition assessment matrix is available (pages 22-41) and identifies the pertinent nutrition assessment data for each nutrition diagnosis. This tool is intended to assist in identifying a list of possible diagnoses based on data collected. The matrix enables the practitioner to identify possible nutrition diagnoses by reading down the list of data to find the identified parameter (e.g., increased BMI), then reading across the matrix to identify possible diagnoses (e.g., NI 1.5, NC 3.3, NB 1.5). This process may be repeated with additional data (e.g., excess energy intake from energy-dense foods: NI 1.5, NI 2.2, NI 2.4, NI 2.5, and NC 3.3), until a list of possible diagnoses is developed. The nutrition diagnostic language reference sheets provide additional detail. It is likely that as the steps in the nutrition care process evolve and as more research emerges there will be changes in the matrix in future versions of this publication.

SUMMARY

Nutrition assessment is the first step in the nutrition care process, but it is used throughout each cycle of the nutrition care process and is not an isolated event. Dietetics practitioners recognize that nutrition assessment is a dynamic process that develops throughout the nutrition care process. For example, a dietetics practitioner may be in the middle of the nutrition education intervention when the client provides a new price of information that may cause a modification of the nutrition diagnosis, PES statement, or even the nutrition intervention.

Future research will continue to shed light on the appropriate data to collect and its application in nutrition assessment with a patient/client or group. Moreover, as the profession utilizes nutrition assessment within the other steps of the nutrition care process, the most valid and reliable assessment data to use in nutrition diagnosis, nutrition intervention, and nutrition monitoring and evaluation will also become evident.

REFERENCES

1. Lacey K, Pritchett E. Nutrition care process and model: ADA adopts road map to quality care and outcomes management. *J Am Diet Assoc.* 2003;103:1061-1072.
2. American Dietetic Association. Pamela Charney, Ainsley Malone, eds. *ADA Pocket Guide to Nutrition Assessment.* Chicago, IL: American Dietetic Association; 2004.

Nutrition Assessment Matrix
Food/Nutrition History Data and Related Nutrition Diagnostic Terminology

Parameter (not all-inclusive)	Nutrition Diagnostic Terminology		
Excess intake of:			
Alcohol; binge drinking	NI 4.3		
Amino acids	NI 52.3		
Bioactive substances	NI 4.2		
Convenience foods, pre-prepared meals, and foods prepared away from home	NI 2.2	NB 2.4	
Energy from energy dense or high fat foods/beverages, TPN or EN	NI 1.5 NC 3.3	NI 2.2	NI 2.4
Fat, foods prepared with added fat	NI 5.4	NI 51.2	NC 2.2
Fat from high-risk lipids (saturated fat, *trans* fat, cholesterol)	NI 51.2		
Fiber	NI 5.4	NI 53.6	NC 2.2
Fluid	NI 3.2		
Foods without vitamins	NI 54.1		
Foods containing vitamins	NI 54.2		
Food prepared with added fat of a nondesirable type	NI 51.3		
Food in a defined time period	NB 1.5		
Iron	NI 5.5		
Manganese	NI 5.5		
Mercury	NB 3.1		
Minerals	NI 55.2		
Parenteral or enteral nutrition	NI 1.5		
Phosphorus	NI 5.4	NC 2.2	
Plant foods containing soluble fiber, β-glucan, or plant sterol and stanol esters	NI 4.2		
Protein	NI 4.2 NC 2.2	NI 5.4	NI 52.2
Protein, type	NI 52.3		
Sodium	NI 3.2 NC 2.2	NI 5.4	
Substances that interfere with digestion or absorption	NI 4.2		
Zinc	NI 5.5	55.2	
Associated factors:			
Binge eating patterns	NI 2.2		
Change in way clothes fit	NC 3.2		
Highly variable calorie intake	NI 2.2		
Lipid or dextrose infusions, peritoneal dialysis, or other medical treatments that provide substantial calories	NI 2.4		

Nutrition Assessment Matrix
Food/Nutrition History Data and Related Nutrition Diagnostic Terminology

Parameter (not all-inclusive)	Nutrition Diagnostic Terminology		
Insufficient intake of:			
Carbohydrate	NI 53.1		
Energy	NI 1.4	NI 2.1	NI 5.2
Fiber, soy protein, β-glucan, or plant sterol and stanol esters	NI 4.1	NI 53.5	
Fluid	NI 3.1		
Fat, essential fatty acids	NI 51.1	NI 51.2	
Fat, monounsaturated, polyunsaturated, or Ω-3 fatty acids	NI 51.3		
Food/supplements and nutrients	NI 5.1	NI 5.3	NI 54.1
	NI 55.1	NC 1.2	NB 2.4
	NB 3.2		
Food or food from specific foods/groups due to GI symptoms	NC 1.4	NC 2.1	
Vitamins/micronutrients	NC 2.2	NI 54.1	
Parenteral or enteral nutrition	NI 1.4	NI 2.3	
Protein	NI 2.1	NI 5.2	NI 52.1
Vitamin D intake/sunlight exposure	NI 55.1	NI 54.1	
Associated factors:			
Alterations in food intake from usual	NC 1.2	NC 3.2	
Anorexia, nausea, vomiting	NC 2.2	NI 2.1	
Changes in appetite or taste	NC 2.3	NI 2.1	
Changes in recent food intake level	NC 3.4	NC 3.2	
Decreased appetite	NI 55.2		
Failure to recognize foods	NB 2.6		
Forgets to eat	NB 2.6		
Hunger	NC 3.1	NB 3.2	
Infant coughing, crying, latching on and off, pounding on breasts	NC 1.3		
Infant lethargy	NC 1.3		
Infant with decreased feeding frequency/duration, early cessation of feeding, and/or feeding resistance	NC 1.3		
Infant with fewer than six wet diapers in 24 hours	NC 1.3		
Infant with hunger, lack of satiety after feeding	NC 1.3		
Lack of interest in food	NI 1.4	NI 5.2	NI 55.1
	NI 54.1		
Mother doesn't hear infant swallowing	NC 1.3		
Mother with lack of confidence in ability to breastfeed	NC 1.3		
Mother with small amount of milk when pumping	NC 1.3		
Recent food avoidance and or/lack of interest in food	NI 5.3		
Refusal to eat, chew	NC 3.1	NB 2.6	
Spitting food out or prolonged feeding time	NC 1.2		
Swallowing difficulty	NI 3.1		
Thirst	NI 3.1		

Nutrition Assessment Matrix
Food/Nutrition History Data and Related Nutrition Diagnostic Terminology

Parameter (not all-inclusive)	Nutrition Diagnostic Terminology		
Intake different from recommended:			
Carbohydrate	NI 53.2	NI 53.3	NI 53.4
Carbohydrate, protein, and/or fat intake from enteral and/or parenteral nutrients	NI 2.5		
Food, inappropriate use of	NB 2.6		
Food choices, inappropriate	NI 55.1		
Food group/nutrient imbalance	NB 1.2		
Food intake includes raw eggs; unpasturized milk products; soft cheeses; undercooked meats; wild plants, berries, or mushrooms	NB 3.1		
Food variety, limited	NB 3.2		
Intake that does not support replacement or mitigation of OTC, prescribed drugs, herbals, botanicals, or dietary supplements	NC 2.3		
Medication (over-the-counter or prescribed), herbal, botanical, or dietary supplement intake that is problematic or inconsistent with recommended foods	NC 2.3		
Protein or other supplementation	NI 52.2	NI 52.3	
US Dietary Guidelines, any nutrient	NI 54.2	NB 1.7	
Vitamin/mineral deficiency	NC 3.1	NI 55.1	NI 54.1
Food and nutrient intolerance:			
Allergic reactions to certain carbohydrate foods or food groups	NI 53.3		
Coughing and choking with eating	NC 1.1		
Decreased intake or avoidance of food difficult to form into a bolus	NC 1.2		
Diminished joint mobility or wrist, hand, or digits that impair ability to independently consume food	NI 1.4	NI 53.1	
Diarrhea in response to high refined carbohydrate intake	NI 53.3		
Dropping cups, utensils	NB 2.6		
Dropping food from utensil on repeated attempts to feed	NB 2.6		
Feeling of food "getting stuck"	NC 1.1		
Inability to eat due to foods provided not conducive to self feeding	NB 2.6		
Nausea, vomiting, diarrhea, high gastric residual volume	NI 2.5		
Pain on swallowing	NC 1.1		
Poor lip closure, drooling	NC 1.1	NB 2.6	
Pouching food	NC 1.1		
Prolonged chewing, feeding time	NC 1.1		
Utensil biting	NB 2.6		

Nutrition Assessment Matrix
Food/Nutrition History Data and Related Nutrition Diagnostic Terminology

Parameter (not all-inclusive)	Nutrition Diagnostic Terminology		
Nutrition and health awareness:			
Avoidance of food or calorie-containing beverages	NB 1.5	NC 1.1	
Avoidance of foods of age-appropriate texture	NC 1.2		
Avoidance of foods/food groups	NB 1.2		
Belief that aging can be slowed by dietary limitations	NB 3.2		
Chronic dieting behavior	NI 55.1	NB 1.5	
Cultural or religious practices that limit intake	NI 52.1		
Cultural or religious practices that limit modification of dietary carbohydrate intake	NI 53.2		
Defensiveness, hostility, or resistance to change	NB 1.3		
Denial of hunger	NB 1.5		
Denial of need for food- and nutrition-related changes	NB 1.3		
Eating alone, feeling embarrassed by the amount of food eaten	NB 1.5		
Eating much more rapidly than normal, eating until feeling uncomfortably full, consuming large amounts of food when not feeling hungry	NB 1.5		
Embarrassment or anger at need for self monitoring	NB 1.4	NB 2.3	
Emotional distress, anxiety, or frustration surrounding mealtimes	NB 2.6		
Excessive reliance on nutrition terming and preoccupation with nutrient content of food	NB 1.5		
Expected food/nutrition related outcomes are not achieved	NB 1.6		
Failure to complete any agreed homework	NB 1.6		
Failure to keep appointments/schedule or engage in counseling	NB 1.3	NB 1.6	
Fear of foods or dysfunctional thoughts regarding food or food experiences	NB 1.5		
Feeling disgusted with oneself, depressed, or guilty after overeating	NB 1.5		
Food faddism	NC 3.1	NB 1.2	NB 3.2
Food preoccupation	NB 1.5		
Frustration or dissatisfaction with MNT recommendations	NB 2.5		
Incomplete self-monitoring records	NB 1.4		
Inflexibility with food selection	NB 1.5		
Irrational thoughts about food's affect on the body	NB 1.5		
Knowledge about current fad diets	NB 1.5		
Lack of appreciation of the importance of making recommended nutrition related changes	NB 1.6		
Mealtime resistance	NC 1.1		
Negative body language (note: varies by culture)	NB 1.3		
Pica	NC 3.1	NB 1.2	NB 3.2
Previous failures to effectively change target behavior	NB 1.3		
Prolonged use of substances known to increase vitamin requirements or reduce vitamin absorption	NI 54.1		
Sense of lack of control of overeating during the episode	NB 1.5		
Unwillingness or disinterest in applying nutrition related recommendations	NC 3.3		
Verbalizes unwillingness/disinterest in learning	NB 1.1		
Weight preoccupation	NB 1.5		

Nutrition Assessment Matrix
Food/Nutrition History Data and Related Nutrition Diagnostic Terminology

Parameter (not all-inclusive)	Nutrition Diagnostic Terminology		
Food and nutrient knowledge and skill:			
Food- and nutrition-related knowledge deficit	NI 5.1	NC 1.4	NC 2.2
Inability to apply food- and nutrition-related information	NC 3.3	NB 1.1	
Inability to apply guideline information	NB 1.7		
Inability to change food- or activity-related behavior	NB 2.5		
Inability to interpret data or self management tools	NB 2.3		
Inability to maintain weight or regain of weight	NC 3.3		
Inability to recall agreed upon changes	NB 1.6		
Inability or unwillingness to select, or disinterest in selecting food consistent with guidelines	NB 1.7		
Inaccurate or incomplete understanding/information information related to guidelines or needed changes	NB 1.1	NB 1.7	
Lack of ability to prepare meals	NI 5.3		
Lack of compliance or inconsistent compliance with plan	NB 1.6		
Lack of efficacy to make changes or to overcome barriers to change	NB 1.3		
Limited knowledge of carbohydrate composition of foods or of carbohydrate metabolism	NI 53.3		
Mother has insufficient knowledge of breastfeeding or infant hunger/satiety signals	NC 1.3		
Mother is concerned about breastfeeding/lack of support	NC 1.3		
No prior knowledge of need for food and nutrition-related recommendations	NB 1.1		
Provides inaccurate or incomplete written response to questionnaire/written tool, or is unable to read written tool	NB 1.1		
Relates concerns about previous attempts to learn information	NB 1.1	NB 2.5	
Uncertainty as to how to consistently apply food/nutrition information	NB 1.6		
Uncertainty of how to complete monitoring records	NB 1.4		
Uncertainty regarding appropriate foods to prepare based upon nutrition prescription	NB 2.4		
Uncertainty regarding changes that could/should be made in response to data in self monitoring records	NB 1.4	NB 2.3	
Uncertainty regarding nutrition-related recommendations	NC 3.3		
Use of popular press/internet as source of medical and/or nutrition information	NI 55.1		
Physical activity:			
Decreased or sedentary activity level (due to barriers or other reasons)	NC 3.3	NB 2.1	
Increased physical activity	NI 1.2	NC 3.1	NB 2.2
Excessive physical activity (ignoring family, job; exercising without rest/rehabilitation days or while injured or sick)	NB 1.5	NB 2.2	

Nutrition Assessment Matrix
Food/Nutrition History Data and Related Nutrition Diagnostic
Terminology

Parameter (not all-inclusive)	Nutrition Diagnostic Terminology		
Food availability:			
Economic constraints that limit availability of appropriate foods	NI 2.1 NI 53.4	NI 53.2	NI 53.3
Inability to purchase and transport foods to one's home	NB 2.4		
Intake consistent with estimated or measured energy needs	NC 3.4		
Lack of available foods/products with bioactive substances in markets	NI 4.1		
Lack of facilities or accommodations for breastfeeding in community or at work	NC 1.3		
Ready access to available foods/products with bioactive substance	NI 4.2		
Unfavorable Nutrition Quality of Life (NQOL) rating	NB 2.5		
Other:			
Client desires to implement a Mediterranean-type diet	NI 51.3		
Extreme hunger with or without palpitations, tremor, sweating	NC 3.4		
Intake consistent with estimated or measured energy needs	NC 3.4		
No self-management equipment	NB 1.4		
Normal intake in the face of illness	NC 3.2		
Use of alcohol, narcotics	NC 3.4		

Nutrition Assessment Matrix
Anthropometric Data and Related Nutrition Diagnostic Terminology

Parameter: (not all inclusive)	Findings	Nutrition Diagnostic Terminology		
Anthropometric Data				
Body Mass Index (BMI)	decreased	NI 2.3	NI 5.1	NI 5.2
		NC 3.1	NB 1.5	NB 3.2
BMI	increased	NI 1.5	NC 3.3	NB 1.5
Body fat distribution	changed	NC 3.4		
Body fat percentage	increased	NI 1.5		
Growth	delayed	NI 1.2	NI 1.3	NI 2.3
		NI 5.1	NI 52.2	NI 54.2
		NC 2.1	NB 1.4	NB 3.2
Height	loss	NI 55.1		
Muscle circumference, mid-arm	decreased	NI 1.3	NC 3.1	
Muscle mass	increased	NI 1.2		
Skinfold thickness	increased	NC 3.3		
Waist circumference	increased	NC 3.3		
Wasting		NC 1.4	NI-5.2	
Weight	change, rapid	NC 2.2		
Weight	loss	NI 1.4	NI 2.1	NI 2.3
		NI 2.5	NI 3.1	NI 4.2
		NI 5.3	NI 51.1	NC 2.1
		NC 3.2	NB 2.2	
	unintentional	NI 1.2	NI 5.1	NI 5.2
Weight	decreased	NC 3.1	NB 2.2	
Weight	gain	NI 1.3	NI 1.5	NI 2.2
		NI 3.2	NC 2.3	NC 3.3
		NC 3.4		
	in excess of lean tissue accretion	NI 2.4	NI 2.5	
	interdialytic	NI 5.4		
Weight	failure to gain as planned	NI 2.3	NI 5.2	NI 5.3
		NB 1.6		

Nutrition Assessment Matrix
Biochemical Data, Medical Tests, and Procedures and Related Nutrition Diagnostic Terminology

Parameter (not all-inclusive)	Findings	Nutrition Diagnostic Terminology		
Biochemical data				
3-methyl histidine, urine	increased	NI 52.3		
Albumin, serum	decreased	NI 5.1	NI 5.2	NC 3.4
Alcohol, blood	increased	NI 4.3		
Alpha tocopherol, plasma	decreased	NI 54.1		
Amino acids (specific levels)	increased	NI 52.3	NC 2.1	
Ammonia, serum	increased	NI 52.3	NC 2.2	
Amylase, serum	increased	NI 51.2	NI 51.3	
AST, aspartate aminotransferase	increased	NI 4.3	NC 2.2	NB 2.2
ALT, alanine aminotransferase	increased	NC 2.2		
Bilirubin, total serum	increased	NI 51.2	NI 51.3	NC 2.2
BUN	increased	NI 3.1	NI 5.4	NI 52.2
BUN:creatinine ratio	increased	NI 52.3 NI 2.4	NC 2.2	NB 1.5
Calcium, serum	decreased	NI 2.3		
Calcium, serum ionized	decreased	NI 54.1		
Calcium, serum ionized	increased	NI 542		
Calcium, urine	decreased	NI 55.1		
Chloride, serum	decreased	NB 1.5		
Cholesterol, HDL	decreased	NI 5.4 NI 55.2	NI 51.2	NI 51.3
Cholesterol, LDL	increased	NI 5.4	NI 51.2	NI 51.3
Cholesterol, serum	decreased	NI 1.4 NI 5.1	NI 2.3	NI 4.2
Cholesterol, serum	increased	NI 5.4 NB 1.5	NI 51.2	NI 51.3
Copper	decreased	NI 2.3	NI 55.1	
Cortisol levels	increased	NB 2.2		
C-reactive protein	elevated	NI 5.1	NI 51.3	
Creatinine	elevated	NI 5.4	NC 2.2	
Digestive enzymes	altered	NC 1.4	NC 2.1	
D-xylose	abnormal	NC 1.4	NC 2.1	
Fat, fecal	increased	NI 51.2	NC 1.4	NC 2.1
Ferritin, serum	decreased	NB 2.2		
Ferritin, serum	increased	NI 55.2		
Folic acid, serum	decreased	NI 54.1		
Folic acid, erythrocyte		NI 54.2		
GFR, glomerular filtration rate	decreased	NI 5.4 NC 2.2	NI 52.2	NI 52.3
GGT, gamma-glutamyl transferase	elevated	NI 4.3		
Glucose, blood	increased	NI 1.1 NI 2.4 NI 53.4	NI 1.5 NI 53.2 NC 2.2	NI 2.2 NI 53.3 NC 3.4

Nutrition Assessment Matrix
Biochemical Data, Medical Tests, and Procedures and Related Nutrition Diagnostic Terminology

Parameter (not all-inclusive)	Findings	Nutrition Diagnostic Terminology		
Biochemical data				
Glucose, blood	decreased	NI 53.3 NB 1.5	NI 53.4	NC 2.2
Glutathione reductase, erythrocyte	increased	NI 54.1		
GTT (glucose tolerance test)	abnormal	NI 53.2		
Hematocrit	increased	NB 2.2		
Hemoglobin	decreased	NI 55.1		
Hemoglobin A1c	increased	NI 2.2	NI 53.2	
Hormone levels	fluctuating	NC 3.4		
Homocysteine	increased	NI 54.1		
Hydrogen breath test	abnormal	NC 1.4	NC 2.1	
IGF binding protein	abnormal	NB 2.2		
Immune function	suppressed	NB 2.2		
Iodine, urinary	decreased	NI 55.1		
Iron	decreased	NI 2.3		
Iron binding capacity	decreased	NI 2.3		
Ketones, urine	present	NB 1.5		
Leucopenia	present	NB 1.5		
Lipase	increased	NI 51.2	NI 51.3	
Lipid profile, serum	abnormal	NC 2.2 NB 1.7	NC 3.4	NB 1.5
Liver enzymes	elevated	NI 1.5 NI 4.2 NI 51.3	NI 2.4 NI 5.4 NC 2.2	NI 2.5 NI 51.2 NB 2.2
Magnesium, serum	decreased	NI 5.1	NI 55.1	
Magnesium, serum	increased	NI 55.2		
Mean corpuscular volume	increased	NI 4.3		
N'methyl-nicotanimide	decreased	NI 54.1		
N'methyl-nicotanimide	increased	NI 54.2		
Osmolality, serum	increased	NI 3.1		
Osmolality, serum	decreased	NI 3.2		
Parathyroid hormone	increased	NI 54.1	NI 54.2	
pCO$_2$	abnormal	NI 2.4	NC 2.2	
Phosphorus, serum	decreased	NI 1.5 NI 55.1	NI 5.1	NI 54.1
Phosphorus, serum	increased	NI 2.5	NI 5.4	NI 55.2
pO$_2$	abnormal	NC 2.2		
Potassium, serum	decreased	NI 1.5 NC 2.2	NI 2.5 NB 1.5	NI 5.1
Potassium, serum	increased	NI 5.1	NI 5.4	NC 2.2
Prealbumin	decreased	NI 5.1		
Pyrodoxal 5'phosphate, plasma	decreased	NI 54.1		
Pyrodoxal 5'phosphate, plasma	increased	NI 54.2		

Nutrition Assessment Matrix
Biochemical Data, Medical Tests, and Procedures and Related Nutrition Diagnostic Terminology

Parameter (not all-inclusive)	Findings	Nutrition Diagnostic Terminology		
Biochemical data				
Retinol, serum	decreased	NI 54.1		
Retinol, serum	increased	NI 54.2		
Sodium, serum	decreased	NI 3.2	NC 3.4	NB 1.5
Sodium, serum	increased	NI 3.1		
Stool culture	positive	NC 1.4	NB 3.1	
Thyroid function tests (TSH, T4, T3)	abnormal	NI 1.3	NI 55.2	NB 1.5
Toxicology reports	positive	NB 3.2		
Transketolase activity, erythrocyte	increased	NI 54.1		
Transferrin	increased	NI 4.3		
Triene:tetraene ratio	increased	NI 51.1		
Triglycerides	increased	NI 5.4	NI 51.2	NI 51.3
Vitamin B-12	decreased	NI 54.1		
Vitamin C, plasma	decreased	NI 54.1		
Vitamin K (PT, PTT, INR)	abnormal	NI 2.3	NI 54.1	NI 54.2
Zinc, serum	decreased	NI 2.3	NB 2.2	
Medical tests and procedures				
Gastric-emptying study	abnormal	NC 1.4		
Mineral density, bone	decreased	NI 55.1		
Respiratory quotient	abnormal	NI 1.5	NI 2.3	
Metabolic rate, resting	decreased	NI 1.3		
Metabolic rate, resting	increased	NI 1.1	NI 1.2	
Small-bowel transit time	abnormal	NC 1.4		

Nutrition Assessment Matrix
Physical Examination Data and Related Nutrition Diagnostic Terminology

Parameter (not all-inclusive)	Findings	Nutrition Diagnostic Terminology		
Head and neck				
Eyes:				
Bitot's spots	present	NI 54.1		
Dryness	present	NI 54.2		
Night blindness	present	NI 54.1		
Xerophthalmia	present	NI 54.1		
Tongue:				
Bright red	present	NI 54.1		
Dry or cracked	present	NC 1.2		
Glossitis	present	NI 54.1	NC 2.1	
Extrusion	present	NB 2.6		
Impaired tongue movement	present	NC 1.2		
Frenulum abnormality (infants)	present	NC 1.3		
Magenta	present	NI 54.1		
Mouth and throat:				
Cheilosis	present	NI 54.1	NC 2.1	
Dry mucous membranes, hoarse or wet voice, tongue extrusion	present	NI 2.3 / NC 1.1	NI 3.1 / NB 2.6	NI 54.2 / NB 3.1
Gums, inflamed or bleeding	present	NI 2.3	NI 5.1	NI 54.1
Ketone smell on breath	present	NI 53.1		
Lesions, oral	present	NC 1.2	NC 2.1	
Lips	dry or cracked	NI 54.2	NC 1.2	
Mucosa (mouth and pharynx)	edema	NI 54.1		
Parotid glands	enlarged	NB 1.5		
Stomatitis	present	NI 54.1		
Teeth	missing, caries, damaged enamel, poorly fitting dentures	NI 1.4 / NB 1.2	NI 53.2	NC 1.2
Head:				
Cranial nerve function (V, VII, IX, X, XII)	altered	NC 1.2		
Fontanelle, bulging (in infants)	present	NI 54.2		
Hair, changes, brittle and lifeless	present	NI 55.2	NB 1.5	
Hairs, coiled	present	NI 54.1		
Hair loss	present	NI 1.3 / NI 5.2	NI 2.3 / NI 54.2	NI 5.1
Headache, nausea, and vomiting	present	NI 54.2		
Lanugo hair formation on face and trunk	present	NB 1.5		
Mucosa, nasal	dryness	NI 54.2		
Occipital wasting	present	NI 5.2		
Mental status:				
Confusion	present	NI 54.1		
Concentration	impaired	NB 1.5		

Nutrition Assessment Matrix
Physical Examination Data and Related Nutrition Diagnostic Terminology

Parameter (not all-inclusive)	Findings	Nutrition Diagnostic Terminology		
Gastrointestinal system				
Ascites	present	NI 3.2	NC 2.2	
Bowel sounds	abnormal	NC 1.4	NC 2.1	
Constipation	present	NI 4.2	NI 5.5	NC 1.4
Distention, abdominal	present	NC 1.4	NC 2.1	
Diarrhea	present	NI 2.3	NI 4.2	NI 5.5
Diarrhea in response to carbohydrate feeding	present	NI 53.2		
Nausea	present	NI 2.3		
Upset, stomach	present	NI 54.2		
Vomiting	present	NI 2.3		
Neurologic system				
Motor and gait disturbances	present	NI 54.1		
Neurological changes	present	NI 4.2	NI 52.3	
Vibratory and position sense	decreased	NI 54.1		
Cardiovascular-pulmonary system				
Cardiovascular changes	arrythmias	NI 4.2	NB 1.5	
Edema, pulmonary (crackles or rales)	crackles or rales	NI 3.2		
Spine, limbs and extremities				
Arthralgia; joint effusions	present	NI 54.1		
Bone alterations	fragility	NI 54.2		
Bones	obvious prominence	NI 5.2		
Bones, long	widening at ends	NI 54.1		
Hands and feet	cyanosis	NB 1.5		
Hands and feet	tingling and numbness	NI 54.1		
Injuries	frequent and prolonged	NB 2.2		
Muscle soreness	chronic	NB 2.2		
Nail beds	blue, clubbing	NC 2.2		
Nail beds	pale	NI 2.3	NI 5.1	
Nail changes	present	NI 55.2		
Russell's sign	present	NB 1.5		
Skin				
Acanthosis nigricans	present	NI 2.2		
Calcification of soft tissues (calcinosis)	present	NI 54.2		
Changes consistent with nutrient deficiency/excess	present	NI 51.1	NB 1.7	NB 3.2
Condition	changes	NI 54.2		
Edema, peripheral	present	NI 2.4	NI 2.5	NI 5.2
		NC 2.2	NB 1.5	
Erythema, scaling and peeling of the skin	present	NI 54.2		

Nutrition Assessment Matrix
Physical Examination Data and Related Nutrition Diagnostic Terminology

Parameter (not all-inclusive)	Findings	Nutrition Diagnostic Terminology		
Skin, continued				
Ecchymosis	present	NI 54.1		
Follicular hyperkeratosis	present	NI 54.1		
Jaundice and itching	present	NC 2.2		
Muscle mass	decreased	NI 1.3	NI 2.3	NI 2.5
		NI 5.1	NB 1.5	
Fat, body	decreased	NC 3.2	NC 3.3	
		NB 1.5	NB 2.2	
Fat, body	increased	NC 3.3		
Skin	dry, scaly	NI 2.1	NI 3.1	NI 5.2
		NI 51.1	NB 1.5	
Skin integrity	decreased	NI 2.3	NI 5.1	
Skin lesions	present	NI 51.2	NI 51.3	NI 54.1
Skin turgor	decreased	NI 3.1	NC 1.1	
Skin turgor	increased	NI 2.3	NI 3.2	NI 5.4
Seborrheic dermatitis	present	NI 54.1		
Perifolicular hemorrhages	present	NI 54.1		
Petechiae	present	NI 54.1		
Pressure ulcers (stage II-IV)	present	NI 2.3	NI 5.1	
Wound healing	delayed	NI 5.1	NI 5.2	NI 5.3
		NI 54.1		
Xanthomas	present	NI 51.2	NI 51.3	
Vital signs				
Blood pressure	decreased	NI 5.2	NB 1.5	
Blood pressure	increased	NI 4.2		
Heart rate	decreased	NB 1.5		
Heart rate	increased	NI 1.1	NC 3.2	
Respiratory rate	increased	NI 1.1	NI 1.5	NC 3.2
Shortness of breath	present	NI 3.2	NC 2.2	
Temperature	decreased	NB 1.5		
Temperature	increased	NI 1.1	NC 3.2	
Urine output	decreased	NI 3.1		
Miscellaneous				
Body language (note: varies by culture)	negative	NB 1.3	NB 1.6	

Nutrition Assessment Matrix
Client History Data and Related Diagnostic Terminology

Parameter (not all-inclusive)	Nutrition Diagnostic Terminology		
Social history:			
Abuse, physical, sexual, or emotional	NC 3.3		
Alcohol intake during pregnancy despite knowledge of risk	NI 4.3		
Alcohol intake, excessive	NI 4.3	NC 1.2	
Avoidance of social events at which food is served	NB 1.5		
Change in living/independence	NI 55.1		
Chronic noncompliance	NB 1.3		
Endurance, decreased	NI 1.3		
Environmental conditions, e.g., infants exclusively fed breast milk with limited exposure to sunlight (vitamin D)	NI 54.1		
Geographic latitude and history of Ultraviolet-B exposure/sunscreen use	NI 55.1		
Geographic location and socioeconomic status associated with altered nutrient intake of indigenous phenomenon	NI 5.2		
Giving birth to an infant with fetal alcohol syndrome	NI 4.3		
Hunger associated with inadequate access to food supply	NI 5.3		
Illness or physical disability	NC 3.1	NB 3.2	
Insomnia, change in sleep habits	NC 3.4		
Lack of ability to prepare meals	NI 5.3		
Lack of developmental readiness	NC 1.2		
Lack of funds for purchase of appropriate foods	NI 5.3		
Lack of suitable support system to access food	NB 3.2		
Libido, decreased	NI 1.3		
Lifestyle changes, recent	NB 2.5		
Low cardio-respiratory fitness and/or low muscle strength	NB 2.1		
New medical diagnosis or change in existing diagnosis or condition	NI 4.3 / NB 1.4	NB 1.1 / NB 2.3	NB 1.3 / NB 2.5
Occupation of athlete, dancer, gymnast	NC 3.1		
Physical activity, easy fatigue with increased activity; unable to achieve desired levels	NI 2.3		
Physical disability or limitation	NC 3.3	NB 2.6	
Sight impairment	NB 2.4		
Unrealistic expectations of weight gain or ideal weight	NI 2.4		
Vision problems	NB 3.1		
Personal/Family history:			
Of eating disorders, depression, obsessive-compulsive disorders, anxiety disorders	NB 1.5		
Of hyperlipidemia, atherosclerosis, or pancreatitis	NI 51.2	NI 51.3	

Nutrition Assessment Matrix
Client History Data and Related Diagnostic Terminology

Parameter (not all-inclusive)	Nutrition Diagnostic Terminology		
Medical/Health history:			
AIDS/HIV	NI 1.1	NI 2.1	NI 2.3
	NI 5.1	NI 51.1	NC 3.2
Alcoholism	NC 2.2		
Alzheimer's disease	NI 1.2	NI 3.1	NC 1.2
	NB 2.6		
Anemia	NI 54.1	NI 55.2	NB 1.5
	NI 51.1		
Anxiety disorder	NI 1.5	NI 2.2	NB 2.1
Anxiety/depression	NI 1.3		
Arthritis	NB 2.1		
Asthma	NC 3.4		
Atherosclerosis	NI 51.2		
Biliary disease	NI 51.2	NI 51.3	
Binge eating	NB 2.2		
Breast surgery	NC 1.3		
Bulimia nervosa	NB 2.2		
Burns	NI 1.1	NI 2.3	NI 5.1
	NC 3.2		
Cadidiasis	NC 1.3		
Cancer	NI 54.2	NB 1.2	
Cancer, head, neck, or pharyngeal	NC 1.2		
Cancer (some types)	NI 1.1	NC 3.2	
Candidiasis or thrush	NC 1.3		
Cardiac, neurologic, respiratory changes	NB 3.1		
Cardiovascular disease	NI 3.2	NI 4.1	NI 4.2
	NI 5.3	NI 5.4	NI 51.3
	NI 54.2	NC 2.2	NB 2.3
	NB 1.2	NB 2.3	
Celiac disease	NI 53.1	NI 54.1	NI 55.1
	NC 1.4	NC 2.1	
Cerebral palsy	NI 1.2	NC 1.2	NB 2.4
Chronic fatigue syndrome	NB 2.1		
Chronic obstructive pulmonary disease	NI 1.1	NC 3.2	
Chronic or acute disease or trauma,	NI 5.2		
Cleft lip/palate	NC 1.2	NC 1.3	
Cognitive or emotional impairment	NB 2.3	NB 2.4	
Cold intolerance	NI 1.3		
Constipation, obstructive	NI 53.6		
Crohn's disease	NI 2.3	NI 5.1	
	NC 1.4	NC 2.1	
Cushing's syndrome	NC 3.4		
Cystic fibrosis	NI 51.2		
Dementia	NI 1.2	NI 3.1	NB 2.6
	NB 3.2		
Depression	NI 1.5	NI 2.1	NI 4.3
	NC 3.3	NB 1.5	NB 2.1

Nutrition Assessment Matrix
Client History Data and Related Diagnostic Terminology

Parameter (not all-inclusive)	Nutrition Diagnostic Terminology		
Medical diagnoses, continued:			
Developmental delay	NB 2.6		
Diabetes mellitus	NB 1.2	NI 51.3	NI 53.2
	NI 53.3	NI 53.4	NB 1.4
	NB 2.3		
Diverticulitis	NI 53.6	NC 1.4	
Dysphasia	NC 1.1		
Eating disorder	NI 1.3	NI 53.6	
Encephalopathy, hepatic	NI 5.4		
Falls, unexplained	NI 4.3		
Fatigue	NC 3.4		
Fluorosis	NI 55.2		
Foodborne illness, e.g., bacterial, viral, and parasitic infection,	NB 3.1		
Gastrointestinal stricture	NI 53.6		
Geographic location and socioeconomic status associated with nutrient intake of indigenous phenomenon	NI 5.2		
Headache	NB 3.1		
Hip/long- bone fractures	NI 1.1		
Hyperemia	NI 54.1		
Hyperlipidemia	NI 51.2		
Hypertension	NI 4.2	NI 4.3	NI 5.4
Hyperthyroidism (pre- or untreated)	NI 1.1	NC 3.2	
Hypertriglyceridemia, severe	NI 4.3		
Hypoglycemia	NI 53.3	NI 53.4	
Hypotension	NI 1.3		
Hypothyroidism	NC 3.3		
Hypotonic conditions	NI 1.3		
Illness, recent	NI 5.3		
Inborn errors of metabolism	NI 52.3		
Infection	NI 1.1	NI 53.2	
Inflammatory bowel disease	NI 53.5	NI 55.1	
Irritable bowel syndrome	NI 5.4	NI 53.6	NC 1.4
Kidney stones	NI 55.1		
Lactase deficiency	NI 53.2		
Liver disease	NI 3.2	NI 5.2	NI 5.4
	NI 51.3	NI 53.1	NI 54.2
	NI 55.2	NB 2.3	
Malabsorption, protein and/or nutrient	NI 2.1	NI 52.1	NI 52.2
Maldigestion	NC 1.4		
Malnutrition	NI 1.3	NI 5.2	NI 5.3
	NC 3.1		
Mastitis	NC 1.3		
Mental illness with obsessive compulsive tendencies	NI 53.6		
Mental illness, dementia, confusion	NC 3.1	NB 1.2	NB 1.7
	NB 3.2		

Nutrition Assessment Matrix
Client History Data and Related Diagnostic Terminology

Parameter (not all-inclusive)	Nutrition Diagnostic Terminology		
Medical diagnoses, continued:			
Metabolic syndrome	NI 1.5	NI 2.2	NI 53.3
	NI 53.4		
Multiple sclerosis	NB 2.6		
Nephrotic syndrome	NI 3.2		
Neurological disorders	NB 2.6		
Obesity, morbid	NB 2.1		
Obesity/overweight	NI 1.5	NI 2.2	NI 51.3
	NI 53.3	NI 53.4	NB 1.4
Oral soft issue infection, e.g., candidiasis, leukoplakia	NC 1.2		
Osteomalacia	NI 54.1		
Pancreatic disease	NI 4.3	NI 53.1	
Paralysis	NB 2.6		
Paraplegia	NB 2.4		
Parkinson's disease	NI 1.2		
Pellegra	NI 54.1		
Phytobezoar	NI 53.6		
Poisoning by drugs, medicinals, or biological substances	NB 3.1		
Poisoning from food or poisonous plants	NB 3.1		
Polycystic ovary disease	NI 55.1		
Polyps, colon	NI 55.1		
Prader-Willi syndrome	NI 1.3		
Premature birth	NC 1.3		
Premenstrual syndrome	NI 55.1		
Prolapsing hemorrhoids	NI 53.6		
Psychiatric illness	NC 3.4		
Pulmonary failure	NI 5.3		
Rachitic rosary in children	NI 54.1		
Renal disease, end stage	NI 3.2	NI 5.4	NB 2.3
Rickets	NI 54.1		
Rheumatic conditions	NC 3.4		
Seizure disorder	NI 53.1		
Sepsis or severe infection	NI 51.1	NI 53.2	NI 53.5
Short bowel syndrome	NI 53.6	NI 54.1	NI 55.1
Syndrome of Inappropriate Antidiuretic Hormone (SIADH)	NI 3.2		
Stroke	NB 2.6		
Tardive dyskinesia	NB 2.6		
Thrush or candidiasis	NC 1.3		
Trauma	NI 1.1	NC 3.2	
Tremors	NB 2.6		
Tuberculosis	NI 2.1	NI 51.1	
Ulcer disease	NI 53.5	NI 53.6	
Upper respiratory infections or pneumonia	NC 1.1		
Vagotomy	NC 1.4		
Weight loss	NB 2.6		
Wired jaw	NC 1.2		

Nutrition Assessment Matrix
Client History Data and Related Diagnostic Terminology

Parameter (not all-inclusive)	Nutrition Diagnostic Terminology		
Mental status:			
Concentration difficulty	NI 1.3		
Evidence of addictive, obsessive, or compulsive tendencies	NB 2.2		
History of mood and anxiety disorders, personality disorders, substance abuse disorders	NB 1.5		
Signs and symptoms:			
Abdominal cramping	NI 53.6		
Abdominal pain	NC 2.1		
Achalasia	NC 1.1		
Acute or chronic pain	NI 2.1		
Amenorrhea	NB 2.2		
Angina	NI 51.2		
Anorexia, nausea, vomiting, diarrhea, steatorrhea, constipation, abdominal pain	NC 1.4		
Bloating	NB 3.1		
Body temperature (low with weight loss)	NI 1.3		
Bowel motility, decreased	NI 1.3		
Bradycardia	NI 1.3		
Chills	NB 3.1		
Cholesterol, serum	NI 4.1	NI 4.2	
Contributes to the development of anemia	NI 5.5		
Cramping	NB 3.1		
Diarrhea	NI 5.5	NI 51.2	NI 51.3
	NI 53.6	NC 2.1	NB 3.1
Discomfort or pain associated with intake of foods rich in bioactive substances	NI 4.1	NI 4.2	
Dizziness	NB 3.1		
Engorgement	NC 1.3		
Enteral or parenteral nutrition intolerance	NI 2.5		
Epigastric pain	NI 5.5	NI 51.2	NI 51.3
Estrogen status	NI 55.1		
Failure to thrive	NI 1.3		
Falls, unexplained	NI 4.3		
Feeding tube or venous access in the wrong position or removed	NI 2.3		
Fever	NI 5.1	NB 3.1	
Flatulence, excessive	NI 53.6		
Gastrointestinal disturbances	NI 55.2		
High stool volume or frequency that causes discomfort to the individual	NI 53.6		
Hunger, use of alcohol or drugs that reduce hunger	NI 1.4	NI 2.1	NI 5.2
Muscle weakness	NC 3.4		
Muscle weakness, fatigue, cardiac arrhythmia, dehydration, and electrolyte imbalance	NB 1.5		
Nausea	NI 5.5	NI 53.6	NB 3.1

Nutrition Assessment Matrix
Client History Data and Related Diagnostic Terminology

Parameter (not all-inclusive)	Nutrition Diagnostic Terminology		
Signs and symptoms, continued:			
Oral manifestations of systemic disease	NC 1.2		
Report of always feeling cold	NB 1.5		
Self-induced vomiting, diarrhea, bloating, constipation, flatulence	NB 1.5		
Shortness of breath or dyspnea on exertion or at rest	NI 3.2	NB 2.6	
Steatorrhea	NI 51.2		
Stool volume, low	NI 53.5		
Vomiting	NI 5.5	NI 53.6	NB 3.1
Treatments:			
Bowel resection	NC 1.4	NC 2.1	
Chemotherapy with oral side effects	NC 1.2		
Enteral or parenteral nutrition therapy	NI 52.3		
Esophagostomy or esophageal dilatation	NC 1.4		
Gastrectomy	NC 1.4		
Gastric bypass	NC 1.4	NC 2.1	
Intestinal resection	NI 2.3		
Knee surgery	NB 2.1		
Oral surgery, recent major	NC 1.2		
Ostomy, new	NB 1.4		
Radiation therapy	NC 2.1		
Radiation therapy to oral cavity	NC 1.2		
Rigorous therapy regimen	NB 2.4		
Surgery	NI 1.1	NI 5.3	NC 3.2
Surgery requiring recumbent position	NB 2.6		
Surgery, recent	NB 2.4		
Medications and supplements:			
Insulin or insulin secretagogues	NI 53.4		
Medications that cause somnolence and decreased cognition	NB 2.1		
Medication associated with weight loss	NC 3.2		
Medication, lipid lowering	NI 51.2		
Medications administered in large amounts of fluid	NI 3.2		
Medications affecting absorption or metabolism	NI 5.1		
Medications associated with increased appetite	NC 3.4		
Medications that affect appetite	NC 3.1		
Medications that cause altered glucose levels	NI 53.2	NI 53.3	NI 53.4
Medications that cause anorexia	NI 2.1		
Medications that impact RMR	NC 3.3		
Medications that impair fluid excretion	NI 3.2		
Medications that increase resting energy expenditure	NI 1.1		
Medications that reduce requirements of impair metabolism of energy, protein, fat, or fluid	NI 2.4		

Nutrition Assessment Matrix
Client History Data and Related Diagnostic Terminology

Parameter (not all-inclusive)	Nutrition Diagnostic Terminology
Medications and supplements, continued:	
Medications that reduce thirst	NI 3.1
Medications that require nutrient supplementation that cannot be accomplished with food intake alone	NC 2.3
Medications with known food-medication interactions	NC 2.3
Misuse of laxatives, enemas, diuretics, stimulants, and/or metabolic enhancers	NB 1.5

Nutrition Care Process Step 2. Nutrition Diagnosis
The new component of the Nutrition Care Process

INTRODUCTION

The ADA has identified and defined nutrition diagnoses/problems to be used in the profession of dietetics. Nutrition diagnosis is identifying and labeling an actual occurrence, risk of, or potential for developing a nutritional problem that a dietetics professional is responsible for treating independently. The standardized language of nutrition diagnoses/problems is an integral component in the Nutrition Care Process. In fact, several other professions, including medicine, nursing, physical therapy, and occupational therapy, utilize care processes with defined terms for making nutrition diagnoses specific to their professional scope of practice.

ADA's Standardized Language Task Force developed a conceptual framework for the standardized nutrition language and identified the nutrition diagnoses/problems. The framework outlines the domains within which the nutrition diagnoses/problems fall and the flow of the nutrition care process in relation to the continuum of health, disease, and disability.

The methodology for developing sets of terms such as these included systematically collecting data from multiple sources simultaneously. Data were collected from a select group of ADA recognized leaders and award winners prior to starting the project. A 12-member task force developed the terms with input from groups of community, ambulatory, acute care, and long-term care practitioners and obtained feedback from experts concerning the research supporting the terms and definitions.

The methodology for continued development and refinement of these terms has been identified. As with the ongoing updating of the American Medical Association Current Procedural Terminology (CPT) codes, these will also be published on an annual basis. Additionally, an ADA member, Pamela Charney, PhD, RD, has completed a validation study of the nutrition diagnosis terms. Charney's research was completed in January 2005 and focused on whether dietitians would select the same nutrition diagnostic term when provided various patient care scenarios and whether dietitians agreed on which of the defining characteristics were necessary to identify the presence of a particular nutrition diagnosis. Eight terms were selected for this second analysis: hypometabolism, inadequate bioactive substance intake, imbalance of nutrients, inconsistent carbohydrate intake, altered gastrointestinal (GI) function, food and nutrition related knowledge deficit, not ready for diet/lifestyle change, and undesirable food choices. This version of the nutrition diagnostic terms includes changes to the reference sheets for these nutrition diagnoses based on Dr. Charney's results.

The nutrition diagnostic terms are also being incorporated into two other research studies in the ambulatory setting. The CARLE Enhanced Nutrition Component to the Medicare Demonstration Research Project started collecting nutrition diagnostic term usage in April 2005 and preliminary data analysis is being completed at this time. The nutrition diagnostic terms are being incorporated into a study of obesity and chronic disease with North Carolina Blue Cross and Blue Shield that began in February 2006. Further, another two-part study is underway in which a questionnaire will evaluate the dietitians' perceptions of the most important defining characteristic for all of the nutrition diagnostic terms using methodology similar to Dr. Charney's. The second phase will include a study through the Dietetics Practice Based Research in acute care and other institutional settings where two dietitians will independently select nutrition diagnostic terms and create PES (Problem, Etiology, Signs/Symptoms, see page 45) statements for the same patient. Levels of agreement between dietitians using a real patient will be assessed.

As each of the research studies is completed, findings will be incorporated into future versions of these terms. Future iterations and changes to the nutrition diagnoses/problems and the reference sheet are expected as this standard language evolves. The process for practitioners to submit suggested revisions to the nutrition diagnoses is included in this book on page 268.

ADA will also formally submit these terms to become part of nationally recognized health care databases and in standardized informatics languages, such as the Systematized Nomenclature of Medicine International (SNOMED). ADA has already begun the dialogue with these groups to let them know the direction that the Association is headed and to keep them appraised of progress. Thus far, the feedback from the database and informatics groups has been quite positive, and they have expressed a need for documenting the unique nature of nutrition services.

NUTRITION CARE PROCESS AND NUTRITION DIAGNOSIS

Nutrition diagnosis is a critical step between nutrition assessment and nutrition intervention. The nutrition diagnosis is the identification and labeling of the specific nutrition problem that dietetics professionals are responsible for treating independently.

Naming the nutrition diagnosis, identifying the etiology, and signs and symptoms provides a way to document the link between nutrition assessment and nutrition intervention and set realistic and measurable expected outcomes for each patient/client. Identifying the nutrition diagnosis also assists practitioners in establishing priorities when planning an individual patient/client's nutrition intervention.

A nutrition diagnosis may be temporary, altering as the patient/client's response changes (e.g., excessive carbohydrate intake). Ideally, with nutrition intervention, the nutrition diagnosis would be resolved and go away. Nutrition diagnosis differs from medical diagnosis. Medical diagnosis is a disease or pathology of specific organs or body systems (e.g., diabetes) and does not change as long as the condition exists.

CATEGORIES OF NUTRITION DIAGNOSTIC TERMINOLOGY

The 62 nutrition diagnoses/problems have been given labels that are clustered into three domains: intake, clinical, and behavioral-environmental. Each domain represents unique characteristics that contribute to nutritional health. Within each domain are classes and, in some cases, subclasses of nutrition diagnoses.

A definition of each follows:

The **Intake** domain lists actual problems related to intake of energy, nutrients, fluids, or bioactive substances through oral diet, or nutrition support (cntcral or parenteral nutrition).

Class: Energy Balance (1)—Actual or estimated changes in energy (kcal).
Class: Oral or Nutrition Support Intake (2)—Actual or estimated food and beverage intake from oral diet or nutrition support compared with patient/client's goal.
Class: Fluid Intake (3)—Actual or estimated fluid intake compared with patient/client's goal.
Class: Bioactive Substances Intake (4)—Actual or observed intake of bioactive substances, including single or multiple functional food components, ingredients, dietary supplements, and alcohol.
Class: Nutrient Intake (5)—Actual or estimated intake of specific nutrient groups or single nutrients as compared with desired levels.
        Sub-Class: Fat and Cholesterol (51)
        Sub-Class: Protein (52)
        Sub-Class: Carbohydrate and Fiber (53)
        Sub-Class: Vitamin (54)
        Sub-Class: Mineral (55)

The **Clinical** domain is nutritional findings/problems identified as related to medical or physical conditions.

Class: Functional (1)—Change in physical or mechanical functioning that interferes with or prevents desired nutritional consequences.
Class: Biochemical (2)—Change in the capacity to metabolize nutrients as a result of medications, surgery, or as indicated by altered lab values.
Class: Weight (3)—Chronic weight or changed weight status when compared with usual or desired body weight.

The **Behavioral-Environmental** domain includes nutritional findings/problems identified that relate to knowledge, attitudes/beliefs, physical environment, access to food, and food safety.

Class: Knowledge and Beliefs (1)—Actual knowledge and beliefs as reported, observed, or documented.
Class: Physical Activity and Function (2)—Actual physical activity, self-care, and quality of life problems as reported, observed, or documented.
Class: Food Safety and Access (3)—Actual problems with food access or food safety.

Examples of nutrition diagnoses and their definitions include:

INTAKE DOMAIN ▪ Energy Balance

Inadequate energy intake NI-1.4

Energy intake that is less than energy expenditure, established reference standards, or recommendations based on physiological needs. Exception: when the goal is weight loss or during end-of-life care.

CLINICAL DOMAIN ▪ Functional

Swallowing difficulty NC-1.1

Impaired movement of food and liquid from the mouth to the stomach.

| Not ready for diet/lifestyle change NB-1.3 | Lack of perceived value of nutrition-related behavior change compared to costs (consequences or effort required to make changes); conflict with personal value system; antecedent to behavior change. |

NUTRITION DIAGNOSIS STATEMENTS (OR PES)

The nutrition diagnosis is summarized into a structured sentence named the *nutrition diagnosis statement*. This statement, also called a *PES statement* is composed of three distinct components: the problem (P), the etiology (E), and the signs and symptoms (S). The practitioner obtains the etiology and the signs and symptoms during the nutrition assessment phase of the nutrition care process. The nutrition diagnosis is derived from the synthesis of nutrition assessment data, and the wording is obtained from the nutrition diagnoses reference sheets (see pages 59-185).

The generic format for the nutrition diagnosis statement is:

Problem (P) *related to* etiology (E) *as evidenced by* signs and symptoms (S).

Where:

The **Problem or Nutrition Diagnosis Label** describes alterations in the patient/client's nutrition status that dietetics professionals are responsible for treating independently. A nutrition diagnosis allows the dietetics professional to identify realistic and measurable outcomes, formulate nutrition interventions, and monitor and evaluate change.	The **Etiology** (Cause/Contributing Risk Factors) are those factors contributing to the existence, or maintenance of pathophysiological, psychosocial, situational, developmental, cultural, and/or environmental problems. It is linked to the nutrition diagnosis label by the words "related to." Identifying the etiology will lead to the selection of a nutrition intervention aimed at resolving the underlying cause of the nutrition problem whenever possible.	The **Signs/Symptoms** (Defining Characteristics) consist of objective (signs) and/or subjective (symptoms) data used to determine whether the patient/client has the nutrition diagnosis specified. It is linked to the etiology by the words "as evidenced by." The clear identification of quantifiable data in the signs and symptoms will serve as the basis for monitoring and evaluating nutrition outcomes

A well-written nutrition diagnostic statement is:

• Simple, clear, and concise
• Specific to the patient/client or group
• Related to a single patient/client nutrition-related problem
• Accurately related to an etiology
• Based on reliable and accurate nutrition assessment data

Specific questions dietetics practitioners should use in evaluating the PES they have developed are:

- Can the RD resolve or improve the nutrition diagnosis?
  - Can the practitioner envision a nutrition intervention that would address the etiology and thus resolve or improve the problem?
  - If not, is the nutrition intervention targeted to reducing or eliminating the signs and symptoms?
- Does the nutrition assessment data support the nutrition diagnosis, etiology, and signs and symptoms?
- Is the etiology listed the "root cause" that can be address by the RD in the intervention?
  - (Ask Why 5 times) Why does this problem exist, why, why, why, why?
- Will measuring the signs and symptoms tell the practitioner if the problem is resolved or improved?
- Are the signs and symptoms specific enough that the practitioner can measure/evaluate changes at the next visit to document resolution or improvement of the nutrition diagnosis?
- When all things are equal and the practitioner has a choice between stating the PES statement using two nutrition diagnosis labels in different domains, choose the intake nutrition diagnosis.

Examples of nutrition diagnosis statements (PES) are:

Diagnosis or Problem		Etiology		Signs and/or Symptoms
Excessive fat intake	*Related to*	Frequent consumption of fast-food meals	*As evidenced by*	Increasing serum cholesterol level
Excessive energy intake	*Related to*	Unchanged dietary intake and restricted mobility while fracture healing	*As evidenced by*	5# weight gain during last 3 weeks due to consumption of 500 kcal/day more than estimated needs
Disordered eating pattern	*Related to*	Harmful belief about food and nutrition (that kcals are not absorbed after using laxatives)	*As evidenced by*	Use of laxatives after meals
Altered GI function (constipation)	*Related to*	Undesirable food choices	*As evidenced by*	Inadequate fiber and fluid intake and excessive intake of refined carbohydrates

NUTRITION DIAGNOSIS REFERENCE SHEET

A reference sheet is available for each nutrition diagnosis. Reference sheets contain four distinct components: nutrition diagnosis label, definition of nutrition diagnosis label, examples of common etiologies, and signs/symptoms. Following is a description of the four components of the reference sheet.

The **Problem or Nutrition Diagnosis Label** describes alterations in the patient/client's nutrition status that dietetics professionals are responsible for treating independently. Nutrition diagnosis differs from medical diagnosis in that a nutrition diagnosis changes as the patient/client response changes. The medical diagnosis does not change as long as the disease or condition exists. A nutrition diagnosis allows the dietetics professional to identify realistic and measurable outcomes, formulate nutrition interventions, and monitor and evaluate change.

The **Definition** of Nutrition Diagnosis Label briefly describes the Nutrition Diagnosis Label to differentiate a discrete problem area.

The **Etiology** (Cause/Contributing Risk Factors) are those factors contributing to the existence, or maintenance of pathophysiological, psychosocial, situational, developmental, cultural, and/or environmental problems. It is linked to the Nutrition Diagnosis Label by the words *related to*.

The **Signs/Symptoms** (Defining Characteristics) consist of subjective and/or objective data used to determine whether the patient/client has the nutrition diagnosis specified. It is linked to the etiology by the words *as evidenced by*.

The signs and symptoms are gathered in Step 1 of the nutrition care process: nutrition assessment. There are five categories of nutrition assessment data used to cluster the information on the nutrition diagnosis reference sheet—biochemical data, medical tests, and procedures; anthropometric measurements; physical exam findings; food/nutrition history; and client history. Within each nutrition assessment category, potential indicators associated with the specific nutrition diagnosis are listed on the reference sheet.

Example
Swallowing Difficulty NC-1.1

Nutrition Assessment Category	Potential Indicator of this Nutrition Diagnosis
Physical Exam Finding	• Evidence of dehydration, e.g., dry mucous membranes, poor skin turgor

These reference sheets, beginning on page 59, will assist practitioners with consistently and correctly identifying the nutrition diagnoses.

SUMMARY

Nutrition diagnosis is the critical link in the nutrition care process between nutrition assessment and nutrition intervention. Nutrition interventions can then be clearly targeted to address either the etiology (E) or signs and symptoms (S) of the specific nutrition diagnosis/problem identified. Using a standardized terminology for identifying the nutrition diagnosis/problem will make one aspect of the critical thinking of dietetics professionals visible to other professionals as well as provide a clear method of communicating among dietetics professionals. Implementation of a standard language throughout the profession, with tools to assist practitioners, is making this new language a success. Ongoing study and evaluation is critical as the standardized language is utilized by the profession.

REFERENCES

1. American Dietetic Association. *Nutrition Diagnosis: A Critical Step in the Nutrition Care Process.* Chicago, IL: American Dietetic Association; 2006.
2. Lacey K, Pritchett E. Nutrition care process and model: ADA adopts road map to quality care and outcomes management. *J Am Diet Assoc.* 2003;103:1061-1072.
3. Mathieu J, Foust M, Ouellette P. Implementing nutrition diagnosis, step two in the nutrition care process and model: Challenges and lesions learned in two health care facilities. *J Am Diet Assoc.* 2005;105:1636-1640.

INTAKE   NI

Defined as "actual problems related to intake of energy, nutrients, fluids, bioactive substances through oral diet or nutrition support"

Energy Balance (1)
Defined as "actual or estimated changes in energy (kcal)"

- ☐ Hypermetabolism   NI-1.1
  (Increased energy needs)
- ☐ Increased energy expenditure   NI-1.2
- ☐ Hypometabolism   NI-1.3
  (Decreased energy needs)
- ☐ Inadequate energy intake   NI-1.4
- ☐ Excessive energy intake   NI-1.5

Oral or Nutrition Support Intake (2)
Defined as "actual or estimated food and beverage intake from oral diet or nutrition support compared with patient goal"

- ☐ Inadequate oral food/   NI-2.1
  beverage intake
- ☐ Excessive oral food/   NI-2.2
  beverage intake
- ☐ Inadequate intake from   NI-2.3
  enteral/parenteral nutrition
- ☐ Excessive intake from   NI-2.4
  enteral/parenteral nutrition
- ☐ Inappropriate infusion of   NI-2.5
  enteral/parenteral nutrition
  (use with caution)

Fluid Intake (3)
Defined as "actual or estimated fluid intake compared with patient goal"

- ☐ Inadequate fluid intake   NI-3.1
- ☐ Excessive fluid intake   NI-3.2

Bioactive Substances (4)
Defined as "actual or observed intake of bioactive substances, including single or multiple functional food components, ingredients, dietary supplements, alcohol"

- ☐ Inadequate bioactive   NI-4.1
  substance intake
- ☐ Excessive bioactive   NI-4.2
  substance intake
- ☐ Excessive alcohol intake   NI-4.3

Nutrient (5)
Defined as "actual or estimated intake of specific nutrient groups or single nutrients as compared with desired levels"

- ☐ Increased nutrient needs   NI-5.1
  (specify) _____
- ☐ Evident protein-energy   NI-5.2
  malnutrition
- ☐ Inadequate protein-   NI-5.3
  energy intake
- ☐ Decreased nutrient needs   NI-5.4
  (specify) _____
- ☐ Imbalance of nutrients   NI-5.5

Fat and Cholesterol (51)
- ☐ Inadequate fat intake   NI-51.1
- ☐ Excessive fat intake   NI-51.2
- ☐ Inappropriate intake   NI-51.3
  of food fats
  (specify) _____

Protein (52)
- ☐ Inadequate protein intake   NI-52.1
- ☐ Excessive protein intake   NI-52.2
- ☐ Inappropriate intake   NI-52.3
  of amino acids
  (specify) _____

Carbohydrate and Fiber (53)
- ☐ Inadequate carbohydrate   NI-53.1
  intake
- ☐ Excessive carbohydrate   NI-53.2
  intake
- ☐ Inappropriate intake of   NI-53.3
  types of carbohydrate
  (specify) _____
- ☐ Inconsistent   NI-53.4
  carbohydrate intake
- ☐ Inadequate fiber intake   NI-53.5
- ☐ Excessive fiber intake   NI-53.6

Vitamin (54)
- ☐ Inadequate vitamin   NI-54.1
  intake *(specify)* _____
- ☐ Excessive vitamin   NI-54.2
  intake *(specify)* _____
  - ☐ A   ☐ C
  - ☐ Thiamin   ☐ D
  - ☐ Riboflavin   ☐ E
  - ☐ Niacin   ☐ K
  - ☐ Folate   ☐ Other _____

Mineral (55)
- ☐ Inadequate mineral intake   NI-55.1
  (specify)
  - ☐ Calcium   ☐ Iron
  - ☐ Potassium   ☐ Zinc
  - ☐ Other _____
- ☐ Excessive mineral intake   NI-55.2
  (specify)
  - ☐ Calcium   ☐ Iron
  - ☐ Potassium   ☐ Zinc
  - ☐ Other _____

CLINICAL   NC

Defined as "nutritional findings/problems identified as related to medical or physical conditions"

Functional (1)
Defined as "change in physical or mechanical functioning that interferes with or prevents desired nutritional consequences"

- ☐ Swallowing difficulty   NC-1.1
- ☐ Chewing (masticatory) difficulty   NC-1.2
- ☐ Breastfeeding difficulty   NC-1.3
- ☐ Altered GI function   NC-1.4

Biochemical (2)
Defined as "change in capacity to metabolize nutrients as a result of medications, or surgery, or as indicated by altered lab values"

- ☐ Impaired nutrient utilization   NC-2.1
- ☐ Altered nutrition-related   NC-2.2
  laboratory values
- ☐ Food-medication interaction   NC-2.3

Weight (3)
Defined as "chronic weight or changed weight status when compared with usual or desired body weight"

- ☐ Underweight   NC-3.1
- ☐ Involuntary weight loss   NC-3.2
- ☐ Overweight/obesity   NC-3.3
- ☐ Involuntary weight gain   NC-3.4

BEHAVIORAL-ENVIRONMENTAL   NB

Defined as "nutritional findings/problems identified that relate to knowledge, attitudes/beliefs, physical environment, access to food, or food safety"

Knowledge and Beliefs (1)
Defined as "actual knowledge and beliefs as related, observed or documented"

- ☐ Food- and nutrition-related   NB-1.1
  knowledge deficit
- ☐ Harmful beliefs/attitudes   NB-1.2
  about food- or nutrition-
  related topics *(use with caution)*
- ☐ Not ready for diet/   NB-1.3
  lifestyle change
- ☐ Self-monitoring deficit   NB-1.4
- ☐ Disordered eating pattern   NB-1.5
- ☐ Limited adherence to nutrition-   NB-1.6
  related recommendations
- ☐ Undesirable food choices   NB-1.7

Physical Activity and Function (2)
Defined as "actual physical activity, self-care, and quality-of-life problems as reported, observed, or documented"

- ☐ Physical inactivity   NB-2.1
- ☐ Excessive exercise   NB-2.2
- ☐ Inability or lack of desire   NB-2.3
  to manage self-care
- ☐ Impaired ability to   NB-2.4
  prepare foods/meals
- ☐ Poor nutrition quality of life   NB-2.5
- ☐ Self-feeding difficulty   NB-2.6

Food Safety and Access (3)
Defined as "actual problems with food access or food safety"

- ☐ Intake of unsafe food   NB-3.1
- ☐ Limited access to food   NB-3.2

Date Identified	Date Resolved

Problem _____

Etiology _____

Signs/Symptoms _____

Problem _____

Etiology _____

Signs/Symptoms _____

Problem _____

Etiology _____

Signs/Symptoms _____

NUTRITION DIAGNOSIS TERMS AND DEFINITIONS

Nutrition Diagnostic Term	Term Number	Definition	Reference Sheet Page Numbers
DOMAIN: INTAKE	NI	**Actual problems related to intake of energy, nutrients, fluids, bioactive substances through oral diet or nutrition support (enteral or parenteral nutrition).**	
Class: Energy Balance (1)		Actual or estimated changes in energy (kcal) balance.	
Hypermetabolism (Increased energy needs)	NI-1.1	Resting metabolic rate (RMR) more than predicted requirements due to stress, trauma, injury, sepsis, or disease. Note: RMR is the sum of metabolic processes of active cell mass related to the maintenance of normal body functions and regulatory balance during rest.	59-60
Increased energy expenditure	NI-1.2	Resting metabolic rate (RMR) more than predicted requirements due to body composition, medications, endocrine, neurologic, or genetic changes. Note: RMR is the sum of metabolic processes of active cell mass related to the maintenance of normal body functions and regulatory balance during rest.	61
Hypometabolism (Decreased energy needs)	NI-1.3	Resting metabolic rate (RMR) less than predicted requirements due to body composition, medications, endocrine, neurologic, or genetic changes.	62-63
Inadequate energy intake	NI-1.4	Energy intake that is less than energy expenditure, established reference standards, or recommendations based on physiological needs. Exception: when the goal is weight loss or during end-of-life care.	64-65
Excessive energy intake	NI-1.5	Energy intake that exceeds energy expenditure, established reference standards, or recommendations based on physiological needs. Exception: when weight gain is desired.	66-67

NUTRITION DIAGNOSIS TERMS AND DEFINITIONS

Nutrition Diagnostic Term	Term Number	Definition	Reference Sheet Page Numbers
Class: *Oral or Nutrition Support Intake (2)*		Actual or estimated food and beverage intake from oral diet or nutrition support compared with patient goal.	
Inadequate oral food/beverage intake	NI-2.1	Oral food/beverage intake that is less than established reference standards or recommendations based on physiological needs. Exception: when recommendation is weight loss or during end-of-life care.	68-69
Excessive oral food/beverage intake	NI-2.2	Oral food/beverage intake that exceeds energy expenditure, established reference standards, or recommendations based on physiological needs. Exception: when weight gain is desired.	70-71
Inadequate intake from enteral/parenteral nutrition	NI-2.3	Enteral or parenteral infusion that provides fewer calories or nutrients compared to establish reference standards or recommendations based on physiological needs. Exception: when recommendation is for weight loss or during end-of-life care.	72-74
Excessive intake from enteral/parenteral nutrition	NI-2.4	Enteral or parenteral infusion that provides more calories or nutrients compared to established reference standards or recommendations based on physiological needs	75-76
Inappropriate infusion of enteral/parenteral nutrition USE WITH CAUTION ONLY AFTER DISCUSSION WITH OTHER MEMBERS IF THE HEALTH CARE TEAM	NI-2.5	Enteral or parenteral infusion that provides either fewer or more calories and/or nutrients or is of the wrong composition or type, parental nutrition that is not warranted because the patient is able to tolerate an enteral intake, or is unsafe because of the potential for sepsis or other complications	77-78

51

Edition: 2007

NUTRITION DIAGNOSIS TERMS AND DEFINITIONS

Nutrition Diagnostic Term	Term Number	Definition	Reference Sheet Page Numbers
Class: *Fluid Intake (3)*			
Inadequate fluid intake	NI-3.1	Actual or estimated fluid intake compared with patient goal.	
Excessive fluid intake	NI-3.2	Lower intake of fluid-containing foods or substances compared to established reference standards or recommendations based on physiological needs	79-80
		Higher intake of fluid compared to established reference standards or recommendations based on physiological needs	81-82
Class: *Bioactive Substances (4)*			
Inadequate bioactive substance intake	NI-4.1	Actual or observed intake of bioactive substances, including single or multiple functional food components, ingredients, dietary supplements, alcohol.	
Excessive bioactive substance intake	NI-4.2	Lower intake of bioactive substances or foods containing bioactive substances compared to established reference standards or recommendations based on physiological needs	83-84
		Higher intake of bioactive substances other than traditional nutrients, such as functional foods, bioactive food components, dietary supplements, or food concentrates compared to established reference standards or recommendations based on physiological needs	85-86
Excessive alcohol intake	NI-4.3	Intake more than the suggested limits for alcohol	87-88
Class: *Nutrient (5)*			
Increased nutrient needs (specify)	NI-5.1	Actual or estimated intake of specific nutrient groups or single nutrients as compared with desired levels.	
		Increased need for a specific nutrient compared to established reference standards or recommendations based on physiological needs	89-90

Edition: 2007

52

NUTRITION DIAGNOSIS TERMS AND DEFINITIONS

Nutrition Diagnostic Term	Term Number	Definition	Reference Sheet Page Numbers
Evident protein-energy malnutrition	NI-5.2	Inadequate intake of protein and/or energy over prolonged periods of time resulting in loss of fat stores and/or muscle wasting	91-92
Inadequate protein-energy intake	NI-5.3	Inadequate intake of protein and/or energy compared to established reference standards or recommendations based on physiological needs of short or recent duration	93-94
Decreased nutrient needs (specify)	NI-5.4	Decreased need for a specific nutrient compared to established reference standards or recommendations based on physiological needs	95-96
Imbalance of nutrients	NI-5.5	An undesirable combination of ingested nutrients, such that the amount of one nutrient ingested interferes with or alters absorption and/or utilization of another nutrient	97-98
Sub-Class: Fat and Cholesterol (51)			
Inadequate fat intake	NI-51.1	Lower fat intake compared to established reference standards or recommendations based on physiological needs. Exception: when recommendation is for weight loss or during end-of-life care.	99-100
Excessive fat intake	NI-51.2	Higher fat intake compared to established reference standards or recommendations based on physiological needs	101-102
Inappropriate intake of food fats (specify)	NI-51.3	Intake of wrong type or quality of food fats compared to established reference standards or recommendations based on physiological needs	103-104
Sub-Class: Protein (52)			
Inadequate protein intake	NI-52.1	Lower intake of protein-containing foods or substances compared to established reference standards or recommendations based on physiological needs	105-106

53

Edition: 2007

NUTRITION DIAGNOSIS TERMS AND DEFINITIONS

Nutrition Diagnostic Term	Term Number	Definition	Reference Sheet Page Numbers
Excessive protein intake	NI-52.2	Intake more than the recommended level of protein compared to established reference standards or recommendations based on physiological needs	107-108
Inappropriate intake of amino acids (specify)	NI-52.3	Intake that is more or less than recommended level and/or type of amino acids compared to established reference standards or recommendations based on physiological needs	109-110
Sub-Class: *Carbohydrate and Fiber (53)*			
Inadequate carbohydrate intake	NI-53.1	Lower intake of carbohydrate-containing foods or substances compared to established reference standards or recommendations based on physiological needs	111
Excessive carbohydrate intake	NI-53.2	Intake more than the recommended level and type of carbohydrate compared to established reference standards or recommendations based on physiological needs	112-113
Inappropriate intake of types of carbohydrate (specify)	NI-53.3	Intake or the type or amount of carbohydrate that is more or less than the established reference standards or recommendations based on physiological needs	114-115
Inconsistent carbohydrate intake	NI-53.4	Inconsistent timing of carbohydrate intake throughout the day, day to day, or a pattern of carbohydrate intake that is not consistent with recommended pattern based on physiological needs	116-117
Inadequate fiber intake	NI-53.5	Lower intake of fiber-containing foods or substances compared to established reference standards or recommendations based on physiological needs	118-119
Excessive fiber intake	NI-53.6	Higher intake of fiber-containing foods or substances compared to recommendations based on patient/client condition	120-121

54

Edition: 2007

NUTRITION DIAGNOSIS TERMS AND DEFINITIONS

Nutrition Diagnostic Term	Term Number	Definition	Reference Sheet Page Numbers
Sub-Class: Vitamin (54)			
Inadequate vitamin intake (specify)	NI-54.1	Lower intake of vitamin-containing foods or substances compared to established reference standards or recommendations based on physiological needs	122-124
Excessive vitamin intake (specify)	NI-54.2	Higher intake of vitamin-containing foods or substances compared to established reference standards or recommendations based on physiological needs	125-126
Sub-Class: Mineral (55)			
Inadequate mineral intake (specify)	NI-55.1	Lower intake of mineral-containing foods or substances compared to established reference standards or recommendations based on physiological needs	127-128
Excessive mineral intake (specify)	NI-55.2	Higher intake of mineral from foods, supplements, medications, or water, compared to established reference standards or recommendations based on physiological needs	129-130
DOMAIN: CLINICAL	NC	**Nutritional findings/problems identified that relate to medical or physical conditions.**	
Class: Functional (1)		Change in physical or mechanical functioning that interferes with or prevents desired nutritional consequences.	
Swallowing difficulty	NC-1.1	Impaired movement of food and liquid from the mouth to the stomach	131-132
Chewing (masticatory) difficulty	NC-1.2	Impaired ability to manipulate or masticate food for swallowing	133-135
Breastfeeding difficulty	NC-1.3	Inability to sustain nutrition through breastfeeding	136-137
Altered GI function	NC-1.4	Changes in ability to digest or absorb nutrients	138-139

Edition: 2007

NUTRITION DIAGNOSIS TERMS AND DEFINITIONS

Nutrition Diagnostic Term	Term Number	Definition	Reference Sheet Page Numbers
Class: Biochemical (2)			
Impaired nutrient utilization	NC-2.1	Change in capacity to metabolize nutrients as a result of medications, surgery, or as indicated by altered lab values.	140-141
Altered nutrition-related laboratory values (specify)	NC-2.2	Changes in ability to absorb or metabolize nutrients and bioactive substances	142-143
Food-medication interaction	NC-2.3	Undesirable/harmful interaction(s) between food and over-the-counter (OTC) medications, prescribed medications, herbals, botanicals, and/or dietary supplements that diminishes, enhances, or alters effect of nutrients and/or medications	144-145
Class: Weight (3)		Chronic weight or changed weight status when compared with usual or desired body weight.	
Underweight	NC-3.1	Low body weight compared to established reference standards or recommendations	146-147
Involuntary weight loss	NC-3.2	Decrease in body weight that is not planned or desired	148-149
Overweight/obesity	NC-3.3	Increased adiposity compared to established reference standards or recommendations	150-151
Involuntary weight gain	NC-3.4	Weight gain more than that which is desired or expected	152-153

Edition: 2007

NUTRITION DIAGNOSIS TERMS AND DEFINITIONS

Nutrition Diagnostic Term	Term Number	Definition	Reference Sheet Page Numbers
DOMAIN: BEHAVIORAL-ENVIRONMENTAL	NB	**Nutritional findings/problems identified that relate to knowledge, attitudes/beliefs, physical environment, access to food, or food safety.**	
Class: Knowledge and Beliefs (1)			
Food- and nutrition-related knowledge deficit	NB-1.1	Actual knowledge and beliefs as reported, observed, or documented	154-155
	NB-1.1	Incomplete or inaccurate knowledge about food, nutrition, or nutrition-related information and guidelines, e.g., nutrient requirements, consequences of food behaviors, life stage requirements, nutrition recommendations, diseases and conditions, physiological function, or products	154-155
Harmful beliefs/attitudes about food or nutrition-related topics USE WITH CAUTION TO BE SENSITIVE TO PATIENT CONCERNS	NB-1.2	Beliefs/attitudes and practices about food, nutrition, and nutrition-related topics that are incompatible with sound nutrition principles, nutrition care, or disease/condition	156-157
Not ready for diet/lifestyle change	NB-1.3	Lack of perceived value of nutrition-related behavior change compared to costs (consequences or effort required to make changes); conflict with personal value system; antecedent to behavior change	158-159
Self-monitoring deficit	NB-1.4	Lack of data recording to track personal progress	160-161
Disordered eating pattern	NB-1.5	Beliefs, attitudes, thoughts, and behaviors related to food, eating, and weight management, including classic eating disorders as well as less severe, similar conditions that negatively impact health	162-165
Limited adherence to nutrition-related recommendations	NB-1.6	Lack of nutrition-related changes as per intervention agreed upon by client or population	166-167
Undesirable food choices	NB-1.7	Food and/or beverage choices that are inconsistent with US Recommended Dietary Intake, *US Dietary Guidelines*, or with the Food Guide Pyramid or with targets defined in the nutrition prescription or nutrition care process	168-169

57

Edition: 2007

NUTRITION DIAGNOSIS TERMS AND DEFINITIONS

Nutrition Diagnostic Term	Term Number	Definition	Reference Sheet Page Numbers
Class: *Physical Activity and Function (2)*			
Physical inactivity	NB-2.1	Actual physical activity, self-care, and quality-of-life problems as reported, observed, or documented	170-171
Excessive exercise	NB-2.2	Low level of activity or sedentary behavior to the extent that it reduces energy expenditure and impacts health	172-173
Inability or lack of desire to manage self care	NB-2.3	An amount of exercise that exceeds that which is necessary to improve health and/or athletic performance	174-175
Impaired ability to prepare foods/meals	NB-2.4	Lack of capacity or unwillingness to implement methods to support healthful food- and nutrition-related behavior	176-177
Poor nutrition quality of life	NB-2.5	Cognitive or physical impairment that prevents preparation of foods/meals	178-179
Self feeding difficulty	NB-2.6	Diminished Nutrition Quality of Life scores related to food impact, self-image, psychological factors social/interpersonal, physical, or self-efficacy	180-181
Class: *Food Safety and Access (3)*		Impaired ability to place food in mouth	
Intake of unsafe food	NB-3.1	Actual problems with food access or food safety.	182-183
Limited access to food	NB-3.2	Intake of food and/or fluids intentionally or unintentionally contaminated with toxins, poisonous products, infectious agents, microbial agents, additives, allergens, and/or agents of bioterrorism	184-185
		Diminished ability to acquire food from sources (e.g., shopping, gardening, meal delivery) due to financial constraints, physical impairment, caregiver support, or unsafe living conditions (e.g., crime hinders travel to grocery store). Limitation to food because of concerns about weight or aging.	

HYPERMETABOLISM (NI-1.1)

Definition

Resting metabolic rate (RMR) more than predicted requirements due to stress, trauma, injury, sepsis, or disease. Note: RMR is the sum of metabolic processes of active cell mass related to the maintenance of normal body functions and regulatory balance during rest.

Etiology (Cause/Contributing Risk Factors)

Factors gathered during the nutrition assessment process that contribute to the existence or the maintenance of pathophysiological, psychosocial, situational, developmental, cultural, and/or environmental problems:

- Catabolic illness
- Infection
- Sepsis

Signs/Symptoms (Defining Characteristics)

A typical cluster of subjective and objective signs and symptoms gathered during the nutrition assessment process that provide evidence that a problem exists; quantify the problem and describe its severity.

Nutrition Assessment Category	Potential Indicators of this Nutrition Diagnosis (one or more must be present)
Biochemical Data, Medical Tests and Procedures	• Blood glucose elevated and difficult to control • Measured RMR > estimated or expected RMR
Anthropometric Measurements	
Physical Examination Findings	• Fever • Increased heart rate • Increased respiratory rate
Food/Nutrition History	
Client History	• Conditions associated with a diagnosis or treatment, e.g., AIDS/HIV, burns, chronic obstructive pulmonary disease, hip/long bone fracture, infection, surgery, trauma, hyperthyroidism (pre- or untreated), some cancers (specify) • Medications associated with ↑ RMR

INTAKE DOMAIN • Energy Balance

HYPERMETABOLISM (NI-1.1)

References:

1. Bitz C, Toubro S, Larsen TM, Harder H, Rennie KL, Jebb SA, Astrup A. Increased 24 hour energy expenditure in Type 2 diabetes mellitus. *Diabetes Care.* 2004;27:2416-21.
2. Dickerson RN, Roth-Yousey L. Medication effects on metabolic rate: A systematic review. *J Am Diet Assoc.* 2005;105:835-843.
3. Frankenfield D, Roth-Yousey L, Compher C. Comparison of predictive equations to measured resting metabolic rate in healthy nonobese and obese individuals, a systematic review. *J Am Diet Assoc.* 2005;105:775-789.

Edition: 2007

INCREASED ENERGY EXPENDITURE (NI-1.2)

Definition

Resting metabolic rate (RMR) more than predicted requirements due to body composition, medications, endocrine, neurologic, or genetic changes. Note: RMR is the sum of metabolic processes of active cell mass related to the maintenance of normal body functions and regulatory balance during rest.

Etiology (Cause/Contributing Risk Factors)

Factors gathered during the nutrition assessment process that contribute to the existence or the maintenance of pathophysiological, psychosocial, situational, developmental, cultural, and/or environmental problems:

- Anabolism or growth
- Voluntary or involuntary physical activity/movement

Signs/Symptoms (Defining Characteristics)

A typical cluster of subjective and objective signs and symptoms gathered during the nutrition assessment process that provide evidence that a problem exists; quantify the problem and describe its severity.

Nutrition Assessment Category	Potential Indicators of this Nutrition Diagnosis (one or more must be present)
Biochemical Data, Medical Tests and Procedures	
Anthropometric Measurements	• Unintentional weight loss of ≥ 10% in 6 months, ≥ 5% in 1 month • Evidence of need for accelerated or catch-up growth or weight gain in children; absence of normal growth • Increased proportional lean body mass
Physical Examination Findings	• Measured RMR > estimated or expected RMR
Food/Nutrition History	• Increased physical activity, e.g., endurance athlete
Client History	• Conditions associated with a diagnosis or treatment, e.g., Parkinson's disease, cerebral palsy, Alzheimer's disease, other dementia

References:

1. Frankenfield D, Roth-Yousey L, Compher C. Comparison of predictive equations to measured resting metabolic rate in healthy nonobese and obese individuals, a systematic review. *J Am Diet Assoc.* 2005;105:775-789.

Edition: 2007

HYPOMETABOLISM (NI-1.3)

Definition
Resting metabolic rate (RMR) less than predicted requirements due to body composition, medications, endocrine, neurologic, or genetic changes.

Etiology (*Cause/Contributing Risk Factors*)
Factors gathered during the nutrition assessment process that contribute to the existence or the maintenance of pathophysiological, psychosocial, situational, developmental, cultural, and/or environmental problems:

- Loss of lean body mass, weight loss
- Medications, e.g., midazolam, propranalol, glipizide
- Endocrine changes, e.g., hypothyroidism

Signs/Symptoms (*Defining Characteristics*)
A typical cluster of subjective and objective signs and symptoms gathered during the nutrition assessment process that provide evidence that a problem exists; quantify the problem and describe its severity.

Nutrition Assessment Category	Potential Indicators of this Nutrition Diagnosis (one or more must be present)
Biochemical Data, Medical Tests and Procedures	• Increased TSH, decreased T4, T3 (hypothyroidism) • Measured RMR < estimated or expected RMR
Anthropometric Data	• Decreased weight or mid-arm muscle circumference • Weight gain (e.g., hypothyroidism) • Growth stunting or failure, based on National Center for Health Statistics (NCHS) growth standards
Physical Exam Findings	• Decreased or normal adipose and muscle mass • Respiratory rate, decreased • Hair loss
Food/Nutrition History	

Edition: 2007

HYPOMETABOLISM (NI-1.3)

Client History	• Conditions associated with a diagnosis or treatment, e.g., hypothyroidism, anorexia nervosa, malnutrition, failure to thrive, Prader-Willi syndrome, hypotonic conditions • Bradycardia, hypotension, decreased bowl motility, low body temperature (in significant weight loss) • Cold intolerance, decreased endurance, difficulty concentrating, decreased libido, feelings of anxiety/depression

References:

1. Brozek J. Starvation and nutritional rehabilitation; a quantitative case study. *J Am Diet Assoc.* 1952;28:917-926.
2. Collins S. Using middle upper arm circumference to assess severe adult malnutrition during famine. *JAMA.* 1996;276:391-395.
3. Detzer MJ, Leitenberg H, Poehlman ET, Rosen JC, Silberg NT, Vara LS. Resting metabolic rate in women with bulimia nervosa: a cross sectional and treatment study. *Am J Clin Nutr.* 1994;60:327-332.
4. Dickerson RN, Roth-Yousey L. Medication effects on metabolic rate: A systematic review. *J Am Diet Assoc.* 2005;105:835-43.
5. Frankenfield D, Roth-Yousey L, Compher C. Comparison of predictive equations to measured resting metabolic rate in healthy nonobese and obese individuals, a systematic review. *J Am Diet Assoc.* 2005;105:775-89.
6. Kerruish KP, O'Conner JO, Humphries IRJ, Kohn MR, Clarke SD, Briody JN, Thomson EJ, Wright KA, Gaskin KJ, Baur LA. Body composition in adolescents with anorexia nervosa. *Am J Clin Nutr.* 2002;75:31-37.
7. Mollinger LA, Spurr GB, el Ghatil AZ, Barboriak JS, Rooney CB, Davidoff DD. Daily energy expenditure and basil metabolic rates of patients with spinal cord injury. *Arch Phys Med Rehabil.* 1985;66:420-426.
8. Obarzanek E, Lesem MD, Jimerson DC. Resting metabolic rate of anorexia nervosa patients during weight gain. *Am J Clin Nutr.* 1994;60:666-675.
9. Pavlovic M, Zavalic M, Corovic N, Stilinovic L, Malinar M. Loss of body mass in ex prisoners of war. *Eur J Clin Nutr.* 1993;47:808-814.

INTAKE DOMAIN • Energy Balance

INADEQUATE ENERGY INTAKE (NI-1.4)

Definition

Energy intake that is less than energy expenditure, established reference standards, or recommendations based on physiological needs Exception: when the goal is weight loss or during end-of-life care.

Etiology (*Cause/Contributing Risk Factors*)

Factors gathered during the nutrition assessment process that contribute to the existence or the maintenance of pathophysiological, psychosocial, situational, developmental, cultural, and/or environmental problems:

- Pathologic or physiological causes that result in increased energy requirements or decreased ability to consume sufficient energy, e.g., increased nutrient needs due to prolonged catabolic illness
- Lack of access to food or artificial nutrition, e.g., economic constraints, cultural, or religious practices restricting food given to elderly and/or children
- Food- and nutrition-related knowledge deficit
- Psychological causes, e.g., depression or disordered eating

Signs/Symptoms (*Defining Characteristics*)

A typical cluster of subjective and objective signs and symptoms gathered during the nutrition assessment process that provide evidence that a problem exists; quantify the problem and describe its severity.

Nutrition Assessment Category	Potential Indicators of this Nutrition Diagnosis (one or more must be present)
Biochemical Data, Medical Tests and Procedures	• ↓ Cholesterol
Anthropometric Measurements	
Physical Examination Findings	• Weight loss • Poor dentition

INTAKE DOMAIN - Energy Balance

INADEQUATE ENERGY INTAKE (NI-1.4)

Food/Nutrition History	Reports or observations of:
	• Insufficient energy intake from diet compared to needs based on estimated or measured resting metabolic rate
	• Restriction or omission of energy-dense foods from diet
	• Food avoidance and/or lack of interest in food
	• Inability to independently consume foods/fluids (diminished joint mobility of wrist, hand, or digits)
	• Parenteral or enteral nutrition insufficient to meet needs based on estimated or measured resting metabolic rate
Client History	• Excessive consumption of alcohol or other drugs that reduce hunger

References:

1   National Academy of Sciences, Institute of Medicine. *Dietary Reference Intakes for Energy, Carbohydrate, Fiber, Fat, Fatty Acids, Cholesterol, Protein, and Amino Acids.* Washington, DC: National Academy Press; 2002.

Edition: 2007

65

EXCESSIVE ENERGY INTAKE (NI-1.5)

Definition

Energy intake that exceeds energy expenditure, established reference standards, or recommendations based on physiological needs. Exception: when weight gain is desired.

Etiology (*Cause/Contributing Risk Factors*)

Factors gathered during the nutrition assessment process that contribute to the existence or the maintenance of pathophysiological, psychosocial, situational, developmental, cultural, and/or environmental problems:

- Harmful beliefs/attitudes about food, nutrition, and nutrition-related topics
- Food- and nutrition-related knowledge deficit
- Lack of access to healthful food choices, e.g., healthful food choices not provided as an option by caregiver or parent, homeless
- Lack of value for behavior change, competing values
- Mental illness, depression
- Medications that increase appetite, e.g., steroids, antidepressants
- Overfeeding of parenteral/enteral nutrition (TPN/EN)
- Unwilling or uninterested in reducing energy intake
- Failure to adjust for lifestyle changes and decreased metabolism (e.g., aging)
- Resolution of prior hypermetabolism without reduction in intake

Signs/Symptoms (*Defining Characteristics*)

A typical cluster of subjective and objective signs and symptoms gathered during the nutrition assessment process that provide evidence that a problem exists; quantify the problem and describe its severity.

Edition: 2007

INTAKE DOMAIN • Energy Balance

EXCESSIVE ENERGY INTAKE (NI-1.5)

Nutrition Assessment Category	Potential Indicators of this Nutrition Diagnosis (one or more must be present)
Biochemical Data, Medical Tests and Procedures	• Overfeeding of TPN/EN (usually seen early after initiation of feeding) • Hyperglycemia • Hypokalemia < 3.5 mEq/L • Hypophosphatemia < 1.0 mEq/L • Abnormal liver function tests • Respiratory quotient >1.0
Anthropometric Measurements	• Body fat percentage > 25% for men and > 32% for women • BMI > 25 • Weight gain
Physical Exam Findings	• Increased body adiposity • Overfeeding TPN/EN • Increased respiratory rate
Food/Nutrition History	• Observations or reports of intake of high caloric density or large portions of foods/beverages • Observations, reports or calculation of TPN/EN above estimated or measured (e.g., indirect calorimetry) energy expenditure
Client History	• Conditions associated with a diagnosis or treatment of, e.g., obesity, overweight, metabolic syndrome, depression, or anxiety disorder

References:
1. McClave SA, Lowen CC, Kleber MJ, McConnell JW, Jung LY, Goldsmith LJ. Clinical use of the respiratory quotient obtained from indirect calorimetry. *JPEN J Parenter Enteral Nutr.* 2003;27:21-26.
2. McClave SA, Lowen CC, Kleber MJ, Nicholson JF, Jimmerson SC, McConnell JW, Jung LY. Are patients fed appropriately according to their caloric requirements? *JPEN J Parenter Enteral Nutr.* 1998;22:375-381.
3. Overweight and Obesity: Health Consequences. www.surgeongeneral.gov/topics/obesity/calltoaction/fact_consequences.htm. Accessed August 28, 2004.

Edition: 2007

67

INADEQUATE ORAL FOOD/BEVERAGE INTAKE (NI-2.1)

Definition

Oral food/beverage intake that is less than established reference standards or recommendations based on physiological needs. Exception: when the goal is weight loss or during end-of-life care.

Etiology (*Cause/Contributing Risk Factors*)

Factors gathered during the nutrition assessment process that contribute to the existence or the maintenance of pathophysiological, psychosocial, situational, developmental, cultural, and/or environmental problems:

- Physiological causes, e.g., increased nutrient needs due to prolonged catabolic illness
- Lack of access to food, e.g., economic constraints, cultural or religious practices, restricting food given to elderly and/or children
- Food- and nutrition-related knowledge deficit concerning sufficient oral food/beverage intake
- Psychological causes, e.g., depression or disordered eating

Signs/Symptoms (*Defining Characteristics*)

A typical cluster of subjective and objective signs and symptoms gathered during the nutrition assessment process that provide evidence that a problem exists; quantify the problem and describe its severity.

Nutrition Assessment Category	Potential Indicators of this Nutrition Diagnosis (one or more must be present)
Biochemical Data, Medical Tests and Procedures	
Anthropometric Measurements	• Weight loss, insufficient growth velocity
Physical Examination Findings	• Dry skin, mucous membranes, poor skin turgor
Food/Nutrition History	Reports or observations of: • Insufficient intake of energy or high-quality protein from diet when compared to requirements • Economic constraints that limit food availability • Anorexia, nausea, or vomiting • Change in appetite or taste

Edition: 2007

INADEQUATE ORAL FOOD/BEVERAGE INTAKE (NI-2.1)

Client History
• Conditions associated with a diagnosis or treatment of catabolic illness such as AIDS, tuberculosis, anorexia nervosa, sepsis or infection from recent surgery, depression, acute or chronic pain • Protein and/or nutrient malabsorption • Excessive consumption of alcohol or other drugs that reduce hunger • Medications that cause anorexia

References:

1. National Academy of Sciences, Institute of Medicine. *Dietary Reference Intakes for Energy, Carbohydrate, Fiber, Fat, Fatty Acids, Cholesterol, Protein, and Amino Acids.* Washington, DC: National Academy Press; 2002.

2. National Academy of Sciences, Institute of Medicine. *Dietary Reference Intakes for Water, Potassium, Sodium, Chloride, and Sulfate.* Washington, DC: National Academy Press; 2002.

Edition: 2007

EXCESSIVE ORAL FOOD/BEVERAGE INTAKE (NI-2.2)

Definition

Oral food/beverage intake that exceeds energy expenditure, established reference standards, or recommendations based on physiological needs. Exception: when weight gain is desired.

Etiology (*Cause/Contributing Risk Factors*)

Factors gathered during the nutrition assessment process that contribute to the existence or the maintenance of pathophysiological, psychosocial, situational, developmental, cultural, and/or environmental problems:

- Harmful beliefs/attitudes about food, nutrition, and nutrition-related topics
- Food- and nutrition-related knowledge deficit
- Lack of access to healthful food choices, e.g., healthful food choices not provided as an option by caregiver or parent, homeless
- Lack of value for behavior change, competing values
- Inability to limit or refuse offered foods
- Lack of food planning, purchasing, and preparation skills
- Loss of appetite awareness
- Medications that increase appetite, e.g., steroids, antidepressants
- Unwilling or uninterested in reducing intake

Signs/Symptoms (*Defining Characteristics*)

A typical cluster of subjective and objective signs and symptoms gathered during the nutrition assessment process that provide evidence that a problem exists; quantify the problem and describe its severity.

Nutrition Assessment Category	Potential Indicators of this Nutrition Diagnosis (one or more must be present)
Biochemical Data, Medical Tests and Procedures	• Variable high blood glucose levels • Abnormal Hgb A1C • Resting metabolic rate measurement reflecting excess intake, e.g., respiratory quotient >1.0
Anthropometric Measurements	• Weight gain not attributed to fluid retention or normal growth
Physical Exam Findings	• Evidence of acanthosis nigricans

Edition: 2007

EXCESSIVE ORAL FOOD/BEVERAGE INTAKE (NI-2.2)

Food/Nutrition History	Reports or observations of:
	• Intake of high caloric-density foods/beverages (juice, soda, or alcohol) at meals and/or snacks
	• Intake of large portions of foods/beverages, food groups, or specific food items
	• Intake that exceeds estimated or measured energy needs
	• Highly variable daily energy intake
	• Binge eating patterns
	• Frequent, excessive fast food or restaurant intake
Client History	• Conditions associated with a diagnosis or treatment of, e.g., obesity, overweight, or metabolic syndrome, depression, anxiety disorder

References:

1. Overweight and Obesity: Health Consequences. www.surgeongeneral.gov/topics/obesity/calltoaction/fact_consequences.htm. Accessed August 28, 2004.Position of the American Dietetic Association: Weight management. *J Am Diet Assoc.* 2002;102:1145-1155.
2. Position of the American Dietetic Association: Total diet approach to communicating food and nutrition information. *J Am Diet Assoc.* 2002;102:100-108.
3. Position of the American Dietetic Association: The role of dietetics professionals in health promotion and disease prevention. *J Am Diet Assoc.* 2002;102:1680-1687.

Edition: 2007

INADEQUATE INTAKE FROM ENTERAL/PARENTERAL (EN/TPN) NUTRITION (NI-2.3)

Definition

Enteral or parenteral infusion that provides fewer calories or nutrients compared to established reference standards or recommendations based on physiological needs. Exception: when recommendation is for weight loss or during end-of-life care.

Etiology (*Cause/Contributing Risk Factors*)

Factors gathered during the nutrition assessment process that contribute to the existence or the maintenance of pathophysiological, psychosocial, situational, developmental, cultural, and/or environmental problems:

- Altered absorption or metabolism of nutrients, e.g., medications
- Food- and nutrition-related knowledge deficit (patient/client, caregiver, supplier)-- incorrect formula/formulation given, e.g., wrong enteral feeding, missing component of TPN
- Lack of, compromised, or incorrect access for delivering EN/TPN
- Increased biological demand of nutrients, e.g., accelerated growth, wound healing, chronic infection, multiple fractures
- Intolerance of EN/TPN
- Infusion volume not reached or schedule for infusion interrupted

Signs/Symptoms (*Defining Characteristics*)

A typical cluster of subjective and objective signs and symptoms gathered during the nutrition assessment process that provide evidence that a problem exists; quantify the problem and describe its severity.

Edition: 2007

INADEQUATE INTAKE FROM ENTERAL/PARENTERAL (EN/TPN) NUTRITION (NI-2.3)

Nutrition Assessment Category	Potential Indicators of this Nutrition Diagnosis (one or more must be present)

Biochemical Data, Medical Tests and Procedures	• Cholesterol < 160 mg/dL (4.16 mmol/L)
	• Metabolic cart/indirect calorimetry measurement, e.g., respiratory quotient < 0.7
	• Vitamin/mineral abnormalities
	  • Calcium < 9.2 mg/dL (2.3 mmol/L)
	  • Vitamin K—Prolonged prothrombin time (PT), partial thromboplastin time (PTT)
	  • Copper < 70 µg/dL (11 µmol/L)
	  • Zinc < 78 µg/dL (12 µmol/L)
	  • Iron < 50 µg/dL(nmol/L); iron-binding capacity < 250 µg/dL (44.8 µmol/L)

Anthropometric Measurements	• Growth failure, based on National Center for Health Statistics (NCHS) growth standards and fetal growth failure • Insufficient maternal weight gain • Lack of planned weight gain • Unintentional weight loss of ≥5% in 1 month or ≥10% in 6 months (not attributed to fluid) in adults • Any weight loss in infants or children • Underweight (BMI < 18.5)
Physical Exam Findings	• Clinical evidence of vitamin/mineral deficiency (e.g., hair loss, bleeding gums, pale nail beds, neurologic changes) • Evidence of dehydration, e.g., dry mucous membranes, poor skin turgor • Loss of skin integrity, delayed wound healing, or pressure ulcers • Loss of muscle mass and/or subcutaneous fat • Nausea, vomiting, diarrhea
Food/Nutrition History	Reports or observations of: • Inadequate EN/TPN volume compared to estimated or measured (indirect calorimetry) requirements
Client History	• Conditions associated with a diagnosis or treatment, e.g., intestinal resection, Crohn's disease, HIV/AIDS, burns, pre-term birth, malnutrition • Feeding tube or venous access in wrong position or removed • Altered capacity for desired levels of physical activity or exercise, easy fatigue with increased activity

73

INADEQUATE INTAKE FROM ENTERAL/PARENTERAL (EN/TPN) NUTRITION (NI-2.3)

References:

1. McClave SA, Spain DA, Skolnick JL, Lowen CC, Kieber MJ, Wickerham PS, Vogt JR, Looney SW. Achievement of steady state optimizes results when performing indirect calorimetry. *JPEN J Parenter Enteral Nutr*. 2003;27:16-20.
2. McClave SA, Lowen CC, Kieber MJ, McConnell JW, Jung LY, Goldsmith LJ. Clinical use of the respiratory quotient obtained from indirect calorimetry. *JPEN J Parenter Enteral Nutr*. 2003;27:21-26.
3. McClave SA, Snider HL. Clinical use of gastric residual volumes as a monitor for patients on enteral tube feeding. *JPEN J Parenter Enteral Nutr*. 2002;26(Suppl):S43-S48; discussion S49-S50.
4. McClave SA, DeMeo MT, DeLegge MH, DiSario JA, Heyland DK, Maloney JP, Metheny NA, Moore FA, Scolapio JS, Spain DA, Zaloga GP. North American Summit on Aspiration in the Critically Ill Patient: consensus statement. *JPEN J Parenter Enteral Nutr*. 2002;26(Suppl):S80-S85.
5. McClave SA, McClain CJ, Snider HL. Should indirect calorimetry be used as part of nutritional assessment? *J Clin Gastroenterol*. 2001;33:14-19.
6. McClave SA, Sexton LK, Spain DA, Adams JL, Owens NA, Sullins MB, Blandford BS, Snider HL. Enteral tube feeding in the intensive care unit: factors impeding adequate delivery. *Crit Care Med*. 1999;27:1252-1256.
7. McClave SA, Lowen CC, Kieber MJ, Nicholson JF, Jimmerson SC, McConnell JW, Jung LY. Are patients fed appropriately according to their caloric requirements? *JPEN J Parenter Enteral Nutr*. 1998;22:375-381.
8. Spain DA, McClave SA, Sexton LK, Adams JL, Blanford BS, Sullins ME, Owens NA, Snider HL. Infusion protocol improves delivery of enteral tube feeding in the critical care unit. *JPEN J Parenter Enteral Nutr*. 1999;23:288-292.

EXCESSIVE INTAKE FROM ENTERAL OR PARENTERAL NUTRITION (NI-2.4)

Definition

Enteral or parenteral infusion that provides more calories or nutrients compared to established reference standards or recommendations based on physiological needs.

Etiology (Cause/Contributing Risk Factors)

Factors gathered during the nutrition assessment process that contribute to the existence or the maintenance of pathophysiological, psychosocial, situational, developmental, cultural, and/or environmental problems:

- Physiological causes, e.g., decreased needs related to low activity levels with critical illness or organ failure
- Food- and nutrition-related knowledge deficit on the part of the caregiver, patient/client, or clinician

Signs/Symptoms (Defining Characteristics)

A typical cluster of subjective and objective signs and symptoms gathered during the nutrition assessment process that provide evidence that a problem exists; quantify the problem and describe its severity.

Nutrition Assessment Category	Potential Indicators of this Nutrition Diagnosis (one or more must be present)
Biochemical Data, Medical Tests and Procedures	- Elevated BUN:creatinine ratio (protein) - Hyperglycemia (carbohydrate) - Hypercapnia - Elevated liver enzymes
Anthropometric Measurements	- Weight gain in excess of lean tissue accretion
Physical Examination Findings	- Edema with excess fluid administration
Food/Nutrition History	Reports or observations of: - Documented intake from enteral or parenteral nutrients that is consistently above recommended intake for carbohydrate, protein, and fat (e.g., 36 kcal/kg for well, active adults, 25 kcal/kg or as measured by indirect calorimetry for critically ill adults, 0.8 g/kg protein for well adults, 1.5 g/kg protein for critically ill adults, 1.2 g/kg lipid for adults, or 3 g/kg for children)*

* When entering weight (i.e., gram) information into the medical record, use institution or Joint Commission on Accreditation of Healthcare Organizations' approved abbreviation list.

Edition: 2007

75

EXCESSIVE INTAKE FROM ENTERAL OR PARENTERAL NUTRITION (NI-2.4)

Client History	• Use of drugs that reduce requirements or impair metabolism of energy, protein, fat, or fluid. • Unrealistic expectations of weight gain or ideal weight

References:

1. National Academy of Sciences, Institute of Medicine. *Dietary Reference Intakes for Energy, Carbohydrate, Fiber, Fat, Fatty Acids, Cholesterol, Protein, and Amino Acids.* Washington, DC: National Academy Press, 2002.
2. National Academy of Sciences, Institute of Medicine. *Dietary Reference Intakes for Water, Potassium, Sodium, Chloride, and Sulfate.* Washington, DC: National Academy Press, 2004.
3. Aarsland A, Chinkes D, Wolfe RR. Hepatic and whole-body fat synthesis in humans during carbohydrate overfeeding. *Am J Clin Nutr.* 1997;65:1774-1782.
4. McClave SA, Lowen CC, Kleber MJ, Nicholson JF, Jimmerson SC, McConnell JW, Jung LY. Are patients fed appropriately according to their caloric requirements? *JPEN J Parenter Enteral Nutr.* 1998;22:375-381.
5. McClave SA, Lowen CC, Kleber MJ, McConnell JW, Jung LY, Goldsmith LJ. Clinical use of the respiratory quotient obtained from indirect calorimetry. *JPEN J Parenter Enteral Nutr.* 2003;27:21-26.
6. Wolfe RR, O'Donnell TF Jr, Stone MD, Richmand DA, Burke JF. Investigation of factors determining the optimal glucose infusion rate in total parenteral nutrition. *Metabolism.* 1980;29:892-900.
7. Jensen GL, Mascioli EA, Seidner DL, Istfan NW, Domnitch AM, Selleck K, Babayan VK, Blackburn GL, Bistrian BR. Parenteral infusion of long- and medium-chain triglycerides and reticuloendothelial system function in man. *JPEN J Parenter Enteral Nutr.* 1990;14:467-471.

Edition: 2007

INAPPROPRIATE INFUSION OF ENTERAL OR PARENTERAL NUTRITION (NI-2.5)

Use with caution—only after discussion with other health team members

Definition

Enteral or parenteral infusion that provides either fewer or more calories and/or nutrients or is of the wrong composition or type, parenteral or enteral nutrition that is not warranted because the patient/client is able to tolerate an enteral intake, or is unsafe because of the potential for sepsis or other complications.

Etiology (*Cause/Contributing Risk Factors*)

Factors gathered during the nutrition assessment process that contribute to the existence or the maintenance of pathophysiological, psychosocial, situational, developmental, cultural, and/or environmental problems:

• Physiological causes, e.g., improvement in patient/client status, allowing return to total or partial oral diet; changes in the course of disease resulting in changes in nutrient requirements

• Product or knowledge deficit on the part of the caregiver or clinician

• End-of-life care if patient/client or family do not desire nutrition support

Signs/Symptoms (*Defining Characteristics*)

A typical cluster of subjective and objective signs and symptoms gathered during the nutrition assessment process that provide evidence that a problem exists; quantify the problem and describe its severity.

Nutrition Assessment Category	Potential Indicators of this Nutrition Diagnosis (one or more must be present)
Biochemical Data, Medical Tests and Procedures	• Abnormal liver function tests in patient/client on long-term (more than 3-6 weeks) feeding • Abnormal levels of markers specific for various nutrients, e.g., hyperphosphatemia in patient/client receiving feedings with a high phosphorus content, hypokalemia in patient/client receiving feedings with low potassium content
Anthropometric Measurements	• Weight gain in excess of lean tissue accretion • Weight loss
Physical Examination Findings	• Edema with excess fluid administration • Loss of subcutaneous fat and muscle stores

77

INAPPROPRIATE INFUSION OF ENTERAL OR PARENTERAL NUTRITION (NI-2.5)

Food/Nutrition History	Reports or observations of:
	• Documented intake from enteral or parenteral nutrients that is consistently more or less than recommended intake for carbohydrate, protein, and/or fat– especially related to patient/client's ability to consume an oral diet that meets needs at this point in time
	• Documented intake of other nutrients that is consistently more or less than recommended
	• Nausea, vomiting, diarrhea, high gastric residual volume
Client History	• History of enteral or parenteral nutrition intolerance
	• Complications such as fatty liver in the absence of other causes

References:

1. Aarsland A, Chinkes D, Wolfe RR. Hepatic and whole-body fat synthesis in humans during carbohydrate overfeeding. *Am J Clin Nutr.* 1997;65:1774-1782.
2. McClave SA, Lowen CC, Kleber MJ, Nicholson JF, Jimmerson SC, McConnell JW, Jung LY. Are patients fed appropriately according to their caloric requirements? *JPEN J Parenter Enteral Nutr.* 1998;22:375-381.
3. McClave SA, Lowen CC, Kleber MJ, McConnell JW, Jung LY, Goldsmith LJ. Clinical use of the respiratory quotient obtained from indirect calorimetry. *JPEN J Parenter Enteral Nutr.* 2003;27:21-26.
4. National Academy of Sciences, Institute of Medicine. *Dietary Reference Intakes for Energy, Carbohydrate, Fiber, Fat, Fatty Acids, Cholesterol, Protein, and Amino Acids.* Washington, DC: National Academy Press; 2002.
5. National Academy of Sciences, Institute of Medicine. *Dietary Reference Intakes for Water, Potassium, Sodium, Chloride, and Sulfate.* Washington DC: National Academy Press; 2004.
6. National Academy of Sciences, Institute of Medicine. *Dietary Reference Intakes for Calcium, Phosphorus, Magnesium, Vitamin D, and Fluoride.* Washington, DC: National Academy Press; 1997.
7. National Academy of Sciences, Institute of Medicine. *Dietary Reference Intakes for Vitamin C, Vitamin E, Selenium, and Carotenoids.* Washington, DC: National Academy Press; 2000.
8. Wolfe RR, O'Donnell TF, Jr., Stone MD, Richmand DA, Burke JF. Investigation of factors determining the optimal glucose infusion rate in total parenteral nutrition. *Metabolism.* 1980;29:892-900.

INADEQUATE FLUID INTAKE (NI-3.1)

Definition

Lower intake of fluid-containing foods or substances compared to established reference standards or recommendations based on physiological needs.

Etiology (*Cause/Contributing Risk Factors*)

Factors gathered during the nutrition assessment process that contribute to the existence or the maintenance of pathophysiological, psychosocial, situational, developmental, cultural, and/or environmental problems:

- Physiological causes, e.g., increased fluid needs due to climate/temperature change; increased exercise or conditions leading to increased fluid losses; fever causing increased insensible losses, decreased thirst sensation, use of drugs that reduce thirst
- Lack of access to fluid, e.g., economic constraints, cultural or religious practices, unable to access fluid independently such as elderly or children
- Food- and nutrition-related knowledge deficit
- Psychological causes, e.g., depression or disordered eating; dementia resulting in decreased recognition of thirst

Signs/Symptoms (*Defining Characteristics*)

A typical cluster of subjective and objective signs and symptoms gathered during the nutrition assessment process that provide evidence that a problem exists; quantify the problem and describe its severity.

Nutrition Assessment Category	Potential Indicators of this Nutrition Diagnosis (one or more must be present)
Biochemical Data, Medical Tests and Procedures	• Plasma or serum osmolality greater than 290 mOsm/kg • ↑ BUN, ↑ Na
Anthropometric Measurements	• Acute weight loss
Physical Examination Findings	• Dry skin and mucous membranes, poor skin turgor • Urine output <30mL/hr
Food/Nutrition History	Reports or observations of: • Insufficient intake of fluid compared to requirements • Thirst • Difficulty swallowing

Edition: 2007

INADEQUATE FLUID INTAKE (NI-3.1)

Client History
• Conditions associated with a diagnosis or treatment of, e.g., Alzheimer's disease or other dementia resulting in decreased recognition of thirst, diarrhea
• Use of drugs that reduce thirst

References:

1. National Academy of Sciences, Institute of Medicine. *Dietary Reference Intakes for Water, Potassium, Sodium, Chloride, and Sulfate*, Washington, DC: National Academy Press; 2004.
2. Grandjean AC, Campbell, SM. *Hydration: Fluids for Life*. Monograph Series. Washington DC: International Life Sciences Institute North America; 2004.
3. Grandjean AC, Reimers KJ, Buyckx ME: Hydration: Issues for the 21st Century. *Nutr Rev.* 2003;61:261-271.

80

EXCESSIVE FLUID INTAKE (NI-3.2)

Definition
Higher intake of fluid compared to established reference standards or recommendations based on physiological needs.

Etiology (Cause/Contributing Risk Factors)
Factors gathered during the nutrition assessment process that contribute to the existence or the maintenance of pathophysiological, psychosocial, situational, developmental, cultural, and/or environmental problems:

- Physiological causes, e.g., decreased fluid losses due to kidney, liver or cardiac failure; diminished water and sodium losses due to changes in exercise or climate, syndrome of inappropriate antidiuretic hormone (SIADH)
- Food- and nutrition-related knowledge deficit
- Psychological causes, e.g., depression or disordered eating

Signs/Symptoms (Defining Characteristics)
A typical cluster of subjective and objective signs and symptoms gathered during the nutrition assessment process that provide evidence that a problem exists; quantify the problem and describe its severity.

Nutrition Assessment Category	Potential Indicators of this Nutrition Diagnosis (one or more must be present)
Biochemical Data, Medical Tests and Procedures	• Lowered plasma osmolarity (270-280 mOsm/kg), only if positive fluid balance is in excess of positive salt balance • Decreased serum sodium in SIADH
Anthropometric Measurements	• Weight gain
Physical Examination Findings	• Edema in the skin of the legs, sacral area, or diffusely; weeping of fluids from lower legs • Ascites • Pulmonary edema as evidenced by shortness of breath; orthopnea; crackles or rales
Food/Nutrition History	Reports or observations of: • Fluid intake in excess of recommended intake • Excessive salt intake

81

Edition: 2007

EXCESSIVE FLUID INTAKE (NI-3.2)

Client History	• Conditions associated with a diagnosis or treatment, e.g., end-stage renal disease, nephrotic syndrome, heart failure, or liver disease
	• Nausea, vomiting, anorexia, headache, muscle spasms, convulsions, coma (SIADH)
	• Shortness of breath or dyspnea with exertion or at rest
	• Providing medications in large amounts of fluid
	• Use of drugs that impair fluid excretion

References:

1. National Academy of Sciences, Institute of Medicine. *Dietary Reference Intakes for Water, Potassium, Sodium, Chloride, and Sulfate.* Washington DC. National Academy Press; 2004.
2. Schirer, R.W. ed. *Renal and Electrolyte Disorders.* Philadelphia, PA: Lipincott Williams and Willkins; 2003.
3. SIADH: http://www.nlmnih.gov/medlineplus/ency/article/000394.htm. Accessed: May 30, 2006.

INTAKE DOMAIN • Bioactive Substances

INADEQUATE BIOACTIVE SUBSTANCE INTAKE (NI-4.1)

Definition

Lower intake of bioactive substances or foods containing bioactive substances compared to established reference standards or recommendations based on physiological needs.

Etiology (*Cause/Contributing Risk Factors*)

Factors gathered during the nutrition assessment process that contribute to the existence or the maintenance of pathophysiological, psychosocial, situational, developmental, cultural, and/or environmental problems:

- Food- and nutrition-related knowledge deficit
- Limited access to a food that contains the substance
- Altered GI function, e.g., pain or discomfort

Signs/Symptoms (*Defining Characteristics*)

A typical cluster of subjective and objective signs and symptoms gathered during the nutrition assessment process that provide evidence that a problem exists; quantify the problem and describe its severity.

Nutrition Assessment Category	Potential Indicators of this Nutrition Diagnosis (one or more must be present)
Biochemical Data, Medical Tests and Procedures	
Anthropometric Measurements	
Physical Exam Findings	

Food/Nutrition History	Reports or observations of:
	• Low intake of plant foods containing:
	  • Soluble fiber, e.g., psyllium (↓ total and LDL cholesterol)
	  • Soy protein (↓ total and LDL cholesterol)
	  • β-glucan, e.g., whole oat products (↓ total and LDL cholesterol)
	  • Plant sterol and stanol esters, e.g., fortified margarines (↓ total and LDL cholesterol)
	• Lack of available foods/products with bioactive substance in markets

83

Edition: 2007

INTAKE DOMAIN • Bioactive Substances

INADEQUATE BIOACTIVE SUBSTANCE INTAKE (NI-4.1)

Client History	• Conditions associated with a diagnosis or treatment, e.g., cardiovascular disease, elevated cholesterol
	• Discomfort or pain associated with intake of foods rich in bioactive substances, e.g., soluble fiber, β-glucan, soy protein

References:

1.   Position of the American Dietetic Association: Functional foods. *J Am Diet Assoc.* 2004;104:814-826.

Edition: 2007

EXCESSIVE BIOACTIVE SUBSTANCE INTAKE (NI-4.2)

Definition

Higher intake of bioactive substances other than traditional nutrients, such as functional foods, bioactive food components, dietary supplements, food concentrates compared to established reference standards or recommendations based on physiological needs.

Etiology (Cause/Contributing Risk Factors)

Factors gathered during the nutrition assessment process that contribute to the existence or the maintenance of pathophysiological, psychosocial, situational, developmental, cultural, and/or environmental problems:

- Food- and nutrition-related knowledge deficit
- Contamination, misname, mislabel, misuse, recent brand change, recent dose increase, recent formulation change of substance consumed
- Frequent intake of foods containing bioactive substances
- Altered GI function, e.g., pain or discomfort

Signs/Symptoms (Defining Characteristics)

A typical cluster of subjective and objective signs and symptoms gathered during the nutrition assessment process that provide evidence that a problem exists; quantify the problem and describe its severity.

Nutrition Assessment Category	Potential Indicators of this Nutrition Diagnosis (one or more must be present)
Biochemical Data, Medical Tests and Procedures	• Lab values indicating excessive intake of the specific substance, such as rapid decrease in cholesterol from intake of stanol or sterol esters and a statin drug and related dietary changes or medications • Increased hepatic enzyme reflecting hepatocellular damage
Anthropometric Measurements	• Weight loss as a result of malabsorption or maldigestion
Physical Exam Findings	• Constipation or diarrhea related to excessive intake • Neurologic changes, e.g., anxiety, mental status changes • Cardiovascular changes, e.g., heart rate, EKG changes, blood pressure

Edition: 2007

EXCESSIVE BIOACTIVE SUBSTANCE INTAKE (NI-4.2)

Food/Nutrition History	Reports or observations of:
	• High intake of plant foods containing:
	• Soy protein (↓ total and LDL cholesterol)
	• β-glucan, e.g., whole oat products (↓ total and LDL cholesterol)
	• Plant sterol and stanol esters, e.g., fortified margarines (↓ total and LDL cholesterol) or other foods based on dietary substance, concentrate, metabolite, constituent, extract, or combination
	• Substances that interfere with digestion or absorption of foodstuffs
	• Ready access to available foods/products with bioactive substance, e.g., as from dietary supplement vendors
	• Attempts to use supplements or bioactive substances for weight loss, to treat constipation, or to prevent or cure chronic or acute disease
Client History	• Conditions associated with a diagnosis or treatment, e.g., cardiovascular disease, elevated cholesterol, hypertension,
	• Discomfort or pain associated with intake of foods rich in bioactive substances, e.g., soluble fiber, β-glucan, soy protein

References:

1. National Academy of Sciences, Institute of Medicine. *Dietary Supplements: A framework for evaluating safety.* Washington, DC: National Academy Press; 2004.
2. Position of the American Dietetic Association: Functional foods. *J Am Diet Assoc.* 2004;104:814-826.

EXCESSIVE ALCOHOL INTAKE (NI-4.3)

Definition

Intake more than the suggested limits for alcohol.

Etiology (Cause/Contributing Risk Factors)

Factors gathered during the nutrition assessment process that contribute to the existence or the maintenance of pathophysiological, psychosocial, situational, developmental, cultural, and/or environmental problems:

- Harmful beliefs/attitudes about food, nutrition, and nutrition-related topics
- Food- and nutrition-related knowledge deficit
- Lack of value for behavior change, competing values
- Alcohol addiction

Signs/Symptoms (Defining Characteristics)

A typical cluster of subjective and objective signs and symptoms gathered during the nutrition assessment process that provide evidence that a problem exists; quantify the problem and describe its severity.

Nutrition Assessment Category	Potential Indicators of this Nutrition Diagnosis (one or more must be present)
Biochemical Data, Medical Tests and Procedures	• Elevated aspartate aminotransferase (AST), gamma-glutamyl transferase (GGT), carbohydrate-deficient transferrin, mean corpuscular volume, blood alcohol levels
Anthropometric Measurements	
Physical Exam Findings	
Food/Nutrition History	Reports or observations of: • Intake of > 2 drinks*/day (men) • Intake of > 1 drink*/day (women) • Binge drinking • Consumption of any alcohol when contraindicated *1 drink = 5 oz wine, 12 oz beer, 1 oz distilled alcohol

Edition: 2007

EXCESSIVE ALCOHOL INTAKE (NI-4.3)

Client History	• Conditions associated with a diagnosis or treatment, e.g., severe hypertriglyceridemia, elevated blood pressure, depression, liver disease, pancreatitis
	• New medical diagnosis or change in existing diagnosis or condition
	• History of excessive alcohol intake
	• Giving birth to an infant with fetal alcohol syndrome
	• Drinking during pregnancy despite knowledge of risk
	• Unexplained falls

References:

1. Position of the American Dietetic Association: The role of dietetics professionals in health promotion and disease prevention. *J Am Diet Assoc.* 2002;102:1680-1687.

Edition: 2007

INCREASED NUTRIENT NEEDS (SPECIFY) (NI-5.1)

Definition

Increased need for a specific nutrient compared to established reference standards or recommendations based on physiological needs.

Etiology (Cause/Contributing Risk Factors)

Factors gathered during the nutrition assessment process that contribute to the existence or the maintenance of pathophysiological, psychosocial, situational, developmental, cultural, and/or environmental problems:

- Altered absorption or metabolism of nutrient, e.g., from medications
- Compromise of organs related to GI function, e.g., pancreas, liver
- Decreased functional length of intestine, e.g., short-bowel syndrome
- Decreased or compromised function of intestine, e.g., celiac disease, Crohn's disease
- Food- and nutrition-related knowledge deficit
- Increased demand for nutrient, e.g., accelerated growth, wound healing, chronic infection

Signs/Symptoms (Defining Characteristics)

A typical cluster of subjective and objective signs and symptoms gathered during the nutrition assessment process that provide evidence that a problem exists; quantify the problem and describe its severity.

Nutrition Assessment Category	Potential Indicators of this Nutrition Diagnosis (one or more must be present)
Biochemical Data, Medical Tests and Procedures	• Decreased cholesterol < 160 mg/dL, albumin, prealbumin, C-reactive protein, indicating increased stress and increased metabolic needs • Electrolyte/mineral (e.g., potassium, magnesium, phosphorus) abnormalities • Urinary or fecal losses of specific or related nutrient (e.g., fecal fat, d-xylose test) • Vitamin and/or mineral deficiency
Anthropometric Measurements	• Growth failure, based on National Center for Health Statistics (NCHS) growth standards and fetal growth failure • Unintentional weight loss of ≥5% in 1 month or ≥10% in 6 months • Loss of muscle mass, subcutaneous fat • Underweight (BMI < 18.5)

Edition: 2007

INCREASED NUTRIENT NEEDS (SPECIFY) (NI-5.1)

Physical Examination Findings	• Clinical evidence of vitamin/mineral deficiency (e.g., hair loss, bleeding gums, pale nail beds) • Loss of skin integrity, delayed wound healing, or pressure ulcers
Food/Nutrition History	Reports or observations of: • Inadequate intake of foods/supplement containing needed nutrient as compared to estimated requirements • Intake of foods that do not contain sufficient quantities of available nutrient (e.g., overprocessed, overcooked, or stored improperly) • Food- and nutrition-related knowledge deficit (e.g., lack of information, incorrect information or noncompliance with intake of needed nutrient)
Client History	• Fever • Conditions associated with a diagnosis or treatment, e.g., intestinal resection, Crohn's disease, HIV/AIDS, burns, pre-term birth, malnutrition • Medications affecting absorption or metabolism of needed nutrient

References:

1. Beyer P. Gastrointestinal disorders: Roles of nutrition and the dietetics practitioner. *J Am Diet Assoc.* 1998;98:272-277.
2. Position of the American Dietetic Association and Dietitians of Canada: Nutrition intervention in the care of persons with human immunodeficiency virus infection. *J Am Diet Assoc.* 2004;104:1425-1441.

EVIDENT PROTEIN–ENERGY MALNUTRITION (NI-5.2)

Definition

Inadequate intake of protein and/or energy over prolonged periods of time resulting in loss of fat stores and/or muscle wasting.

Etiology (*Cause/Contributing Risk Factors*)

Factors gathered during the nutrition assessment process that contribute to the existence or the maintenance of pathophysiological, psychosocial, situational, developmental, cultural, and/or environmental problems:

- Physiological causes, e.g., altered nutrient needs due to prolonged catabolic illness, malabsorption
- Lack of access to food, e.g., economic constraints, cultural or religious practices, restricting food given to elderly and/or children
- Food- and nutrition-related knowledge deficit, e.g., avoidance of high-quality protein foods
- Psychological causes, e.g., depression or eating disorders

Signs/Symptoms (*Defining Characteristics*)

A typical cluster of subjective and objective signs and symptoms gathered during the nutrition assessment process that provide evidence that a problem exists; quantify the problem and describe its severity.

Nutrition Assessment Category	Potential Indicators of this Nutrition Diagnosis (one or more must be present)
Biochemical Data, Medical Tests and Procedures	• Normal serum albumin level (uncomplicated malnutrition) • Albumin < 3.4 mg/dL (disease/trauma related malnutrition)
Anthropometric Measurements	• BMI < 18.5 indicates underweight • Failure to thrive, e.g., failure to attain desirable growth rates • Inadequate maternal weight gain • Weight loss of > 10% in 6 months • Underweight with muscle wasting • Normal or slightly underweight, stunted growth in children

Edition: 2007

EVIDENT PROTEIN–ENERGY MALNUTRITION (NI-5.2)

Physical Exam Findings	• Uncomplicated malnutrition: Thin, wasted appearance; severe muscle wasting; minimal body fat; sparse, thin, dry, easily pluckable hair; dry, thin skin; obvious bony prominences, occipital wasting; lowered body temperature, blood pressure, heart rate; changes in hair or nails consistent with insufficient protein intake
	• Disease/trauma related malnutrition: Thin to normal appearance, with peripheral edema, ascites, or anasarca; edema of the lower extremities; some muscle wasting with retention of some body fat; dyspigmentation of hair (flag sign) and skin
	• Delayed wound healing
Food/Nutrition History	Reports or observations of:
	• Insufficient energy intake from diet compared to estimated or measured RMR
	• Insufficient intake of high-quality protein when compared to requirements
	• Food avoidance and/or lack of interest in food
Client History	• Chronic or acute disease or trauma, geographic location and socioeconomic status associated with altered nutrient intake of indigenous phenomenon
	• Severe protein and/or nutrient malabsorption (e.g., extensive bowel resection)
	• Excessive consumption of alcohol or other drugs that reduce hunger
	• Enlarged fatty liver

References:
1. Wellcome Trust Working Party. Classification of infantile malnutrition. *Lancet.* 1970;2:302-303.
2. Seres DS, Resurrection, LB. Kwashiorkor: Dysmetabolism versus malnutrition. *Nutr Clin Pract.* 2003;18:297-301.
3. Jelliffe DB, Jelliffe EF. Causation of kwashiorkor: Toward a multifactoral consensus. *Pediatrics.* 1992;90:110-113.
4. Centers for Disease Control and Prevention web site: http://www.cdc.gov/nccdphp/dnpa/bmi/bmi-adult.htm. Accessed October 5, 2004.
5. Fuhrman MP, Charney P, Mueller CM. Hepatic proteins and nutrition assessment. *J Am Diet Assoc.* 2004;104:1258-1264.
6. U.S. Department of Health and Human Services. *The International Classification of Diseases, 9th Revision, 4th Ed.* Washington DC: Publication No. (PHS) 91-1260, 1991.

INADEQUATE PROTEIN–ENERGY INTAKE (NI-5.3)

Definition

Inadequate intake of protein and/or energy compared to established reference standards or recommendations based on physiological needs of short or recent duration.

Etiology *(Cause/Contributing Risk Factors)*

Factors gathered during the nutrition assessment process that contribute to the existence or the maintenance of pathophysiological, psychosocial, situational, developmental, cultural, and/or environmental problems:

- Short-term physiological causes, e.g., increased nutrient needs due to catabolic illness, malabsorption
- Recent lack of access to food, e.g., economic constraints, cultural or religious practices, restricting food given or food selected
- Food- and nutrition-related knowledge deficit, e.g., avoidance of all fats for new dieting pattern
- Recent onset of psychological causes, e.g., depression or eating disorders

Signs/Symptoms *(Defining Characteristics)*

A typical cluster of subjective and objective signs and symptoms gathered during the nutrition assessment process that provide evidence that a problem exists; quantify the problem and describe its severity.

Nutrition Assessment Category	Potential Indicators of this Nutrition Diagnosis (one or more must be present)
Biochemical Data, Medical Tests and Procedures	• Normal albumin (in the setting of normal liver function despite decrease protein-energy intake)
Anthropometric Measurements	• Inadequate maternal weight gain (mild but not severe) • Weight loss of 5%-7% during past 3 months in adults, any weight loss in children • Normal or slightly underweight • Growth failure in children
Physical Exam Findings	• Slow wound healing in pressure ulcer or surgical patient/client

Edition: 2007

INTAKE DOMAIN • Nutrient

INADEQUATE PROTEIN–ENERGY INTAKE (NI-5.3)

Food/Nutrition History	Reports or observations of: • Insufficient energy intake from diet compared to estimated or measured RMR or recommended levels • Restriction or omission of food groups such as dairy or meat group foods (protein); bread or milk group foods (energy) • Recent food avoidance and/or lack of interest in food • Lack of ability to prepare meals
Client History	• Conditions associated with a diagnosis or treatment of mild protein–energy malnutrition, recent illness, e.g., pulmonary or cardiac failure, flu, infection, surgery • Nutrient malabsorption (e.g., bariatric surgery, diarrhea, steatorrhea) • Excessive consumption of alcohol or other drugs that reduce hunger • Patient/client reports of hunger in the face of inadequate access to food supply • Patient/client reports lack of ability to prepare meals • Patient/client reports lack of funds for purchase of appropriate foods

References:

1. Centers for Disease Control and Prevention web site: http://www.cdc.gov/nccdphp/dnpa/bmi/bmi-adult.htm. Accessed October 5, 2004.
2. Fuhrman MP, Charney P, Mueller CM. Hepatic proteins and nutrition assessment. *J Am Diet Assoc.* 2004;104:1258-1264.
3. U.S. Department of Health and Human Services. *The International Classification of Diseases, 9th Revision, 4th Ed.* Washington DC: Publication No. (PHS) 91-1260, 1991.

DECREASED NUTRIENT NEEDS (SPECIFY) (NI-5.4)

Definition

Decreased need for a specific nutrient compared to established reference standards or recommendations based on physiological needs.

Etiology (*Cause/Contributing Risk Factors*)

Factors gathered during the nutrition assessment process that contribute to the existence or the maintenance of pathophysiological, psychosocial, situational, developmental, cultural, and/or environmental problems:

- Renal dysfunction
- Liver dysfunction
- Altered cholesterol metabolism/regulation
- Heart failure
- Food intolerances, e.g., irritable bowel syndrome

Signs/Symptoms (*Defining Characteristics*)

A typical cluster of subjective and objective signs and symptoms gathered during the nutrition assessment process that provide evidence that a problem exists; quantify the problem and describe its severity.

Nutrition Assessment Category	Potential Indicators of this Nutrition Diagnosis (one or more must be present)
Biochemical Data, Medical Tests and Procedures	• Cholesterol > 200 mg/dL (5.2 mmol/L), LDL cholesterol > 100 mg/dL (2.59 mmol/L), HDL cholesterol < 40 mg/dL (1.036 mmol/L), triglycerides > 150 mg/dL (1.695 mmol/L) • Phosphorus > 5.5 mg/dL (1.78 mmol/L) • Glomerular filtration rate (GFR) < 90 mL/min/1.73 m^2 • Elevated BUN, creatinine, potassium • Liver function tests indicating severe liver disease
Anthropometric Measurements	• Interdialytic weight gain greater than expected
Physical Exam Findings	• Edema/fluid retention
Food/Nutrition History	Reports or observations of: • Intake higher than recommended for fat, phosphorus, sodium, protein, fiber

95

DECREASED NUTRIENT NEEDS (SPECIFY) (NI-5.4)

| Client History | • Conditions associated with a diagnosis or treatment that require a specific type and/or amount of nutrient, e.g., cardiovascular disease (fat), early renal disease (protein, phos), ESRD (phos, sodium, potassium, fluid), advanced liver disease (protein), heart failure (sodium, fluid), irritable bowel disease/Crohn's flare up (fiber)
• Diagnosis of hypertension, confusion related to liver disease |

References:

1. Aparicio M, Chauveau P, Combe C. Low protein diets and outcomes of renal patients. *J Nephrol.* 2001;14:433-439.
2. Beto JA, Bansal VK. Medical nutrition therapy in chronic kidney failure: Integrating clinical practice guidelines. *J Am Diet Assoc.* 2004;104:404-409.
3. Cupisti A, Morelli E, D'Alessandro C, Lupetti S, Barsotti G. Phosphate control in chronic uremia: don't forget diet. *J Nephrol.* 2003;16:29-33.
4. Durose CL, Holdsworth M, Watson V, Przygrodzka F. Knowledge of dietary restrictions and the medical consequences of noncompliance by patients on hemodialysis are not predictive of dietary compliance. *J Am Diet Assoc.* 2004;104:35-41.
5. Floch MH, Narayan R. Diet in the irritable bowel syndrome. *Clin Gastroenterol.* 2002;35:S45-S52.
6. Kato J, Kobune M, Nakamura T, Kurojwa G, Takada K, Takimoto R, Sato Y, Fujikawa K, Takahashi M, Takayama T, Ikeda T, Niitsu Y. Normalization of elevated hepatic 8-hydroxy-2'-deoxyguanosine levels in chronic hepatitis C patients by phlebotomy and low iron diet. *Cancer Res.* 2001;61:8697-8702.
7. Lee SH, Molassiotis A. Dietary and fluid compliance in Chinese hemodialysis patients. *Int J Nurs Stud.* 2002;39:695-704.
8. Poduval RD, Wolgemuth C, Ferrell J, Hammes MS. Hyperphosphatemia in dialysis patients: is there a role for focused counseling? *J Ren Nutr.* 2003;13:219-223.
9. Tandon N, Thakur V, Guptan RK, Sarin SK. Beneficial influence of an indigenous low-iron diet on serum indicators of iron status in patients with chronic liver disease. *Br J Nutr.* 2000;83:235-239.
10. Zrinyi M, Juhasz M, Balla J, Katona E, Ben T, Kakuk G, Pall D. Dietary self-efficacy: determinant of compliance behaviours and biochemical outcomes in haemodialysis patients. *Nephrol Dial Transplant.* 2003;19:1869-1873.

Edition: 2007

IMBALANCE OF NUTRIENTS (NI-5.5)

Definition

An undesirable combination of ingested nutrients, such that the amount of one nutrient ingested interferes with or alters absorption and/or utilization of another nutrient.

Etiology (Cause/Contributing Risk Factors)

Factors gathered during the nutrition assessment process that contribute to the existence or the maintenance of pathophysiological, psychosocial, situational, developmental, cultural, and/or environmental problems:

- Consumption of high-dose nutrient supplements
- Food- and nutrition-related knowledge deficit
- Harmful beliefs/attitudes about food, nutrition, and nutrition-related information
- Food faddism

Signs/Symptoms (Defining Characteristics)

A typical cluster of subjective and objective signs and symptoms gathered during the nutrition assessment process that provide evidence that a problem exists; quantify the problem and describe its severity.

Nutrition Assessment Category	Potential Indicators of this Nutrition Diagnosis (one or more must be present)
Biochemical Data, Medical Tests and Procedures	
Anthropometric Data	
Physical Exam Findings	
Food/Nutrition History	Reports or observations of: • High intake of iron supplements (↓ zinc absorption) • High intake of zinc supplements (↓ copper status) • High intake of manganese (↓ iron status)

97

IMBALANCE OF NUTRIENTS (NI-5.5)

Client History	
	• Diarrhea or constipation (iron supplements)
	• Epigastric pain, nausea, vomiting, diarrhea (zinc supplements)
	• Contributes to the development of anemia (manganese supplements)

References:

1. National Academy of Sciences, Institute of Medicine. *Dietary Reference Intakes for Vitamin A, Vitamin K, Arsenic, Boron, Chromium, Copper, Iodine, Iron, Manganese, Molybdenum, Nickel, Silicon, Vanadium, Zinc.* Washington, DC: National Academy Press; 2001.
2. National Academy of Sciences, Institute of Medicine. *Dietary Reference Intakes for Calcium, Phosphorus, Magnesium, Vitamin D, and Fluoride.* Washington, DC: National Academy Press; 1997.

Edition: 2007

INADEQUATE FAT INTAKE (NI-51.1)

Definition

Lower fat intake compared to established reference standards or recommendations based on physiological needs. Exception: when the goal is weight loss or during end-of-life care.

Etiology (*Cause/Contributing Risk Factors*)

Factors gathered during the nutrition assessment process that contribute to the existence or the maintenance of pathophysiological, psychosocial, situational, developmental, cultural, and/or environmental problems:

- Inappropriate food choices, e.g., economic constraints, cultural or religious practices, restricting food given to elderly and/or children, specific food choices
- Food- and nutrition-related knowledge deficit, e.g., prolonged adherence to a very–low-fat diet
- Psychological causes, e.g., depression or disordered eating

Signs/Symptoms (*Defining Characteristics*)

A typical cluster of subjective and objective signs and symptoms gathered during the nutrition assessment process that provide evidence that a problem exists; quantify the problem and describe its severity.

Nutrition Assessment Category	Potential Indicators of this Nutrition Diagnosis (one or more must be present)
Biochemical Data, Medical Tests and Procedures	• Triene: tetraene ratio > 0.2
Anthropometric Measurements	• Weight loss if insufficient calories consumed
Physical Examination Findings	• Rough, scaly skin consistent with essential fatty acid deficiency
Food/Nutrition History	Reports or observations of: • Intake of essential fatty acid–containing foods consistently providing less than 10% of energy
Client History	• Conditions associated with a diagnosis or treatment of, e.g., prolonged catabolic illness (e.g., AIDS, tuberculosis, anorexia nervosa, sepsis or severe infection from recent surgery) • Severe fat malabsorption with bowel resection, pancreatic insufficiency, or hepatic disease accompanied by steatorrhea

Edition: 2007

INTAKE DOMAIN ▪ Fat and Cholesterol

INADEQUATE FAT INTAKE (NI-51.1)

References:

1. National Academy of Science, Institute of Medicine. *Dietary Reference Intakes for Energy, Carbohydrate, Fiber, Fat, Fatty Acids, Cholesterol, Protein, and Amino Acids*. Washington, DC: National Academy Press; 2002.

EXCESSIVE FAT INTAKE (NI-51.2)

Definition

Higher fat intake compared to established reference standards or recommendations based on physiological needs.

Etiology (Cause/Contributing Risk Factors)

Factors gathered during the nutrition assessment process that contribute to the existence or the maintenance of pathophysiological, psychosocial, situational, developmental, cultural, and/or environmental problems:

- Food- and nutrition-related knowledge deficit
- Harmful beliefs/attitudes about food, nutrition, and nutrition-related topics
- Lack of access to healthful food choices, e.g., healthful food choices not provided as an option by caregiver or parent, homeless
- Changes in taste and appetite or preference
- Lack of value for behavior change, competing values

Signs/Symptoms (Defining Characteristics)

A typical cluster of subjective and objective signs and symptoms gathered during the nutrition assessment process that provide evidence that a problem exists; quantify the problem and describe its severity.

Nutrition Assessment Category	Potential Indicators of this Nutrition Diagnosis (one or more must be present)
Biochemical Data, Medical Tests and Procedures	• Cholesterol > 200 mg/dL (5.2 mmol/L), LDL cholesterol > 100 mg/dL (2.59 mmol/L), HDL cholesterol < 40 mg/dL (1.036 mmol/L), triglycerides > 150 mg/dL (1.695 mmol/L) • Elevated serum amylase and/or lipase • Elevated LFTs, T. Bili • Triene-tetraene ratio > 0.4 • Fecal fat > 7g/24 hours
Anthropometric Measurements	
Physical Exam Findings	• Evidence of xanthomas • Evidence of skin lesions

101

EXCESSIVE FAT INTAKE (NI-51.2)

Food/Nutrition History	Reports or observations of:
	• Frequent or large portions of high-fat foods
	• Frequent food preparation with added fat
	• Frequent consumption of high risk lipids (i.e., saturated fat, *trans* fat, cholesterol)
	• Report of foods containing fat more than diet prescription
	• Inadequate intake of essential lipids
Client History	• Conditions associated with a diagnosis or treatment, e.g., hyperlipidemia, cystic fibrosis, angina, artherosclerosis, pancreatic, liver, and biliary diseases, post-transplantation
	• Medication, e.g., pancreatic enzymes, cholesterol- or other lipid-lowering medications
	• Diarrhea, cramping, steatorrhea, epigastric pain
	• Family history of hyperlipidemia, atherosclerosis, or pancreatitis

References:

1. National Academy of Sciences, Institute of Medicine. *Dietary Reference Intakes for Energy, Carbohydrate, Fiber, Fat, Fatty Acids, Cholesterol, Protein, and Amino Acids.* Washington, DC: National Academy Press; 2002.
2. Position of the American Dietetic Association. Weight management. *J Am Diet Assoc.* 2002;102:1145-1155.
3. Position of the American Dietetic Association. Total diet approach to communicating food and nutrition information. *J Am Diet Assoc.* 2002;102:100-108.
4. Position of the American Dietetic Association. The role of dietetics professionals in health promotion and disease prevention. *J Am Diet Assoc.* 2002;102:1680-1687.

Edition: 2007

INAPPROPRIATE INTAKE OF FOOD FATS (SPECIFY) (NI-51.3)

Definition

Intake of wrong type or quality of food fats compared to established reference standards or recommendations based on physiological needs.

Etiology (*Cause/Contributing Risk Factors*)

Factors gathered during the nutrition assessment process that contribute to the existence or the maintenance of pathophysiological, psychosocial, situational, developmental, cultural, and/or environmental problems:

- Food- and nutrition-related knowledge deficit
- Harmful beliefs/attitudes about food, nutrition, and nutrition-related topics
- Lack of access to healthful food choices, e.g., healthful food choices not provided as an option by caregiver or parent, homeless
- Changes in taste and appetite or preference
- Lack of value for behavior change, competing values

Signs/Symptoms (*Defining Characteristics*)

A typical cluster of subjective and objective signs and symptoms gathered during the nutrition assessment process that provide evidence that a problem exists; quantify the problem and describe its severity.

Nutrition Assessment Category	Potential Indicators of this Nutrition Diagnosis (one or more must be present)
Biochemical Data, Medical Tests and Procedures	• Cholesterol > 200 mg/dL (5.2 mmol/L), LDL cholesterol > 100 mg/dL (2.59 mmol/L), HDL cholesterol < 40 mg/dL (1.036 mmol/L), triglycerides > 150 mg/dL (1.695 mmol/L) • Elevated serum amylase and/or lipase • Elevated LFTs, T. Bili, C-reactive protein
Anthropometric Measurements	
Physical Exam Findings	• Evidence of xanthomas • Evidence of skin lesions

103

INTAKE DOMAIN • Fat and Cholesterol

INAPPROPRIATE INTAKE OF FOOD FATS (SPECIFY) (NI-51.3)

Food/Nutrition History	Reports or observations of: • Frequent food preparation with added fat that is not of desired type for condition • Frequent consumption of fats that are undesirable for condition (i.e., saturated fat, *trans* fat, cholesterol, Ω-6 fatty acids) • Inadequate intake of monounsaturated, polyunsaturated, or Ω-3 fatty acids • Desire to implement a Mediterranean-type diet
Client History	• Conditions associated with a diagnosis or treatment of diabetes, cardiac diseases, obesity, liver or biliary disorders • Diarrhea, cramping, steatorrhea, epigastric pain • Family history of diabetes-related heart disease, hyperlipidemia, atherosclerosis, or pancreatitis

References:

1. de Lorgeril M, Salen P, Martin J-L, Monjaud I, Delaye J, Mamelle N. Mediterranean diet, traditional risk factors, and the rate of cardiovascular complications after myocardial infarction. Final report of the Lyon Diet Heart Study. *Circulation.* 1999; 99:779-785.
2. Franz MJ, Bantle JP, Beebe CA, Brunzell JD, Chiasson J-L, Garg A, Holzmeister LA, Hoogwerf B, Mayer-Davis E, Mooradian AD, Purnell JQ, Wheeler M. Technical review. Evidence-based nutrition principles and recommendations for the treatment and prevention of diabetes and related complications. *Diabetes Care.* 2002;202:148-198.
3. Knoops KTB, de Grott LCPGM, Kromhout D, Perrin A-E, Varela) M-V, Menotti A, van Staveren WA. Mediterranean diet, lifestyle factors, and 10-year mortality in elderly European men and women. *JAMA.* 2004;292:1433-1439,
4. Kris-Etherton PM, Harris WS, Appel LJ, for the Nutrition Committee. AHA scientific statement. Fish consumption, fish oil, omega-3 fatty acids, and cardiovascular disease. *Circulation.* 2002;106:2747-2757.
5. Panagiotakos DB, Pitsavos C, Polychronopoulos E, Chrysohoou C, Zampelas A, Trichopoulou A. Can a Mediterranean diet moderate the development and clinical progression of coronary heart disease? A systematic review. *Med Sci Monit.* 2004;10:RA193-RA198.
6. Position of the American Dietetic Association. Weight management. *J Am Diet Assoc.* 2002;102:1145-1155.
7. Position of the American Dietetic Association. Total diet approach to communicating food and nutrition information. *J Am Diet Assoc.* 2002;102:100-108.
8. Position of the American Dietetic Association. The role of dietetics professionals in health promotion and disease prevention. *J Am Diet Assoc.* 2002;102:1680-1687.
9. Zhao G, Etherton TD, Martin KR, West SG, Gilles PJ, Kris-Etherton PM. Dietary alpha-linolenic acid reduces inflammatory and lipid cardiovascular risk factors in hypercholesterolemic men and women. *J Nutr.* 2004;134:2991-2997.

INTAKE DOMAIN - Protein

INADEQUATE PROTEIN INTAKE (NI-52.1)

Definition
Lower intake of protein-containing foods or substances compared to established reference standards or recommendations based on physiological needs.

Etiology *(Cause/Contributing Risk Factors)*
Factors gathered during the nutrition assessment process that contribute to the existence or the maintenance of pathophysiological, psychosocial, situational, developmental, cultural, and/or environmental problems:

- Physiological causes, e.g., increased nutrient needs due to prolonged catabolic illness, malabsorption, age, or condition
- Lack of access to food, e.g., economic constraints, cultural or religious practices, restricting food given to elderly and/or children
- Food- and nutrition-related knowledge deficit
- Psychological causes, e.g., depression or disordered eating

Signs/Symptoms *(Defining Characteristics)*
A typical cluster of subjective and objective signs and symptoms gathered during the nutrition assessment process that provide evidence that a problem exists; quantify the problem and describe its severity.

Nutrition Assessment Category	Potential Indicators of this Nutrition Diagnosis (one or more must be present)
Biochemical Data, Medical Tests and Procedures	
Anthropometric Measurements	
Physical Examination Findings	
Food/Nutrition History	Reports or observation of: • Insufficient intake of protein to meet requirements • Cultural or religious practices that limit protein intake • Economic constraints that limit food availability • Prolonged adherence to a very–low-protein weight-loss diet
Client History	• Conditions associated with a diagnosis or treatment, e.g., severe protein malabsorption such as bowel resection

105

Edition: 2007

INADEQUATE PROTEIN INTAKE (NI-52.1)

References:

1. National Academy of Sciences, Institute of Medicine. *Dietary Reference Intakes for Energy, Carbohydrate, Fiber, Fat, Fatty Acids, Cholesterol, Protein, and Amino Acids.* Washington DC: National Academy Press; 2002.

Edition: 2007

EXCESSIVE PROTEIN INTAKE (NI-52.2)

Definition

Intake more than the recommended level of protein compared to established reference standards or recommendations based on physiological needs.

Etiology (Cause/Contributing Risk Factors)

Factors gathered during the nutrition assessment process that contribute to the existence or the maintenance of pathophysiological, psychosocial, situational, developmental, cultural, and/or environmental problems:

- Liver dysfunction
- Renal dysfunction
- Harmful beliefs/attitudes about food, nutrition, and nutrition-related topics
- Lack of access to specialized protein products
- Metabolic abnormality
- Food faddism

Signs/Symptoms (Defining Characteristics)

A typical cluster of subjective and objective signs and symptoms gathered during the nutrition assessment process that provide evidence that a problem exists; quantify the problem and describe its severity.

Nutrition Assessment Category	Potential Indicators of this Nutrition Diagnosis (one or more must be present)
Biochemical Data, Medical Tests and Procedures	• Altered laboratory values, e.g., ↑ BUN, ↓ glomerular filtration rate (altered renal status)
Anthropometric Measurements	• Growth stunting or failure based on National Center for Health Statistics growth charts (metabolic disorders)
Physical Exam Findings	
Food/Nutrition History	Reports or observations of: • Higher than recommended total protein intake, e.g., early renal disease, advanced liver disease with confusion • Inappropriate supplementation
Client History	• Conditions associated with a diagnosis or treatment, e.g., early renal disease or advanced liver disease with confusion

Edition: 2007

EXCESSIVE PROTEIN INTAKE (NI-52.2)

References:

1. Position of the American Dietetic Association. Food and nutrition misinformation. *J Am Diet Assoc*. 2002;102:260-266.
2. Beto JA, Bansal VK. Medical nutrition therapy in chronic kidney failure: Integrating clinical practice guidelines. *J Am Diet Assoc*. 2004;104:404-409.
3. Brandle E, Sieberth HG, Hautmann RE. Effect of chronic dietary protein intake on the renal function in healthy subjects. *Eur J Clin Nutr*. 1996;50:734-740.
4. Frassetto LA, Todd KM, Morris RC Jr, Sebastian A. Estimation of net endogenous noncarbonic acid production in humans from diet, potassium and protein contents. *Am J Clin Nutr*. 1998;68:576-583.
5. Friedman N, ed. *Absorption and Utilization of Amino Acids, Vol. I*. Boca Raton, FL: CRC Press; 1989: 229-242.
6. Hoogeveen EK, Kostense PJ, Jager A, Heine RJ, Jakobs C, Bouter LM, Donker AJ, Stehower CD. Serum homocysteine level and protein intake are related to risk of microalbuminuria: the Hoorn study. *Kidney Int*. 1998;54:203-209.
7. Rudman D, DiFulco TJ, Galambos JT, Smith RB 3rd, Salam AA, Warren WD. Maximum rate of excretion and synthesis of urea in normal and cirrhotic subjects. *J Clin Invest*. 1973;52:2241-2249.

INAPPROPRIATE INTAKE OF AMINO ACIDS (SPECIFY) (NI-52.3)

Definition

Intake that is more or less than recommended level and/or type of amino acids compared to established reference standards or recommendations based on physiological needs.

Etiology (Cause/Contributing Risk Factors)

Factors gathered during the nutrition assessment process that contribute to the existence or the maintenance of pathophysiological, psychosocial, situational, developmental, cultural, and/or environmental problems:

- Liver dysfunction
- Renal dysfunction
- Harmful beliefs/attitudes about food, nutrition, and nutrition-related topics
- Misused specialized protein products
- Metabolic abnormality
- Food faddism
- Inborn errors of metabolism

Signs/Symptoms (Defining Characteristics)

A typical cluster of subjective and objective signs and symptoms gathered during the nutrition assessment process that provide evidence that a problem exists; quantify the problem and describe its severity.

Nutrition Assessment Category	Potential Indicators of this Nutrition Diagnosis (one or more must be present)
Biochemical Data, Medical Tests and Procedures	• Altered laboratory values, e.g., ↑ BUN, ↓ glomerular filtration rate (altered renal status); increased urinary 3-methyl-histidine • Elevated specific amino acids (inborn errors of metabolism) • Elevated homocysteine or ammonia
Anthropometric Measurements	
Physical Exam Findings	• Physical or neurological changes (inborn errors of metabolism)

109

INTAKE DOMAIN • Protein

INAPPROPRIATE INTAKE OF AMINO ACIDS (SPECIFY) (NI-52.3)

Food/Nutrition History	Reports or observation of:
	• Higher than recommended amino acid intake, e.g., early renal disease, advanced liver disease, inborn error of metabolism
	• Higher than recommended type of amino acids for prescribed parenteral and enteral nutrition therapy
	• Inappropriate amino acid or protein supplementation, as for athletes
	• Higher than recommended type of protein, e.g., excess phenylalanine intake
Client History	• Conditions associated with a diagnosis or treatment of illness that requires PEN therapy
	• History of inborn error of metabolism
	• Uremia, azotemia (renal patients)

References:

1. Beto JA, Bansal VK. Medical nutrition therapy in chronic kidney failure: Integrating clinical practice guidelines. *J Am Diet Assoc.* 2004;104:404-409.
2. Brandle E, Sieberth HG, Hautmann RE. Effect of chronic dietary protein intake on the renal function in healthy subjects. *Eur J Clin Nutr.* 1996;50 :734-740.
3. Cohn RM, Roth KS. Hyperammonia, bane of the brain. *Clin Pediatr.* 2004;43:683.
4. Frassetto LA, Todd KM, Morris RC Jr, Sebastian A. Estimation of net endogenous noncarbonic acid production in humans from diet, potassium and protein contents. *Am J Clin Nutr.* 1998;68:576-583.
5. Friedman N, ed. *Absorption and Utilization of Amino Acids, Vol. I.* Boca Raton, FL: CRC Press; 1989:229-242.
6. Hoogeveen EK, Kostense PJ, Jager A, Heine RJ, Jakobs C, Bouter LM, Donker AJ, Stehower CD. Serum homocysteine level and protein intake are related to risk of microalbuminuria: the Hoorn study. *Kidney Int.* 1998;54:203-209.
7. Position of the American Dietetic Association: Food and nutrition misinformation. *J Am Diet Assoc.* 2002;102:260-266.
8. Rudman D, DiFulco TJ, Galambos JT, Smith RB 3rd, Salam AA, Warren WD. Maximal rate of excretion and synthesis of urea in normal and cirrhotic subjects. *J Clin Invest.* 1973;52:2241-2249.

INTAKE DOMAIN ▪ Carbohydrate and Fiber

INADEQUATE CARBOHYDRATE INTAKE (NI-53.1)

Definition

Lower intake of carbohydrate-containing foods or substances compared to established reference standards or recommendations based on physiological needs.

Etiology (*Cause/Contributing Risk Factors*)

Factors gathered during the nutrition assessment process that contribute to the existence or the maintenance of pathophysiological, psychosocial, situational, developmental, cultural, and/or environmental problems:

- Physiological causes, e.g., increased energy needs due to increased activity level or metabolic change, malabsorption
- Lack of access to food, e.g., economic constraints, cultural or religious practices, restricting food given to elderly and/or children
- Food- and nutrition-related knowledge deficit
- Psychological causes, e.g., depression or disordered eating

Signs/Symptoms (*Defining Characteristics*)

A typical cluster of subjective and objective signs and symptoms gathered during the nutrition assessment process that provide evidence that a problem exists; quantify the problem and describe its severity.

Nutrition Assessment Category	Potential Indicators of this Nutrition Diagnosis (one or more must be present)
Biochemical Data, Medical Tests and Procedures	
Anthropometric Measurements	
Physical Examination Findings	• Ketone smell on breath
Food/Nutrition History	Reports or observation of: • Carbohydrate intake less than recommended amounts • Inability to independently consume foods/fluids, e.g., diminished mobility in hand, wrist, or digits
Client History	• Conditions associated with a diagnosis or treatment, e.g., pancreatic insufficiency, hepatic disease, celiac disease, seizure disorder, or carbohydrate malabsorption

References:

1. National Academy of Sciences, Institute of Medicine. *Dietary Reference Intakes for Energy, Carbohydrate, Fiber, Fat, Fatty Acids, Cholesterol, Protein, and Amino Acids.* Washington, DC: National Academy Press; 2002.

Edition: 2007

EXCESSIVE CARBOHYDRATE INTAKE (NI-53.2)

Definition

Intake more than the recommended level and type of carbohydrate compared to established reference standards or recommendations based on physiological needs.

Etiology (*Cause/Contributing Risk Factors*)

Factors gathered during the nutrition assessment process that contribute to the existence or the maintenance of pathophysiological, psychosocial, situational, developmental, cultural, and/or environmental problems:

- Physiological causes requiring modified carbohydrate intake, e.g., diabetes mellitus, lactase deficiency, sucrase-isomaltase deficiency, aldolase-B deficiency
- Cultural or religious practices that interfere with the ability to reduce carbohydrate intake
- Food- and nutrition-related knowledge deficit, e.g., inability to access sufficient information concerning appropriate carbohydrate intake
- Food and nutrition compliance limitations, e.g., lack of willingness or failure to modify carbohydrate intake in response to recommendations from a dietitian or physician
- Psychological causes, e.g., depression or disordered eating

Signs/Symptoms (*Defining Characteristics*)

A typical cluster of subjective and objective signs and symptoms gathered during the nutrition assessment process that provide evidence that a problem exists; quantify the problem and describe its severity.

Nutrition Assessment Category	Potential Indicators of this Nutrition Diagnosis (one or more must be present)
Biochemical Data, Medical Tests and Procedures	• Hyperglycemia (fasting blood sugar > 126 mg/dL) • Hemoglobin A1C > 6% • Abnormal oral glucose tolerance test (2-hour post load glucose > 200 mg/dL)
Anthropometric Measurements	
Physical Examination Findings	• Dental caries • Diarrhea in response to carbohydrate feeding

EXCESSIVE CARBOHYDRATE INTAKE (NI-53.2)

Food/Nutrition History	Reports or observation of:
	• Cultural or religious practices that do not support modification of dietary carbohydrate intake
	• Economic constraints that limit availability of appropriate foods
	• Carbohydrate intake that is consistently above recommended amounts
Client History	• Conditions associated with a diagnosis or treatment of, e.g., diabetes mellitus, inborn errors of carbohydrate metabolism, lactase deficiency, severe infection, sepsis, or obesity
	• Chronic use of medications that cause hyperglycemia, e.g., steroids
	• Pancreatic insufficiency resulting in reduced insulin production

References:

1. Bowman BA, Russell RM. *Present Knowledge in Nutrition. 8th Ed.* Washington, DC: ILSI Press; 2001.
2. Clement S, Braithwaite SS, Magee MF, Ahmann A, Smith EP, Schafer RG, Hirsch IB, American Diabetes Association Diabetes in Hospitals Writing Committee. Management of diabetes in hospitals. *Diabetes Care.* 2004;27:553-592.
3. National Academy of Sciences, Institute of Medicine. *Dietary Reference Intakes for Energy, Carbohydrate, Fiber, Fat, Fatty Acids, Cholesterol, Protein, and Amino Acids.* Washington, DC: National Academy Press; 2002.
4. The Expert Committee on the Diagnosis and Classification of Diabetes Mellitus. Diagnosis and classification of diabetes mellitus. *Diabetes Care.* 2004;27:S5-S10.

INAPPROPRIATE INTAKE OF TYPES OF CARBOHYDRATES (SPECIFY) (NI-53.3)

Definition

Intake of the type or amount of carbohydrate that is more or less than the established reference standards or recommendations based on physiological needs.

Etiology (Cause/Contributing Risk Factors)

Factors gathered during the nutrition assessment process that contribute to the existence or the maintenance of pathophysiological, psychosocial, situational, developmental, cultural, and/or environmental problems:

- Physiological causes requiring careful use of modified carbohydrate, e.g., diabetes mellitus, metabolic syndrome, hypoglycemia, celiac disease, allergies, obesity
- Cultural or religious practices that interfere with the ability to regulate types of carbohydrate consumed
- Food- and nutrition-related knowledge deficit, e.g., inability to access sufficient information concerning more appropriate carbohydrate types and/or amounts
- Food and nutrition compliance limitations, e.g., lack of willingness or failure to modify carbohydrate intake in response to recommendations from a dietitian, physician, or caregiver
- Psychological causes, e.g., depression or disordered eating

Signs/Symptoms (Defining Characteristics)

A typical cluster of subjective and objective signs and symptoms gathered during the nutrition assessment process that provide evidence that a problem exists; quantify the problem and describe its severity.

Nutrition Assessment Category	Potential Indicators of this Nutrition Diagnosis (one or more must be present)
Biochemical Data, Medical Tests and Procedures	• Hypoglycemia or hyperglycemia documented on regular basis when compared with goal of maintaining glucose levels at or less than 140 mg/dL throughout the day
Anthropometric Measurements	
Physical Examination Findings	

114

INAPPROPRIATE INTAKE OF TYPES OF CARBOHYDRATES (SPECIFY) (NI-53.3)

Food/Nutrition History	Reports or observations of:
	• Diarrhea in response to high intake of refined carbohydrates
	• Economic constraints that limit availability of appropriate foods
	• Carbohydrate intake that is different from recommended types
	• Allergic reactions to certain carbohydrate foods or food groups
	• Limited knowledge of carbohydrate composition of foods or of carbohydrate metabolism
Client History	• Conditions associated with a diagnosis or treatment, e.g., diabetes mellitus, obesity, metabolic syndrome, hypoglycemia
	• Chronic use of medications that cause altered glucose levels, e.g., steroids, antidepressants, antipsychotics

References:

1. Bowman BA, Russell RM. *Present Knowledge in Nutrition. 8th Ed.* Washington, DC: ILSI Press, 2001.
2. Clement S, Braithwaite SS, Magee MF, Ahmann A, Smith EP, Schafer RG, Hirsch IB, American Diabetes Association Diabetes in Hospitals Writing Committee. Management of diabetes in hospitals. *Diabetes Care.* 2004;27:553-592.
3. Franz MJ, Bantle JP, Beebe CA, Brunzell JD, Chiasson J-L, Garg A, Holzmeister LA, Hoogwerf B, Mayer-Davis E, Mooradian AD, Purnell JQ, Wheeler M. Technical review. Evidence-based nutrition principles and recommendations for the treatment and prevention of diabetes and related complications. *Diabetes Care.* 2002;202:148-198.
4. Sheard NF, Clark NG, Brand-Miller JC, Franz MJ, Pi-Sunyer FX, Mayer-Davis E, Kulkarni K, Geil P. A statement by the American Diabetes Association. Dietary carbohydrate (amount and type) in the prevention and management of diabetes. *Diabetes Car.e* 2004;27:2266-2271.
5. Gross LS, Li L, Ford ES, Liu S. Increased consumption of refined carbohydrates and epidemic or type 2 diabetes in the United States: an ecologic assessment. *Am J Clin Nutr.* 2004;79:774-779.
6. French S, Lin B-H, Gutherie JF. National trends in soft drink consumption among children and adolescents age 6 to17 years: prevalence, amounts, and sources, 1977/1978 to 1994/1998. *J Am Diet Assoc.* 2003;103L1326-1331,
7. National Academy of Sciences, Institute of Medicine. *Dietary Reference Intakes for Energy, Carbohydrate, Fiber, Fat, Fatty Acids, Cholesterol, Protein, and Amino Acids.* Washington, DC: National Academy Press; 2002.
8. Teff KL, Elliott SS, Tschöp M, Kieffer TJ, Rader D, Heiman M, Townsend RR, Keim NL, D'Alessio D, Havel PJ. Dietary fructose reduces circulating insulin and leptin, attenuates postprandial suppression of ghrelin, and increases triglycerides in women. *J Clin Endocrinol Metab.* 2004;89:2963-2972.
9. The Expert Committee on the Diagnosis and Classification of Diabetes Mellitus. Diagnosis and classification of diabetes mellitus. *Diabetes Care.* 2004;27:S5-S10.

INCONSISTENT CARBOHYDRATE INTAKE (NI-53.4)

Definition

Inconsistent timing of carbohydrate intake throughout the day, day to day, or a pattern of carbohydrate intake that is not consistent with recommended pattern based on physiological or medication needs.

Etiology (*Cause/Contributing Risk Factors*)

Factors gathered during the nutrition assessment process that contribute to the existence or the maintenance of pathophysiological, psychosocial, situational, developmental, cultural, and/or environmental problems:

- Physiological causes requiring careful timing and consistency in the amount of carbohydrate, e.g., diabetes mellitus, hypoglycemia
- Cultural or religious practices or lifestyle factors that interfere with the ability to regulate timing of carbohydrate consumption
- Food- and nutrition-related knowledge deficit, e.g., inability to access sufficient information concerning more appropriate timing of carbohydrate intake
- Food and nutrition compliance limitations, e.g., lack of willingness or failure to modify carbohydrate timing in response to recommendations from a dietitian, physician, or caregiver
- Psychological causes, e.g., depression or disordered eating

Signs/Symptoms (*Defining Characteristics*)

A typical cluster of subjective and objective signs and symptoms gathered during the nutrition assessment process that provide evidence that a problem exists; quantify the problem and describe its severity.

Nutrition Assessment Category	Potential Indicators of this Nutrition Diagnosis (one or more must be present)
Biochemical Data, Medical Tests and Procedures	• Hypoglycemia or hyperglycemia documented on regular basis associated with inconsistent carbohydrate intake • Wide variations in blood glucose levels
Anthropometric Measurements	
Physical Examination Findings	
Food/Nutrition History	Reports or observations of: • Economic constraints that limit availability of appropriate foods • Carbohydrate intake that is different from recommended types or ingested on an irregular basis

INCONSISTENT CARBOHYDRATE INTAKE (NI-53.4)

Client History	• Conditions associated with a diagnosis or treatment, e.g., diabetes mellitus, obesity, metabolic syndrome, hypoglycemia
	• Use of insulin or insulin secretagogues
	• Chronic use of medications that cause altered glucose levels, e.g., steroids, antidepressants, antipsychotics

References:

1. Bowman BA, Russell RM. *Present Knowledge in Nutrition. 8th Ed.* Washington, DC: ILSI Press; 2001.
2. Clement S, Braithwaite SS, Magee MF, Ahmann A, Smith EP, Schafer RG, Hirsch IB, American Diabetes Association Diabetes in Hospitals Writing Committee. Management of diabetes in hospitals. *Diabetes Care.* 2004;27:553-592.
3. Cryer PE, Davis SN, Shamoon H. Technical review. Hypoglycemia in diabetes. *Diabetes Care.* 2003;26L1902-1912.
4. Franz MJ, Bantle JP, Beebe CA, Brunzell JD, Chiasson J-L, Garg A, Holzmeister LA, Hoogwerf B, Mayer-Davis E, Mooradian AD, Purnell JQ, Wheeler M. Technical review. Evidence-based nutrition principles and recommendations for the treatment and prevention of diabetes and related complications. *Diabetes Care.* 2002;202:148-198.
5. National Academy of Sciences, Institute of Medicine. *Dietary Reference Intakes for Energy, Carbohydrate, Fiber, Fat, Fatty Acids, Cholesterol, Protein, and Amino Acids.* Washington, DC: National Academy Press; 2002.
6. Rabasa-Lhoret R, Garon J, Langelier H, Poisson D, Chiasson J-L. The effects of meal carbohydrate content on insulin requirements in type 1 patients with diabetes treated intensively with the basal bolus (ultralente-regular) insulin regimen. *Diabetes Care.* 1999;22:667-673.
7. Savoca MR, Miller CK, Ludwig DA. Food habits are related to glycemic control among people with type 2 diabetes mellitus. *J Am Diet Assoc.* 2004;104:560-566.
8. The Expert Committee on the Diagnosis and Classification of Diabetes Mellitus. Diagnosis and classification of diabetes mellitus. *Diabetes Care.* 2004;27:S5-S10.
9. Wolever TMS, Hamad S, Chiasson J-L, Josse RG, Leiter LA, Rodger NW, Ross SA, Ryan EA. Day-to-day consistency in amount and source of carbohydrate intake associated with improved glucose control in type 1 diabetes. *J Am Coll Nutr.* 1999; 18:242-247.

117

INADEQUATE FIBER INTAKE (NI-53.5)

Definition

Lower intake of fiber-containing foods or substances compared to established reference standards or recommendations based on physiological needs.

Etiology (*Cause/Contributing Risk Factors*)

Factors gathered during the nutrition assessment process that contribute to the existence or the maintenance of pathophysiological, psychosocial, situational, developmental, cultural, and/or environmental problems:

- Lack of access to fiber-containing foods
- Food- and nutrition-related knowledge deficit
- Psychological causes, e.g., depression or disordered eating
- Prolonged adherence to a low-fiber or low-residue diet
- Difficulty chewing or swallowing high-fiber foods
- Economic constraints that limit availability of appropriate foods
- Inability or unwillingness to purchase or consume fiber-containing foods
- Inappropriate food preparation practices, e.g., reliance on overprocessed, overcooked foods

Signs/Symptoms (*Defining Characteristics*)

A typical cluster of subjective and objective signs and symptoms gathered during the nutrition assessment process that provide evidence that a problem exists; quantify the problem and describe its severity.

Nutrition Assessment Category	Potential Indicators of this Nutrition Diagnosis (one or more must be present)
Biochemical Data, Medical Tests and Procedures	
Anthropometric Measurements	
Physical Examination Findings	
Food/Nutrition History	Reports or observations of: • Insufficient intake of fiber when compared to recommended amounts (38 g/day for men and 25 g/day for women)

INTAKE DOMAIN • Carbohydrate and Fiber

INADEQUATE FIBER INTAKE (NI-53.5)

Client History	• Conditions associated with a diagnosis or treatment, e.g., ulcer disease, inflammatory bowel disease, or short-bowel syndrome treated with a low fiber diet • Low stool volume

References:
1. DiPalma JA. Current treatment options for chronic constipation. *Rev Gastroenterol Disord.* 2004;2:S34-S42.
2. Higgins PD, Johanson JF. Epidemiology of constipation in North America: a systematic review. *Am J Gastroenterol.* 2004;99:750-759.
3. Lembo A, Camilieri M. Chronic constipation. *New Engl J Med.* 2003;349:360-368.
4. National Academy of Sciences, Institute of Medicine. *Dietary Reference Intakes for Energy, Carbohydrate, Fiber, Fat, Fatty Acids, Cholesterol, Protein, and Amino Acids.* Washington, DC: National Academy Press; 2002.
5. Talley NJ. Definition, epidemiology, and impact of chronic constipation. *Rev Gastroenterol Disord.* 2004;2:S3-S10.

Edition: 2007

EXCESSIVE FIBER INTAKE (NI-53.6)

Definition

Higher intake of fiber-containing foods or substances compared to recommendations based on patient/client condition.

Etiology (Cause/Contributing Risk Factors)

Factors gathered during the nutrition assessment process that contribute to the existence or the maintenance of pathophysiological, psychosocial, situational, developmental, cultural, and/or environmental problems:

- Food- and nutrition-related knowledge deficit about desirable quantities of fiber for individual condition
- Harmful beliefs or attitudes about food- or nutrition-related topics, e.g., obsession with bowel frequency and habits
- Lack of knowledge about appropriate fiber intake for condition
- Poor dentition, GI stricture, or dysmotility
- Food preparation or eating patterns that involve only high-fiber foods to the exclusion of other nutrient-dense foods

Signs/Symptoms (Defining Characteristics)

A typical cluster of subjective and objective signs and symptoms gathered during the nutrition assessment process that provide evidence that a problem exists; quantify the problem and describe its severity.

Nutrition Assessment Category	Potential Indicators of this Nutrition Diagnosis (one or more must be present)
Biochemical Data, Medical Tests and Procedures	
Anthropometric Measurements	
Physical Examination Findings	
Food/Nutrition History	Reports or observations of: • Fiber intake higher than tolerated or generally recommended for current medical condition
Client History	• Conditions associated with a diagnosis or treatment, e.g., ulcer disease, irritable bowel syndrome, inflammatory bowel disease, short-bowel syndrome, diverticulitis, obstructive constipation, prolapsing hemorrhoids, gastrointestinal stricture, eating disorders, or mental illness with obsessive-compulsive tendencies • Nausea, vomiting, excessive flatulence, diarrhea, abdominal cramping, high stool volume or frequency that causes discomfort to the individual; obstruction; phytobezoar

Edition: 2007

EXCESSIVE FIBER INTAKE (NI-53.6)

References:
1. DiPalma JA. Current treatment options for chronic constipation. *Rev Gastroenterol Disord.* 2004;2:S34-S42.
2. Higgins PD, Johanson JF. Epidemiology of constipation in North America: a systematic review. *Am J Gastroenterol.* 2004;99:750-759.
3. Lembo A, Camilieri M. Chronic constipation. *New Engl J Med.* 2003;349:360-368.
4. National Academy of Sciences, Institute of Medicine. *Dietary Reference Intakes for Energy, Carbohydrate, Fiber, Fat, Fatty Acids, Cholesterol, Protein, and Amino Acids.* Washington, DC: National Academy Press; 2002.
5. Position of the American Dietetic Association: Health implications of dietary fiber. *J Am Diet Assoc.* 2002;102:993-1000.
6. Talley NJ. Definition, epidemiology, and impact of chronic constipation. *Rev Gastroenterol Disord.* 2004;2:S3-S10.
7. van den Berg H, van der Gaag M, Hendriks H. Influence of lifestyle on vitamin bioavailability. *Int J Vitam Nutr Res.* 2002;72:53-55.
8. Wald A. Irritable bowel syndrome. *Curr Treat Options Gastroenterol.* 1999;2:13-19.

121

INADEQUATE VITAMIN INTAKE (SPECIFY) (NI-54.1)

Definition

Lower intake of vitamin-containing foods or substances compared to established reference standards or recommendations based on physiological needs.

Etiology (*Cause/Contributing Risk Factors*)

Factors gathered during the nutrition assessment process that contribute to the existence or the maintenance of pathophysiological, psychosocial, situational, developmental, cultural, and/or environmental problems:

- Physiological causes, e.g., increased nutrient needs due to prolonged catabolic illness, disease state, malabsorption, or medications
- Lack of access to food, e.g., economic constraints, cultural or religious practices, restricting food given to elderly and/or children
- Food- and nutrition-related knowledge deficit concerning food sources of vitamins
- Psychological causes, e.g., depression or eating disorders

Signs/Symptoms (*Defining Characteristics*)

A typical cluster of subjective and objective signs and symptoms gathered during the nutrition assessment process that provide evidence that a problem exists; quantify the problem and describe its severity.

Edition: 2007

INADEQUATE VITAMIN INTAKE (SPECIFY) (NI-54.1)

Nutrition Assessment Category	Potential Indicators of this Nutrition Diagnosis (one or more must be present)
Biochemical Data, Medical Tests and Procedures	• Vitamin A: serum retinol < 10 μg/dL (0.35 μmol/L) • Vitamin C: plasma concentrations <0.2 mg/dL (11.4 μmol/L) • Vitamin D: ionized calcium < 3.9 mg/dL (0.98 mmol/L) with elevated parathyroid hormone, normal serum calcium, and serum phosphorus < 2.6 mg/dL (0.84 mmol/L) • Vitamin E: plasma alpha-tocopherol < 18 μmol/g (41.8 μmol/L) • Vitamin K: elevated prothrombin time; altered INR (without anticoagulation therapy) • Thiamin: erythrocyte transketolase activity > 1.20 μg/mL/h • Riboflavin: erythrocyte glutathione reductase > 1.2 IU/g hemoglobin • Niacin: N'methyl-nicotinamide excretion <5.8 μmol/day • Vitamin B-6: plasma pryrdoxal 5' phosphate <5 ng/mL (20 nmol/L) • Vitamin B-12: serum concentration < 24.4 ng/dL (180 pmol/L); elevated homocysteine • Folic acid—serum concentration < 0.3 μg/dL (7 nmol/L), red cell folate < 315 nmol/L
Anthropometric Measurements	
Physical Exam Findings	• Vitamin A: night blindness, Bitot's spots, xerophthalmia, follicular hyperkeratosis • Vitamin C: follicular hyperkeratosis, petichiae, ecchymosis, coiled hairs, inflamed and bleeding gums, perifolicular hemorrhages, joint effusions, arthralgia, and impaired wound healing • Vitamin D: widening at ends of long bones • Riboflavin: sore throat, hyperemia, edema of pharyngeal and oral mucous membranes, cheilosis, angular stomatitis, glossitis, magenta tongue, seborrheic dermatitis, and normochromic, normocytin anemia with pure erythrocyte cytoplasia of the bone marrow • Niacin: symmetrical, pigmented rash on areas exposed to sunlight; bright red tongue • Vitamin B-6: seborrheic dermatitis, stomatitis, cheilosis, glossitis, confusion, depression • Vitamin B-12: tingling and numbness in extremities, diminished vibratory and position sense, motor disturbances including gait disturbances

123

INTAKE DOMAIN - Vitamin

INADEQUATE VITAMIN INTAKE (SPECIFY) (NI-54.1)

Food/Nutrition History	Reports or observations of:
	• Dietary history reflects inadequate intake of foods containing specific vitamins as compared to requirements or recommended level
	• Dietary history reflects excessive consumption of foods that do not contain available vitamins, e.g., overprocessed, overcooked, or improperly stored foods
	• Prolonged use of substances known to increase vitamin requirements or reduce vitamin absorption
	• Lack of interest in foods
	• Vitamin/mineral deficiency
Client History	• Conditions associated with a diagnosis or treatment, e.g., malabsorption as a result of celiac disease, short-bowel syndrome, or inflammatory bowel
	• Certain environmental conditions, e.g., infants exclusively fed breast milk with limited exposure to sunlight (Vitamin D)
	• Rachitic rosary in children, rickets, osteomalacia
	• Pellegra

References:

1. National Academy of Sciences, Institute of Medicine. *Dietary Reference Intakes for Vitamin A, Vitamin K, Arsenic, Boron, Chromium, Copper, Iodine, Iron, Manganese, Molybdenum, Nickel, Silicon, Vanadium, and Zinc.* Washington, DC: National Academy Press; 2000.
2. National Academy of Sciences, Institute of Medicine. *Dietary Reference Intakes for Thiamine, Riboflavin, Niacin, Vitamin B5, Folate, Vitamin B12, Pantothenic Acid, Biotin, and Choline* Washington, DC: National Academy Press; 2000.
3. National Academy of Sciences, Institute of Medicine. *Dietary Reference Intakes for Vitamin C, Vitamin E, Selenium, and Carotenoids.* Washington, DC: National Academy Press; 2000.
4. National Academy of Sciences, Institute of Medicine. *Dietary Reference Intakes for Calcium, Phosphorus, Magnesium, Vitamin D, and Fluoride.* Washington, DC: National Academy Press; 1997.

EXCESSIVE VITAMIN INTAKE (SPECIFY) (NI-54.2)

Definition

Higher intake of vitamin-containing foods or substances compared to established reference standards or recommendations based on physiological needs.

Etiology (*Cause/Contributing Risk Factors*)

Factors gathered during the nutrition assessment process that contribute to the existence or the maintenance of pathophysiological, psychosocial, situational, developmental, cultural, and/or environmental problems:

- Physiological causes, e.g., decreased nutrient needs due to prolonged immobility or chronic renal disease
- Access to foods and supplements in excess of needs, e.g., cultural or religious practices, inappropriate food and supplements given to pregnant women, elderly, or children
- Food- and nutrition-related knowledge deficit concerning food and supplemental sources of vitamins
- Psychological causes, e.g., depression or eating disorders
- Accidental overdose from oral and supplemental forms, enteral or parenteral sources

Signs/Symptoms (*Defining Characteristics*)

A typical cluster of subjective and objective signs and symptoms gathered during the nutrition assessment process that provide evidence that a problem exists; quantify the problem and describe its severity.

Nutrition Assessment Category	Potential Indicators of this Nutrition Diagnosis (one or more must be present)
Biochemical Data, Medical Tests and Procedures	• Vitamin D: ionized calcium > 5.4 mg/dL (1.35 mmol/L) with elevated parathyroid hormone, normal serum calcium, and serum phosphorus > 2.6 mg/dL (0.84 mmol/L) • Vitamin K: slowed prothrombin time or altered INR • Niacin: N'methyl-nicotinamide excretion > 7.3 μmol/day • Vitamin B-6: plasma pyrdoxal 5'phosphate > 15.7 ng/mL (94 noml/L) • Vitamin A: serum retinol concentration > 60 μg/dL (2.09 μmol/L)
Anthropometric Measurements	• Vitamin D: growth retardation

EXCESSIVE VITAMIN INTAKE (SPECIFY) (NI-54.2)

Physical Exam Findings	• Vitamin A: changes in the skin and mucous membranes; dry lips (cheilitis); early—dryness of the nasal mucosa and eyes; later—dryness, erythema, scaling and peeling of the skin, hair loss, and nail fragility. Headache, nausea, and vomiting. Infants may have bulging fontanelle; children may develop bone alterations.
	• Vitamin D: elevated serum calcium (hypercalcemia) and phosphorus (hyperphosphatemia) levels; calcification of soft tissues (calcinosis), including the kidney, lungs, heart, and even the tympanic membrane of the ear, which can result in deafness. Headache and nausea. Infants given excessive amounts of vitamin D may have gastrointestinal upset, bone fragility.
	• Vitamin K: hemolytic anemia in adults or severe jaundice in infants have been noted on rare occasions
	• Niacin: histamine release, which causes flushing, aggravation of asthma, or liver disease
Food/Nutrition History	Reports or observations of:
	• History or measured intake reflects excessive intake of foods and supplements containing vitamins as compared to estimated requirements, including fortified cereals, meal replacements, vitamin-mineral supplements, other dietary supplements (e.g., fish liver oils or capsules), tube feeding, and/or parenteral solutions
	• Intake > Tolerable Upper Limit (UL) for vitamin A (as retinol ester, not as β-carotene) is 600 µg/d for infants and toddlers; 900 µg/d for children 4-8 y, 1700 µg/d for children 9-13 y, 2800 for children 14-18 y, and 3000 µg/d for adults
	• Intake more than UL for vitamin D is 25 µg/d for infants and 50 µg/d for children and adults
	• Niacin: clinical, high-dose niacinamide (NA), 1-2 g, three times per day, can have side effects
Client History	• Conditions associated with a diagnosis or treatment, e.g., chronic liver or kidney diseases, heart failure, cancer

References:

1. Allen LH, Haskell M. Estimating the potential for vitamin A toxicity in women and young children. *J Nutr.* 2002;132:S2907-S2919.
2. Croquet V, Pilette C, Lespine A, Vuillemin E, Rousselet MC, Oberti F, Saint Andre JP, Periquet B, Francois S, Ifrah N, Cales P. Hepatic hyper-vitaminosis A: importance of retinyl ester level determination. *Eur J Gastroenerol Hepatol.* 2000;12:361-364.
3. Krasinski SD, Russell RM, Otradovec CL, Sadowski JA, Hartz SC, Jacob RA, McGandy RB. Relationship of vitamin A and vitamin E intake to fasting plasma retinol, retinol-binding protein, retinyl esters, carotene, alpha-tocopherol, and cholesterol among elderly people and young adults: increased plasma retinyl esters among vitamin A-supplement users. *Am J Clin Nutr.* 1989;49:112-120.
4. National Academy of Sciences, Institute of Medicine. *Dietary Reference Intakes for Vitamin A, Vitamin K, Arsenic, Boron, Chromium, Copper, Iodine, Iron, Manganese, Molybdenum, Nickel, Silicon, Vanadium, and Zinc.* Washington, DC: National Academy Press;2000.
5. National Academy of Sciences, Institute of Medicine. *Dietary Reference Intakes for Thiamine, Riboflavin, Niacin, Vitamin B6, Folate, Vitamin B12, Pantothenic Acid, Biotin, and Choline.* Washington, DC: National Academy Press;2000.
6. National Academy of Sciences, Institute of Medicine. *Dietary Reference Intakes for Vitamin C, Vitamin E, Selenium, and Carotenoids.* Washington, DC: National Academy Press;2000.
7. Russell RM. New views on RDAs for older adults. *J Am Diet Assoc.* 1997;97:515-518.

INADEQUATE MINERAL INTAKE (SPECIFY) (NI-55.1)

Definition

Lower intake of mineral-containing foods or substances compared to established reference standards or recommendations based on physiological needs.

Etiology (*Cause/Contributing Risk Factors*)

Factors gathered during the nutrition assessment process that contribute to the existence or the maintenance of pathophysiological, psychosocial, situational, developmental, cultural, and/or environmental problems:

- Physiological causes, e.g., increased nutrient needs due to prolonged catabolic illness, malabsorption, hyperexcretion, nutrient/drug and nutrient/nutrient interaction, growth and maturation
- Lack of access to food, e.g., economic constraints, cultural or religious practices, restricting food given to elderly and/or children
- Food- and nutrition-related knowledge deficit concerning food sources of minerals; misdiagnosis of lactose intolerance/lactase deficiency; perception of conflicting nutrition messages from health professionals; inappropriate reliance on supplements
- Psychological causes, e.g., depression or eating disorders
- Environmental causes, e.g., inadequately tested nutrient bioavailability of fortified foods, beverages, and supplements; inappropriate marketing of fortified foods/beverages/supplements as a substitute for natural food source of nutrient(s)

Signs/Symptoms (*Defining Characteristics*)

A typical cluster of subjective and objective signs and symptoms gathered during the nutrition assessment process that provide evidence that a problem exists; quantify the problem and describe its severity.

Nutrition Assessment Category	Potential Indicators of this Nutrition Diagnosis (one or more must be present)
Biochemical Data, Medical Tests and Procedures	• Calcium: bone mineral content (BMC) below the young adult mean. Hypocalciuria, serum 25(OH)D <32 ng/mL
	• Phosphorus < 2.6 mg/dL (0.84 mmol/L)
	• Magnesium <1.8 mg/dL (0.7 mmol/L)
	• Iron: hemoglobin < 13g/L (2mmol/L) (males); < 12g/L (1.86mmol/L) (females)
	• Iodine: urinary excretion <100µg/L (788 nmol/L)
	• Copper, serum copper < 64 µg/dL (10 µmol/L)
Anthropometric Measurements	• Height loss
Physical Exam Findings	• Calcium: diminished bone mineral density, hypertension, obesity

127

Edition: 2007

INTAKE DOMAIN - Mineral

INADEQUATE MINERAL INTAKE (SPECIFY) (NI-55.1)

Food/Nutrition History	Reports or observations of insufficient mineral intake from diet compared to recommended intake: • Food avoidance and/or elimination of whole food group(s) from diet • Lack of interest in food • Inappropriate food choices and/or chronic dieting behavior • Vitamin/mineral deficiency • Use of popular press/internet as source of medical and/or nutrition information
Client History	• Conditions associated with a diagnosis or treatment, e.g., malabsorption as a result of celiac disease, short bowel syndrome, or inflammatory bowel disease • Polycystic ovary syndrome, premenstrual syndrome, kidney stones, colon polyps • Other significant medical diagnoses and therapies • Estrogen status • Geographic latitude and history of Ultraviolet-B exposure/use of sunscreen • Change in living environment/independence

References:
1. Appel LJ, Moore TJ, Obarzanek E, Vollmer WM, Svetkey LP, Sacks FM, Bray GA, Vogt TM, Cutler JA, Windhauser MM, Lin P-H, Karanja N. A clinical trial of the effects of dietary patterns on blood pressure. *N Engl J Med.* 1997;336:1117-1124.
2. Heaney RP. Role of dietary sodium in osteoporosis. *J Am Coll Nutr* (in press) 2006.
3. Heaney RP. Nutrients, interactions, and foods. The Importance of Source. In Burckhardt P, Dawson-Hughes B, Heaney RP, Eds. *Nutritional Aspects of Osteoporosis 2nd Ed.* San Diego, CA: Elsevier, 2004:61-76.
4. Heaney RP. Nutrients, interactions, and foods. Serum 25-hydroxy-vitamin D and the health of the calcium economy. In Burckhardt P, Dawson-Hughes B, Heaney RP, Eds. *Nutritional Aspects of Osteoporosis 2nd Ed.* San Diego, CA: Elsevier, 2004:227-244.
5. Heaney RP, Rafferty K, Bierman J. Not all calcium-fortified beverages are equal. *Nutr Today.* 2005;40:39-41.
6. Heaney RP, Dowell MS, Hale CA, Bendich A. Calcium absorption varies within the reference range for serum 25-hydroxyvitamin D. *J Am Coll Nutr.* 2003;22:142-146.
7. Heaney RP, Dowell MS, Rafferty K, Bierman J. Bioavailability of the calcium in fortified soy imitation milk, with some observations on method. *Am J Clin Nutr.* 2000;71:1166-1169.
8. Holick MF. Functions of vitamin D: importance for prevention of common cancers, Type I diabetes and heart Disease. *Nutritional Aspects of Osteoporosis, 2nd Edition.* Burckhardt P, Dawson-Hughes B, Heaney RP, eds. San Diego, CA:Elsevier Inc.;2004:181-201
9. Massey LK, Whiting SJ. Dietary salt, urinary calcium, and bone loss. *J Bone Miner Res.* 1996; 11:731-736.
10. Suarez FL, Savaiano D, Arbisi P, Levitt MD. Tolerance to the daily ingestion of two cups of milk by individuals claiming lactose intolerance. *Am J Clin Nutr.* 1997;65:1502-1506.
11. Thys-Jacobs S, Donovan D, Papadopoulos A, Sarrel P. Bilezikian JP. Vitamin D and calcium dysregulation in the polycystic ovarian syndrome. *Steroids.1999;* 64:430-435.
12. Thys-Jacobs S, Starkey P, Bernstein D, Tian J. Calcium carbonate and the premenstrual syndrome: Effects on premenstrual and menstrual symptomatology. *Am J Obstet Gynecol.* 1998;179:444-452.
13. Zemel MB, Thompson W, Milstead A, Morris K, Campbell P. Calcium and dairy acceleration of weight and fat loss during energy restriction in obese adults. *Obesity Res.* 2004;12:582-590.

EXCESSIVE MINERAL INTAKE (SPECIFY) (NI-55.2)

Definition

Higher intake of mineral from foods, supplements, medications or water, compared to established reference standards or recommendations based on physiological needs.

Etiology (Cause/Contributing Risk Factors)

Factors gathered during the nutrition assessment process that contribute to the existence or the maintenance of pathophysiological, psychosocial, situational, developmental, cultural, and/or environmental problems:

- Food- and nutrition-related knowledge deficit
- Harmful beliefs/attitudes about food, nutrition, and nutrition-related topics
- Food faddism
- Accidental oversupplementation
- Overconsumption of a limited variety of foods
- Lack of knowledge about management of diagnosed genetic disorder altering mineral homeostasis [hemochromatosis (iron), Wilson's disease (copper)]
- Lack of knowledge about management of diagnosed disease state requiring mineral restriction [cholestatic liver disease (copper and manganese), renal insufficiency (phosphorus, magnesium, potassium)]

Signs/Symptoms (Defining Characteristics)

A typical cluster of subjective and objective signs and symptoms gathered during the nutrition assessment process that provide evidence that a problem exists; quantify the problem and describe its severity.

Nutrition Assessment Category	Potential Indicators of this Nutrition Diagnosis (one or more must be present)
Biochemical Data, Medical Tests and Procedures	Changes in appropriate laboratory values, such as: • ↑ TSH (iodine supplementation) • ↓ HDL (zinc supplementation) • ↑ serum ferritin and transferrin saturation (iron overload) • Hyperphosphatemia • Hypermagnesemia

Edition: 2007

EXCESSIVE MINERAL INTAKE (SPECIFY) (NI-55.2)

Anthropometric Measurements	
Physical Exam Findings	• Hair and nail changes (selenium)
Food/Nutrition History	Reports or observations of: • High intake of foods or supplements containing mineral compared to DRIs • Decreased appetite (zinc supplementation)
Client History	• GI disturbances (iron, magnesium, copper, zinc, selenium) • Copper deficiency anemia (zinc) • Liver damage (copper, iron), enamel or skeletal fluorosis (fluoride)

References:

1. Bowman BA, Russell RM, eds. *Present Knowledge in Nutrition. 8th Ed.* Washington, DC: ILSI Press; 2001.
2. National Academy of Sciences, Institute of Medicine. *Dietary Reference Intakes for Vitamin A, Vitamin K, Arsenic, Boron, Chromium, Copper, Iodine, Iron, Manganese, Molybdenum, Nickel, Silicon, Vanadium, Zinc.* Washington, DC: National Academy Press; 2001.
3. National Academy of Sciences, Institute of Medicine. *Dietary Reference Intakes for Calcium, Phosphorus, Magnesium, Vitamin D, and Fluoride.* Washington, DC: National Academy Press; 1997.
4. Position of the American Dietetic Association: Food and nutrition misinformation. *J Am Diet Assoc.* 2002;102:260-266.

SWALLOWING DIFFICULTY (NC–1.1)

Definition

Impaired movement of food and liquid from the mouth to the stomach.

Etiology (Cause/Contributing Risk Factors)

Factors gathered during the nutrition assessment process that contribute to the existence or the maintenance of pathophysiological, psychosocial, situational, developmental, cultural, and/or environmental problems:

- Mechanical causes, e.g., inflammation, surgery, stricture, or oral, pharyngeal and esophageal tumors
- Motor causes, e.g., neurological or muscular disorders, such as, cerebral palsy, stroke, multiple sclerosis, scleroderma, prematurity

Signs/Symptoms (Defining Characteristics)

A typical cluster of subjective and objective signs and symptoms gathered during the nutrition assessment process that provide evidence that a problem exists; quantify the problem and describe its severity.

Nutrition Assessment Category	Potential Indicators of this Nutrition Diagnosis (one or more must be present)
Biochemical Data, Medical Tests and Procedures	• Radiological findings, e.g., abnormal swallowing studies
Anthropometric Measurements	
Physical Exam Findings	• Evidence of dehydration, e.g., dry mucous membranes, poor skin turgor
Food/Nutrition History	Reports or observations of: • Coughing, choking, prolonged chewing, pouching of food, regurgitation, facial expression changes during eating, prolonged feeding time, drooling, noisy wet upper airway sounds, feeling of "food getting stuck," pain while swallowing • Decreased food intake • Avoidance of foods • Mealtime resistance
Client History	• Conditions associated with a diagnosis or treatment, e.g., dysphagia, achalasia • Repeated upper respiratory infections and or pneumonia

CLINCAL DOMAIN • Functional

SWALLOWING DIFFICULTY (NC-1.1)

References:

1. Braunwald E, Fauci AS, Kasper DL, Hauser SL, Longo DL, Jameson JL, ed. *Harrison's Principles of Internal Medicine. 15th Edition.* New York, NY: McGraw-Hill; 2001.

Edition: 2007

CLINCAL DOMAIN • Functional

CHEWING (MASTICATORY) DIFFICULTY (NC-1.2)

Definition

Impaired ability to bite or chew food in preparation for swallowing.

Etiology (Cause/Contributing Risk Factors)

Factors gathered during the nutrition assessment process that contribute to the existence or the maintenance of pathophysiological, psychosocial, situational, developmental, cultural, and/or environmental problems:

- Craniofacial malformations
- Oral surgery
- Neuromuscular dysfunction
- Partial or complete edentulism
- Soft tissue disease (primary or oral manifestations of a systemic disease)
- Xerostomia

Signs/Symptoms (Defining Characteristics)

A typical cluster of subjective and objective signs and symptoms gathered during the nutrition assessment process that provide evidence that a problem exists; quantify the problem and describe its severity.

Nutrition Assessment Category	Potential Indicators of this Nutrition Diagnosis (one or more must be present)
Biochemical Data, Medical Tests and Procedures	
Anthropometric Measurements	
Physical Exam Findings	• Missing teeth • Alterations in cranial nerves V, VII, IX, X, XII • Dry or cracked lips, tongue • Oral lesions • Impaired tongue movement • Ill-fitting dentures or broken dentures

Edition: 2007

133

CHEWING (MASTICATORY) DIFFICULTY (NC-1.2)

Food/Nutrition History	Reports or observations of: • Decreased intake of food • Alterations in food intake from usual • Decreased intake or avoidance of food difficult to form into a bolus, e.g, nuts, whole pieces of meat, poultry, fish, fruits, vegetables • Avoidance of foods of age-appropriate texture • Spitting food out or prolonged feeding time
Client History	• Conditions associated with a diagnosis or treatment, e.g., alcoholism; Alzheimer's; head, neck or pharyngeal cancer; cerebral palsy; cleft lip/palate; oral soft tissue infections (e.g., candidiasis, leukoplakia); lack of developmental readiness; oral manifestations of systemic disease (e.g., rheumatoid arthritis, lupus, Crohn's disease, penphigus vulgaris, HIV, diabetes) • Recent major oral surgery • Wired jaw • Chemotherapy with oral side effects • Radiation therapy to oral cavity

References:

1. Bailey R, Ledikwe JH, Smiciklas-Wright H, Mitchell DC, Jensen GL. Persistent oral health problems associated with comorbidity and impaired diet quality in older adults. *J Am Diet Assoc.* 2004;104:1273-1276.
2. Chernoff R, ed. Oral health in the elderly. *Geriatric Nutrition.* Gaithersburg, MD: Aspen Publishers; 1999.
3. Dormenval V, Mojon P, Budtz-Jorgensen E. Association between self-assessed masticatory ability, nutritional status and salivary flow rate in hospitalized elderly. *Oral Diseases.* 1999;5:32-38.
4. Hildebrand GH, Dominguez BL, Schork MA, Loesche WJ. Functional units, chewing, swallowing and food avoidance among the elderly. *J Prosthet Dent.* 1997;77:585-595.
5. Hirano H, Ishiyama N, Watanabe I, Nasu I. Masticatory ability in relation to oral status and general health in aging. *J Nutr Health Aging.* 1999;3:48-52.
6. Huhmann M, Touger-Decker R, Byham-Gray L, O'Sullivan-Maillet J, Von Hagen S. Comparison of dysphagia screening by a registered dietitian in acute stroke patients to speech language pathologist's evaluation. *Top Clin Nutr.* 2004;19:239-249.
7. Kademani D, Glick M. Oral ulcerations in individuals infected with human immunodeficiency virus: clinical presentations, diagnosis, management and relevance to disease progression. *Quintessence International.* 1998;29:1103-1108.
8. Keller HH, Ostbye T, Bright-See E. Predictors of dietary intake in Ontario seniors. *Can J Public Health.* 1997;88:303-309.
9. Krall E, Hayes C, Garcia R. How dentition status and masticatory function affect nutrient intake. *J Am Dent Assoc.* 1998;129:1261-1269.
10. Joshipura K, Willett WC, Douglass CW. The impact of edentulousness on food and nutrient intake. *J Am Dent Assoc.* 1996;127:459-467.
11. Mackle T, Touger-Decker R, O'Sullivan Maillet J, Holland, B. Registered Dietitians' use of physical assessment parameters in practice. *J Am Diet Assoc.* 2004;103:1632-1638.
12. Mobley C, Saunders M. Oral health screening guidelines for nondental healthcare providers. *J Amer Diet Assoc.* 1997;97:S123-S126.
13. Morse D. Oral and pharyngeal cancer. In: R Touger-Decker et al eds. *Nutrition and Oral Medicine.* Totowa NJ: Humana Press, Inc; 2005, 205.222.
14. Moynihan P, Butler T, Thomason J, Jepson N. Nutrient intake in partially dentate patients: the effect of prosthetic rehabilitation. *J Dent.* 2000;28:557-563.
15. Position of the American Dietetic Association: Oral health and nutrition. *J Am Diet Assoc.* 2003;103:615-625.
16. Sayhoun NR Lin CL, Krall E. Nutritional status of the older adult is associated with dentition status. *J Am Diet Assoc.* 2003;103:61-66.

CHEWING (MASTICATORY) DIFFICULTY (NC-1.2)

18. Sheiham A, Steele JG. The impact of oral health on stated ability to eat certain foods; finding from the national diet and nutrition survey of older people in Great Britain. *Gerodontology.* 1999;16:11-20.
19. Ship J, Duffy V, Jones J, Langmore S. Geriatric oral health and its impact on eating. *J Am Geriatr Soc.* 1996;44:456-464.
20. Touger-Decker R. Clinical and laboratory assessment of nutrition status. *Dent Clin North America.* 2003;47:259-278.
21. Touger-Decker R, Sirois D, Mobley C (eds). *Nutrition and Oral Medicine.* Totowan, NJ: Humana Press; 2004.
22. Walls AW, Steele JG, Sheiham A, Marcenes W, Moynihan PJ. Oral health and nutrition in older people. *J Public Health Dent.* 2000;60:304-307.

Edition: 2007

BREASTFEEDING DIFFICULTY (NC-1.3)

Definition

Inability to sustain infant nutrition through breastfeeding.

Etiology (*Cause/Contributing Risk Factors*)

Factors gathered during the nutrition assessment process that contribute to the existence or the maintenance of pathophysiological, psychosocial, situational, developmental, cultural, and/or environmental problems:

Infant:

- Difficulty latching on, e.g., tight frenulum
- Poor sucking ability
- Oral pain
- Malnutrition/malabsorption
- Lethargy, sleepiness
- Irritability
- Swallowing difficulty

Mother:

- Painful breasts, nipples
- Breast or nipple abnormality
- Mastitis
- Perception of inadequate milk supply
- Lack of social, cultural, or environmental support

Signs/Symptoms (*Defining Characteristics*)

A typical cluster of subjective and objective signs and symptoms gathered during the nutrition assessment process that provide evidence that a problem exists; quantify the problem and describe its severity.

Nutrition Assessment Category	Potential Indicators of this Nutrition Diagnosis (one or more must be present)
Biochemical Data, Medical Tests and Procedures	• Laboratory evidence of dehydration (infant)
Anthropometric Measurements	• Any weight loss or poor weight gain (infant)
Physical Exam Findings	• Frenulum abnormality (infant) • Vomiting or diarrhea (infant)

Edition: 2007

CLINCAL DOMAIN - Functional

BREASTFEEDING DIFFICULTY (NC-1.3)

Food/Nutrition History	Reports or observations of (infant):
	• Coughing
	• Crying, latching on and off, pounding on breasts
	• Decreased feeding frequency/duration, early cessation of feeding, and/or feeding resistance
	• Lethargy
	• Hunger, lack of satiety after feeding
	• Fewer than six wet diapers in 24 hours
	Reports or observations of (mother):
	• Small amount of milk when pumping
	• Lack of confidence in ability to breastfeed
	• Doesn't hear infant swallowing
	• Concerns regarding mother's choice to breastfeed/lack of support
	• Insufficient knowledge of breastfeeding or infant hunger/satiety signals
	• Lack of facilities or accommodations at place of employment or in community for breastfeeding
Client History	• Conditions associated with a diagnosis or treatment of (infant), e.g., cleft lip/palate, thrush, premature birth, malabsorption, infection
	• Conditions associated with a diagnosis or treatment of (mother), e.g., mastitis, candidiasis, engorgement, history of breast surgery

References:
1. Barron SP, Lane HW, Hannan TE, Struempler B, Williams JC. Factors influencing duration of breast feeding among low-income women. *J Am Diet Assoc.* 1988;88:1557-1561.
2. Bryant C, Coreil J, D'Angelo SL, Bailey DFC, Lazarov MA. A strategy for promoting breastfeeding among economically disadvantaged women and adolescents. *NAACOGs Clin Issu Perinat Womens Health Nurs.* 1992;3:723-730.
3. Bentley ME, Caulfield LE, Gross SM, Bronner Y, Jensen J, Kessler LA, Paige DM. Sources of influence on intention to breastfeed among African-American women at entry to WIC. *J Hum Lact.* 1999;15:27-34.
4. Moreland JC, Lloyd L, Braun SB, Heins JN. A new teaching model to prolong breastfeeding among Latinos. *J Hum Lact.* 2000;16:337-341.
5. Position of the American Dietetic Association: Breaking the barriers to breastfeeding. *J Am Diet Assoc.* 2001;101:1213-1220.
6. Wooldrige MS, Fischer C. Colic, "overfeeding" and symptoms of lactose malabsorption in the breast-fed baby. *Lancet.* 1988;2:382-384.

137

Edition: 2007

CLINCAL DOMAIN • Functional

ALTERED GASTROINTESTINAL (GI) FUNCTION (NC-1.4)

Definition

Changes in ability to digest or absorb nutrients.

Etiology (*Cause/Contributing Risk Factors*)

Factors gathered during the nutrition assessment process that contribute to the existence or the maintenance of pathophysiological, psychosocial, situational, developmental, cultural, and/or environmental problems:

- Alterations in GI anatomical structure, e.g., gastric bypass, Roux En Y
- Changes in the GI tract motility, e.g., gastroparesis
- Compromised GI tract function, e.g., celiac disease, Crohn's disease, infection, radiation therapy
- Compromised function of related GI organs, e.g., pancreas, liver
- Decreased functional length of the GI tract, e.g., short-bowel syndrome

Signs/Symptoms (*Defining Characteristics*)

A typical cluster of subjective and objective signs and symptoms gathered during the nutrition assessment process that provide evidence that a problem exists; quantify the problem and describe its severity.

Nutrition Assessment Category	Potential Indicators of this Nutrition Diagnosis (one or more must be present)
Biochemical Data, Medical Tests and Procedures	• Abnormal digestive enzyme and fecal fat studies • Abnormal hydrogen breath test, d-xylose test, stool culture, and gastric emptying and/or small bowel transit time • Endoscopic or colonoscopic examination results, biopsy results
Anthropometric Measurements	• Wasting due to malnutrition in severe cases
Physical Exam Findings	• Decreased muscle mass • Abdominal distension • Increased (or sometimes decreased) bowel sounds

Edition: 2007

138

CLINCAL DOMAIN • Functional

ALTERED GASTROINTESTINAL (GI) FUNCTION (NC-1.4)

Food/Nutrition History	Reports or observations of: • Avoidance or limitation of total intake or intake of specific foods/food groups due to GI symptoms, e.g., bloating, cramping, pain, diarrhea, steatorrhea (greasy, floating, foul-smelling stools) especially following ingestion of food • Food- and nutrition-related knowledge deficit, e.g., lack of information, incorrect information or noncompliance with modified diet or medication schedule
Client History	• Anorexia, nausea, vomiting, diarrhea, steatorrhea, constipation, abdominal pain • Conditions associated with a diagnosis or treatment, e.g., malabsorption, maldigestion, steatorrhea, constipation, diverticulitis, Crohn's disease, inflammatory bowel disease, cystic fibrosis, celiac disease, irritable bowel syndrome, infection • Surgical procedures, e.g., esophagectomy, dilatation, gastrectomy, vagotomy, gastric bypass, bowel resections

References:
1. Braunwald E, Fauci AS, Kasper DL, Longo DL, Jameson JL, ed. *Harrison's Principles of Internal Medicine. 15th Edition*. New York, NY: McGraw-Hill; 2001.

139

Edition: 2007

IMPAIRED NUTRIENT UTILIZATION (NC-2.1)

Definition

Changes in ability to absorb or metabolize nutrients and bioactive substances.

Etiology (*Cause/Contributing Risk Factors*)

Factors gathered during the nutrition assessment process that contribute to the existence or the maintenance of pathophysiological, psychosocial, situational, developmental, cultural, and/or environmental problems:

- Alterations in gastrointestinal anatomical structure
- Compromised function of the GI tract
- Compromised function of related GI organs, e.g., pancreas, liver
- Decreased functional length of the GI tract
- Metabolic disorders

Signs/Symptoms (*Defining Characteristics*)

A typical cluster of subjective and objective signs and symptoms gathered during the nutrition assessment process that provide evidence that a problem exists; quantify the problem and describe its severity.

Nutrition Assessment Category	Potential Indicators of this Nutrition Diagnosis (one or more must be present)
Biochemical Data, Medical Tests and Procedures	• Abnormal digestive enzyme and fecal fat studies • Abnormal hydrogen breath test, d-xylose test • Abnormal tests for inborn errors of metabolism
Anthropometric Measurements	• Weight loss of $\geq$ 5% in one month, $\geq$ 10% in six months • Growth stunting or failure
Physical Exam Findings	• Abdominal distension • Increased or decreased bowel sounds • Evidence of vitamin and/or mineral deficiency, e.g., glossitis, cheilosis, mouth lesions

CLINICAL DOMAIN · Biochemical

IMPAIRED NUTRIENT UTILIZATION (NC-2.1)

Food/Nutrition History	Reports or observations of:
	• Avoidance or limitation of total intake or intake of specific foods/food groups due to GI symptoms, e.g., bloating, cramping, pain, diarrhea, steatorrhea (greasy, floating, foul-smelling stools) especially following ingestion of food
Client History	• Diarrhea, steatorrhea, abdominal pain
	• Endoscopic or colonoscopic examination results, biopsy results
	• Conditions associated with a diagnosis or treatment, e.g., malabsorption, maldigestion, cystic fibrosis, celiac disease, Crohn's disease, infection, radiation therapy, inborn errors of metabolism
	• Surgical procedures, e.g., gastric bypass, bowel resection

References:

1. Beyer P. Gastrointestinal disorders: Roles of nutrition and the dietetics practitioner. *J Am Diet Assoc.* 1998;98:272-277.
2. Position of the American Dietetic Association: Health implications of dietary fiber. *J Am Diet Assoc.* 2002;102:993-1000.

141

ALTERED NUTRITION-RELATED LABORATORY VALUES (SPECIFY) (NC-2.2)

Definition

Changes due to body composition, medications, body system changes or genetics, or changes in ability to eliminate byproducts of digestive and metabolic processes.

Etiology (Cause/Contributing Risk Factors)

Factors gathered during the nutrition assessment process that contribute to the existence or the maintenance of pathophysiological, psychosocial, situational, developmental, cultural, and/or environmental problems:

- Kidney, liver, cardiac, endocrine, neurologic, and/or pulmonary dysfunction
- Other organ dysfunction that leads to biochemical changes

Signs/Symptoms (Defining Characteristics)

A typical cluster of subjective and objective signs and symptoms gathered during the nutrition assessment process that provide evidence that a problem exists; quantify the problem and describe its severity.

Nutrition Assessment Category	Potential Indicators of this Nutrition Diagnosis (one or more must be present)
Biochemical Data, Medical Tests and Procedures	• Increased AST, ALT, T. bili, serum ammonia (liver disorders) • Abnormal BUN, Cr, K, phosphorus, glomerular filtration rate (GFR) (kidney disorders) • Altered pO_2 and pCO_2 (pulmonary disorders) • Abnormal serum lipids • Abnormal plasma glucose levels • Other findings of acute or chronic disorders that are abnormal and of nutritional origin or consequence
Anthropometric Measurements	• Rapid weight changes • Other anthropometric measures that are altered
Physical Exam Findings	• Jaundice, edema, ascites, itching (liver disorders) • Edema, shortness of breath (cardiac disorders) • Blue nail beds, clubbing (pulmonary disorders)

CLINCAL DOMAIN - Biochemical

ALTERED NUTRITION-RELATED LABORATORY VALUES (SPECIFY) (NC-2.2)

Food/Nutrition History	Reports or observations of:
	• Anorexia, nausea, vomiting
	• Intake of foods high in or overall excess intake of protein, potassium, phosphorus, sodium, fluid
	• Inadequate intake of micronutrients
	• Food- and nutrition-related knowledge deficit, e.g., lack of information, incorrect information ,or noncompliance with modified diet
Client History	• Conditions associated with a diagnosis or treatment, e.g., renal or liver disease, alcoholism, cardiopulmonary disorders

References:

1. Beto JA, Bansal VK. Medical nutrition therapy in chronic kidney failure: integrating clinical practice guidelines. *J Am Diet Assoc.* 2004;104:404-409.
2. Davern II TJ, Scharschmidt BF. Biochemical liver tests. In Feldman M, Scharschmidt BF, Sleisenger MH (eds): *Sleisenger and Fordtran's Gasrointestinal and Liver Disease, ed 6, vol 2,* Philadelphia, PA: WB Saunders; 1998: 1112-1122.
3. Durose CL, Holdsworth M, Watson V, Przygrodzka F. Knowledge of dietary restrictions and the medical consequences of noncompliance by patients on hemodialysis are not predictive of dietary compliance. *J Am Diet Assoc.* 2004;104:35-41.
4. Kassiske BL, Lakatua JD, Ma JZ, Louis TA. A meta-analysis of the effects of dietary protein restriction on the rate of decline in renal function. *Am J Kidney Dis.* 1998;31:954-961.
5. Knight EL, Stampfer MJ, Hankinson SE, Spiegelman D, Curhan GC. The impact of protein intake on renal function decline in women with normal renal function or mild renal insufficiency. *Ann Intern Med.* 2003;138:460-467.
6. Nakao T, Matsumoto, Okada T, Kanazawa Y, Yoshino M, Nagaoka Y, Takeguchi F. Nutritional management of dialysis patients: balancing among nutrient intake, dialysis dose, and nutritional status. *Am J Kidney Dis.* 2003;41:S133-S136.
7. National Kidney Foundation, Inc. Part 5. Evaluation of laboratory measurements for clinical assessment of kidney disease. *Am J Kidney Dis.* 2002;39:S76-S92.
8. National Kidney Foundation, Inc. Guideline 9. Association of level of GFR with nutritional status. *Am J Kidney Dis.* 2002;39:S128-S142.

FOOD–MEDICATION INTERACTION (NC-2.3)

Definition

Undesirable/harmful interaction(s) between food and over-the-counter (OTC) medications, prescribed medications, herbals, botanicals, and/or dietary supplements that diminishes, enhances, or alters effect of nutrients and/or medications.

Etiology (Cause/Contributing Risk Factors)

Factors gathered during the nutrition assessment process that contribute to the existence or the maintenance of pathophysiological, psychosocial, situational, developmental, cultural, and/or environmental problems:

- Combined ingestion or administration of medication and food that results in undesirable/harmful interaction

Signs/Symptoms (Defining Characteristics)

A typical cluster of subjective and objective signs and symptoms gathered during the nutrition assessment process that provide evidence that a problem exists; quantify the problem and describe its severity.

Nutrition Assessment Category	Potential Indicators of this Nutrition Diagnosis (one or more must be present)
Biochemical Data, Medical Tests and Procedures	• Alterations of biochemical tests based on medication affect and patient/client condition
Anthropometric Measurements	• Alterations of anthropometric measurements based on medication affect and patient/client conditions, e.g., weight gain and corticosteroids
Physical Exam Findings	

Food/Nutrition History	Reports or observations of:
	• Intake that is problematic or inconsistent with OTC, prescribed drugs, herbals, botanicals, and dietary supplements, such as:
	   • fish oils and prolonged bleeding
	   • coumadin, vitamin K–rich foods
	   • high-fat diet while on cholesterol lowering medications
	   • iron supplements, constipation and low-fiber diet
	• Intake that does not support replacement or mitigation of OTC, prescribed drugs, herbals, botanicals, and dietary supplements affects such as potassium-wasting diuretics
	• Changes in appetite or taste

144

Edition: 2007

CLINCAL DOMAIN ▪ Biochemical

FOOD–MEDICATION INTERACTION (NC-2.3)

Client History	• Multiple drugs (OTC, prescribed drugs, herbals, botanicals, and dietary supplements) that are known to have food–medication interactions • Medications that require nutrient supplementation that can not be accomplished via food intake, e.g., isoniazid and vitamin B-6

Reference:

1. Position of the American Dietetic Association: Integration of nutrition and pharmacotherapy. *J Am Diet Assoc.* 2003;103:1363-1370.

Edition: 2007

UNDERWEIGHT (NC-3.1)

Definition

Low body weight compared to established reference standards or recommendations.

Etiology (*Cause/Contributing Risk Factors*)

Factors gathered during the nutrition assessment process that contribute to the existence or the maintenance of pathophysiological, psychosocial, situational, developmental, cultural, and/or environmental problems:

- Disordered eating pattern
- Excessive physical activity
- Harmful beliefs/attitudes about food, nutrition, and nutrition-related topics
- Inadequate energy intake
- Increased energy needs
- Limited access to food

Signs/Symptoms (*Defining Characteristics*)

A typical cluster of subjective and objective signs and symptoms gathered during the nutrition assessment process that provide evidence that a problem exists; quantify the problem and describe its severity.

Nutrition Assessment Category	Potential Indicators of this Nutrition Diagnosis (one or more must be present)
Biochemical Data, Medical Tests and Procedures	• Measured resting metabolic rate (RMR) measurement higher than expected and/or estimated RMR
Anthropometric Measurements	• Weight for age less than 5th percentile for infants younger than 12 months • Decreased skinfold thickness and MAMC • BMI < 18.5 (most adults) • BMI for older adults (older than 65 years) < 23 • BMI < 5th percentile (children, 2-19 years)
Physical Exam Findings	• Decreased muscle mass, muscle wasting (gluteal and temporal)

146

Edition: 2007

UNDERWEIGHT (NC-3.1)

Food/Nutrition History	Reports or observations of:
	• Inadequate intake of food compared to estimated or measured needs
	• Limited supply of food in home
	• Dieting, food faddism
	• Hunger
	• Refusal to eat
	• Physical activity more than recommended amount
	• Vitamin/mineral deficiency
Client History	• Malnutrition
	• Illness or physical disability
	• Mental illness, dementia, confusion
	• Medications that affect appetite, e.g., stimulants for ADHD
	• Athlete, dancer, gymnast

References:

1. Assessment of nutritional status. In: Kleinman R (ed.). *Pediatric Nutrition Handbook, 5th ed.* Elk Grove Village, IL: American Academy of Pediatrics; 2004:407-423.
2. Beck AM, Ovesen LW. At which body mass index and degree of weight loss should hospitalized elderly patients be considered at nutritional risk? *Clin Nutr.* 1998;17:195-198.
3. Blaum CS, Fries BE, Fiatarone MA. Factors associated with low body mass index and weight loss in nursing home residents. *J Gerontology: Med Sci.* 1995;50A:M162-M168.
4. Position of the American Dietetic Association: Domestic food and nutrition security. *J Am Diet Assoc.* 2002;102:1840-1847.
5. Position of the American Dietetic Association: Addressing world hunger, malnutrition, and food insecurity. *J Am Diet Assoc.* 2003;103:1046-1057.
6. Position of the American Dietetic Association: Nutrition intervention in the treatment of anorexia nervosa, bulimia nervosa, and eating disorder not otherwise specified (EDNOS). *J Am Diet Assoc.* 2001;101:810-819.
7. Schneider SM, Al-Jaouni R, Pivot X, Braulio VB, Rampal P, Hebuerne X. Lack of adaptation to severe malnutrition in elderly patients. *Clin Nutr.* 2002;21:499-504.
8. Spear BA. Adolescent growth and development. *J Am Diet Assoc.* 2002 (suppl);102:S23- S29.

147

INVOLUNTARY WEIGHT LOSS (NC-3.2)

Definition

Decrease in body weight that is not planned or desired.

Etiology (*Cause/Contributing Risk Factors*)

Factors gathered during the nutrition assessment process that contribute to the existence or the maintenance of pathophysiological, psychosocial, situational, developmental, cultural, and/or environmental problems:

- Physiological causes, e.g., increased nutrient needs due to prolonged catabolic illness
- Lack of access to food, e.g., economic constraints, cultural or religious practices, restricting food given to elderly and/or children
- Prolonged hospitalization
- Psychological issues
- Lack of self-feeding ability

Signs/Symptoms (*Defining Characteristics*)

A typical cluster of subjective and objective signs and symptoms gathered during the nutrition assessment process that provide evidence that a problem exists; quantify the problem and describe its severity.

Nutrition Assessment Category	Potential Indicators of this Nutrition Diagnosis (one or more must be present)
Biochemical Data, Medical Tests and Procedures	
Anthropometric Measurements	• Weight loss of 5% within 30 days, 7.5% in 90 days, or 10% in 180 days
Physical Examination Findings	• Fever • Increased heart rate • Increased respiratory rate • Loss of subcutaneous fat and muscle stores

Edition: 2007

CLINCAL DOMAIN ▪ Weight

INVOLUNTARY WEIGHT LOSS (NC-3.2)

Food/Nutrition History	Reports or observations of: • Normal or usual intake in face of illness • Poor intake, change in eating habits, skipped meals • Change in way clothes fit
Client History	• Conditions associated with a diagnosis or treatment, e.g., AIDS/HIV, burns, chronic obstructive pulmonary disease, hip/long bone fracture, infection, surgery, trauma, hyperthyroidism (pre- or untreated), some types of cancer or metastatic disease (specify) • Medications associated with weight loss, such as certain antidepressants or cancer chemotherapy

References:

1. Collins N. Protein-energy malnutrition and involuntary weight loss: Nutritional and pharmacologic strategies to enhance wound healing. *Expert Opin Pharmacother*. 2003;7:1121-1140.
2. Splett PL, Roth-Yousey LL, Vogelzang JL. Medical nutrition therapy for the prevention and treatment of unintentional weight loss in residential healthcare facilities. *J Am Diet Assoc*. 2003;103:352-362.
3. Wallace JL, Schwartz RS, LaCroix AZ, Uhlmann RF, Pearlman RA. Involuntary weight loss in older patients: incidence and clinical significance. *J Am Geriatr Soc*. 1995;43:329-337.

Edition: 2007

OVERWEIGHT/OBESITY (NC-3.3)

Definition

Increased adiposity compared to established reference standards or recommendations.

Etiology (*Cause/Contributing Risk Factors*)

Factors gathered during the nutrition assessment process that contribute to the existence or the maintenance of pathophysiological, psychosocial, situational, developmental, cultural, and/or environmental problems:

- Decreased energy needs
- Disordered eating pattern
- Excess energy intake
- Food- and nutrition-related knowledge deficit
- Not ready for diet/lifestyle change
- Physical inactivity
- Increased psychological/life stress

Signs/Symptoms (*Defining Characteristics*)

A typical cluster of subjective and objective signs and symptoms gathered during the nutrition assessment process that provide evidence that a problem exists; quantify the problem and describe its severity.

Nutrition Assessment Category	Potential Indicators of this Nutrition Diagnosis (one or more must be present)
Biochemical Data, Medical Tests and Procedures	• Measured resting metabolic rate (RMR) measurement less than expected and/or estimated RMR
Anthropometric Measurements	• BMI more than normative standard for age and gender
	• Waist circumference more than normative standard for age and gender
	• Increased skin fold thickness
	• Weight for height more than normative standard for age and gender
Physical Exam Findings	• Increased body adiposity

Edition: 2007

CLINCAL DOMAIN - Weight

OVERWEIGHT/OBESITY (NC-3.3)

Food/Nutrition History	Reports or observations of:
	• Overconsumption of high-fat and/or calorie-density food or beverage
	• Large portions of food (portion size more than twice than recommended)
	• Excessive energy intake
	• Infrequent, low-duration and/or low-intensity physical activity
	• Large amounts of sedentary activities, e.g., TV watching, reading, computer use in both leisure and work/school
	• Uncertainty regarding nutrition-related recommendations
	• Inability to apply nutrition-related recommendations
	• Inability to maintain weight or regain of weight
	• Unwillingness or disinterest in applying nutrition-related recommendations
Client History	• Conditions associated with a diagnosis or treatment of, e.g., hypothyroidism, metabolic syndrome, eating disorder not otherwise specified, depression
	• Physical disability or limitation
	• History of physical, sexual, or emotional abuse
	• Medications that impact RMR, e.g., midazolam, propranalol, glipizide

References:
1. Crawford S. Promoting dietary change. *Can J Cardiol.* 1995;11(suppl A):14A-15A.
2. Dickerson RN, Roth-Yousey L. Medication effects on metabolic rate: A systematic review. *J Am Diet Assoc.* 2005;105:835-843.
3. Kumanyika SK, Van Horn L, Bowen D, Perri MG, Rolls BJ, Czajkowski SM, Schron E. Maintenance of dietary behavior change. *Health Psychol.* 2000;19(1 suppl):S42-S56.
4. Position of the American Dietetic Association: Weight management. *J Am Diet Assoc.* 2002;102:1145-1155.
5. Position of the American Dietetic Association: Total diet approach to communicating food and nutrition information. *J Am Diet Assoc* 2002;102:100-108.
6. Position of the American Dietetic Association: The role of dietetics professionals in health promotion and disease prevention. *J Am Diet Assoc.* 2002;102:1680-1687.
7. Position of the American Dietetic Association: Nutrition intervention in the treatment of anorexia nervosa, bulimia nervosa, and eating disorder not otherwise specified (EDNOS). *J Am Diet Assoc.* 2001;101:810-819.
8. Shepherd R. Resistance to changes in diet. *Proc Nutr Soc.* 2002;61:267-272.
9. U.S. Preventive Services Task Force. Behavioral counseling in primary care to promote a healthy diet. *Am J Prev Med.* 2003;24:93-100.

151

CLINCAL DOMAIN - Weight

INVOLUNTARY WEIGHT GAIN (NC-3.4)

Definition
Weight gain more than that which is desired or planned.

Etiology (*Cause/Contributing Risk Factors*)
Factors gathered during the nutrition assessment process that contribute to the existence or the maintenance of pathophysiological, psychosocial, situational, developmental, cultural, and/or environmental problems:

- Illness causing unexpected weight gain because of head trauma, immobility, paralysis or related condition
- Chronic use of medications known to cause weight gain, such as use of certain antidepressants, antipsychotics, corticosteroids, certain HIV medications
- Condition leading to excessive fluid weight gains

Signs/Symptoms (*Defining Characteristics*)
A typical cluster of subjective and objective signs and symptoms gathered during the nutrition assessment process that provide evidence that a problem exists; quantify the problem and describe its severity.

Nutrition Assessment Category	Potential Indicators of this Nutrition Diagnosis (one or more must be present)
Biochemical Data, Medical Tests and Procedures	• Decrease in serum albumin, hyponatremia, elevated fasting serum lipid levels, elevated fasting glucose levels, fluctuating hormone levels
Anthropometric Measurements	• Increased weight, any increase in weight more than planned or desired, such as 10% in 6 months • Noticeable change in body fat distribution
Physical Examination Findings	• Fat accumulation, excessive subcutaneous fat stores • Lipodystrophy associated with HIV diagnosis: increase in dorsocervial fat, breast enlargement, increased abdominal girth • Edema • Shortness of breath • Sensitivity to cold, constipation, and hair loss

152

Edition: 2007

CLINCAL DOMAIN - Weight

INVOLUNTARY WEIGHT GAIN (NC-3.4)

Food/Nutrition History	Reports or observations of: • Intake consistent with estimated or measured energy needs • Changes in recent food intake level • Fluid administration above requirements • Use of alcohol, narcotics • Extreme hunger with or without palpitations, tremor, and sweating • Physical inactivity or change in physical activity level
Client History	• Conditions associated with a diagnosis or treatment of asthma, psychiatric illnesses, rheumatic conditions, HIV/AIDS, Cushing's syndrome, obesity, Prader-Willi syndrome • Change in sleep habits, insomnia • Muscle weakness • Fatigue • Medications associated with increased appetite

References:
1. Lichtenstein K, Delaney K, Ward D, Palella F. Clinical factors associated with incidence and prevalence of fat atrophy and accumulation (abstract P64). *Antivir Ther.* 2000;5:61-62
2. Heath KV, Hogg RS, Chan KJ, Harris M, Montessori V, O'Shaughnessy MV, Montaner JS. Lipodystrophy-associated morphological, cholesterol and triglyceride abnormalities in a population-based HIV/AIDS treatment database. *AIDS.* 2001;15:231-239.
3. Safri S, Grunfeld C. Fat distribution and metabolic changes in patients with HIV infection. *AIDS.* 1999;13:2493-2505.
4. Sattler F. Body habitus changes related to lipodystrophy. *Clin Infect Dis.* 2003;36:S84-S90.

153

Edition: 2007

FOOD- AND NUTRITION-RELATED KNOWLEDGE DEFICIT (NB-1.1)

Definition

Incomplete or inaccurate knowledge about food, nutrition, or nutrition-related information and guidelines, e.g., nutrient requirements, consequences of food behaviors, life stage requirements, nutrition recommendations, diseases and conditions, physiological function, or products.

Etiology (Cause/Contributing Risk Factors)

Factors gathered during the nutrition assessment process that contribute to the existence or the maintenance of pathophysiological, psychosocial, situational, developmental, cultural, and/or environmental problems:

- Harmful beliefs/attitudes about food, nutrition, and nutrition-related topics
- Lack of prior exposure to information
- Language or cultural barrier impacting ability to learn information
- Learning disability, neurological or sensory impairment
- Prior exposure to incompatible information
- Prior exposure to incorrect information
- Unwilling or uninterested in learning information

Signs/Symptoms (Defining Characteristics)

A typical cluster of subjective and objective signs and symptoms gathered during the nutrition assessment process that provide evidence that a problem exists; quantify the problem and describe its severity.

Nutrition Assessment Category	Potential Indicators of this Nutrition Diagnosis (one or more must be present)
Biochemical Data, Medical Tests and Procedures	
Anthropometric Measurements	
Physical Exam Findings	

FOOD- AND NUTRITION-RELATED KNOWLEDGE DEFICIT (NB-1.1)

Food/Nutrition History	Reports or observations of:
	• Verbalizes inaccurate or incomplete information
	• Provides inaccurate or incomplete written response to questionnaire/written tool or is unable to read written tool
	• No prior knowledge of need for food- and nutrition-related recommendations
	• Demonstrates inability to apply food- and nutrition-related information, e.g., select food based on nutrition therapy or prepare infant feeding as instructed
	• Relates concerns about previous attempts to learn information
	• Verbalizes unwillingness or disinterest in learning information
Client History	• Conditions associated with a diagnosis or treatment, e.g., mental illness
	• New medical diagnosis or change in existing diagnosis or condition

References:

1. Crawford S. Promoting dietary change. *Can J Cardiol.* 1995;11(suppl A):14A-15A.
2. Kumanyika SK, Van Horn L, Bowen D, Perri MG, Rolls BJ, Czajkowski SM, Schron E. Maintenance of dietary behavior change. *Health Psychol.* 2000;19(1 suppl):S42-S56.
3. Position of the American Dietetic Association: Weight management. *J Am Diet Assoc.* 2002;102:1145-1155.
4. Position of the American Dietetic Association: Total diet approach to communicating food and nutrition information. *J Am Diet Assoc* 2002;102:100-108.
5. Position of the American Dietetic Association: The role of dietetics professionals in health promotion and disease prevention. *J Am Diet Assoc.* 2002;102:1680-1687.
6. Shepherd R. Resistance to changes in diet. *Proc Nutr Soc.* 2002;61:267-272.
7. U.S. Preventive Services Task Force. Behavioral counseling in primary care to promote a healthy diet. *Am J Prev Med.* 2003;24:93-100.

HARMFUL BELIEFS/ATTITUDES ABOUT FOOD OR NUTRITION-RELATED TOPICS (NB-1.2)

Use with caution: Be sensitive to patient concerns.

Definition

Beliefs/attitudes or practices about food, nutrition, and nutrition-related topics that are incompatible with sound nutrition principles, nutrition care, or disease/condition (excluding disordered eating patterns and eating disorders).

Etiology *(Cause/Contributing Risk Factors)*

Factors gathered during the nutrition assessment process that contribute to the existence or the maintenance of pathophysiological, psychosocial, situational, developmental, cultural, and/or environmental problems:

- Disbelief in science-based food and nutrition information
- Exposure to incorrect food and nutrition information
- Eating behavior serves a purpose other than nourishment (e.g., pica)
- Desire for a cure for a chronic disease through the use of alternative therapy

Signs/Symptoms *(Defining Characteristics)*

A typical cluster of subjective and objective signs and symptoms gathered during the nutrition assessment process that provide evidence that a problem exists; quantify the problem and describe its severity.

Nutrition Assessment Category	Potential Indicators of this Nutrition Diagnosis (one or more must be present)
Biochemical Data, Medical Tests and Procedures	
Anthropometric Measurements	
Physical Exam Findings	

Edition: 2007

BEHAVIORAL-ENVIRONMENTAL DOMAIN • Knowledge and Beliefs

HARMFUL BELIEFS/ATTITUDES ABOUT FOOD OR NUTRITION-RELATED TOPICS (NB-1.2)

Food/Nutrition History	Reports or observations of: • Food fetish, pica • Food faddism • Intake that reflects an imbalance of nutrients/food groups • Avoidance of foods/food groups (e.g., sugar, wheat, cooked foods)
Client History	• Conditions associated with a diagnosis or treatment, e.g., obesity, diabetes, cancer, cardiovascular disease, mental illness

References:

1. Chapman GE, Beagan B. Women's perspectives on nutrition, health, and breast cancer. *J Nutr Educ Behav.* 2003;35:135-141.
2. Gonzalez VM, Vitousek KM. Feared food in dieting and non-dieting young women: a preliminary validation of the Food Phobia Survey. *Appetite.* 2004;43:155-173.
3. Jowett SL, Seal CJ, Phillips E, Gregory W, Barton JR, Welfare MR. Dietary beliefs of people with ulcerative colitis and their effect on relapse and nutrient intake. *Clin Nutr.* 2004;23:161-170.
4. Madden H, Chamberlain K. Nutritional health messages in women's magazines: a conflicted space for women readers. *J Health Psychol.* 2004;9:583-597.
5. Peters CL, Shelton J, Sharma P. An investigation of factors that influence the consumption of dietary supplements. *Health Mark Q.* 2003;21:113-135.
6. Position of the American Dietetic Association: Food and nutrition misinformation. *J Am Diet Assoc.* 2002;102:260-266.
7. Povey R, Wellens B, Conner M. Attitudes towards following meat, vegetarian and vegan diets: an examination of the role of ambivalence. *Appetite.* 2001;37:15-26.
8. Putterman E, Linden W. Appearance versus health: does the reason for dieting affect dieting behavior? *J Behav Med.* 2004;27:185-204.
9. Salminen E, Heikkila S, Poussa T, Lagstrom H, Saario R, Salminen S. Female patients tend to alter their diet following the diagnosis of rheumatoid arthritis and breast cancer. *Prev Med.* 2002;34:529-535.

Edition: 2007

NOT READY FOR DIET/LIFESTYLE CHANGE (NB-1.3)

Definition

Lack of perceived value of nutrition-related behavior change compared to costs (consequences or effort required to make changes); conflict with personal value system; antecedent to behavior change.

Etiology (Cause/Contributing Risk Factors)

Factors gathered during the nutrition assessment process that contribute to the existence or the maintenance of pathophysiological, psychosocial, situational, developmental, cultural, and/or environmental problems:

- Harmful beliefs/attitudes about food, nutrition, and nutrition-related topics
- Cognitive deficits or inability to focus on dietary changes
- Lack of social support for implementing changes
- Denial of need to change
- Perception that time, interpersonal, or financial constraints prevent changes
- Unwilling or uninterested in learning information
- Lack of self-efficacy for making change or demoralization from previous failures at change

Signs/Symptoms (Defining Characteristics)

A typical cluster of subjective and objective signs and symptoms gathered during the nutrition assessment process that provide evidence that a problem exists; quantify the problem and describe its severity.

Nutrition Assessment Category	Potential Indicators of this Nutrition Diagnosis (one or more must be present)
Biochemical Data, Medical Tests and Procedures	
Anthropometric Measurements	
Physical Exam Findings	• Negative body language, e.g., frowning, lack of eye contact, defensive posture, lack of focus, fidgeting (Note: Body language varies by culture.)

158

NOT READY FOR DIET/LIFESTYLE CHANGE (NB-1.3)

Food/Nutrition History	Reports or observations of:
	• Denial of need for Food- and nutrition-related changes
	• Inability to understand required changes
	• Failure to keep appointments/schedule follow-up appointments or engage in counseling
	• Previous failures to effectively change target behavior
	• Defensiveness, hostility or resistance to change
	• Lack of efficacy to make change or to overcome barriers to change
Client History	• New medical diagnosis, change in existing diagnosis or condition, or chronic noncompliance

References:

1. Crawford S. Promoting dietary change. *Can J Cardiol.* 1995;11:14A-15A.
2. Greene GW, Rossi SR, Rossi JS, Velicer WF, Fava JS, Prochaska JO. Dietary applications of the Stages of Change Model. *J Am Diet Assoc.* 1999; 99:673-678.
3. Kumanyika SK, Van Horn L, Bowen D, Perri MG, Rolls BJ, Czajkowski SM, Schron E. Maintenance of dietary behavior change. *Health Psychol.* 2000;19:S42-S56.
4. Prochaska JO, Velicer W F. The Transtheoretical Model of behavior change. *Am J Health Promotion.* 1997;12:38-48.
5. Position of the American Dietetic Association: Total diet approach to communicating food and nutrition information. *J Am Diet Assoc.* 2002;102:100-108.
6. Position of the American Dietetic Association: The role of dietetics professionals in health promotion and disease prevention. *J Am Diet Assoc.* 2002;102:1680-1687.
7. Resnicow K, Jackson A, Wang T, De A, McCarty F, Dudley W, Baronowski T. A motivational interviewing intervention to increase fruit and vegetable intake through black churches: Results of the Eat for Life trial. *Am J Public Health.* 2001; 91:1686-1693.
8. Shepherd R. Resistance to changes in diet. *Proc Nutr Soc.* 2002;61:267-272.
9. U.S. Preventive Services Task Force. Behavioral counseling in primary care to promote a healthy diet. *Am J Prev Med.* 2003;24:93-100.

SELF-MONITORING DEFICIT (NB-1.4)

Definition

Lack of data recording to track personal progress.

Etiology (*Cause/Contributing Risk Factors*)

Factors gathered during the nutrition assessment process that contribute to the existence or the maintenance of pathophysiological, psychosocial, situational, developmental, cultural, and/or environmental problems:

- Food- and nutrition-related knowledge deficit
- Lack of social support for implementing changes
- Lack of value for behavior change or competing values
- Perception that lack of resources (e.g., time, financial, or social support) prevent self-monitoring
- Cultural barrier impacting ability to track personal progress
- Learning disability, neurological, or sensory impairment
- Prior exposure to incompatible information
- Not ready for diet/lifestyle change
- Unwilling or uninterested in tracking progress
- Lack of focus and attention to detail, difficulty with time management and/or organization

Signs/Symptoms (*Defining Characteristics*)

A typical cluster of subjective and objective signs and symptoms gathered during the nutrition assessment process that provide evidence that a problem exists; quantify the problem and describe its severity.

Nutrition Assessment Category	Potential Indicators of this Nutrition Diagnosis (one or more must be present)
Biochemical Data, Medical Tests and Procedures	• Recorded data inconsistent with biochemical data, e.g., dietary intake is not consistent with biochemical data
Anthropometric Measurements	
Physical Exam Findings	

Edition: 2007

SELF-MONITORING DEFICIT (NB-1.4)

Food/Nutrition History	Reports or observations of:
	• Incomplete self-monitoring records, e.g., glucose, food, fluid intake, weight, physical activity, ostomy output records
	• Food intake data inconsistent with weight status or growth pattern data
	• Embarrassment or anger regarding need for self-monitoring
	• Uncertainty of how to complete monitoring records
	• Uncertainty regarding changes that could/should be made in response to data in self-monitoring records
	• No self-management equipment, e.g., no blood glucose monitor, pedometer
Client History	• Diagnoses associated with self-monitoring, e.g., diabetes mellitus, obesity, new ostomy
	• New medical diagnosis or change in existing diagnosis or condition

References:

1. American Diabetes Association. Tests of glycemia in diabetes. *Diabetes Care.* 2004;27:S91-S93.
2. Baker RC, Kirschenbaum DS. Weight control during the holidays: highly consistent self-monitoring as a potentially useful coping mechanism. *Health Psychol.* 1998;17:367-370.
3. Berkowitz RI, Wadden TA, Tershakovec AM. Behavior therapy and sibutramine for treatment of adolescent obesity. *JAMA.* 2003;289:1805-1812.
4. Crawford S. Promoting dietary change. *Can J Cardiol.* 1995;11(suppl A):14A-15A.
5. Jeffery R, Drewnowski A, Epstein L, Stunkard A, Wilson G, Wing R. Long-term maintenance of weight loss: current status. *Health Psychol.* 2000;19:5-16.
6. Kumanyika SK, Van Horn L, Bowen D, Perri MG, Rolls BJ, Czajkowski SM, Schron E. Maintenance of dietary behavior change. *Health Psychol.* 2000;19(1 suppl):S42-S56.
7. Lichtman SW, Pisarska K, Berman ER, Pestone M, Dowling H, Offenbacher E, Weisel H, Heshka S, Matthews DE, Heymsfield SB. Discrepancy between self-reported and actual caloric intake and exercise in obese subjects. *N Engl J Med.* 1992;327:1893-1898.
8. Wadden, TA. Characteristics of successful weight loss maintainers. In: Allison DB, Pi-Sunyer FX, eds. *Obesity Treatment: Establishing Goals, Improving Outcomes, and Reviewing the Research Agenda.* New York: Plenum Press; 1995:103-111.

Edition: 2007

DISORDERED EATING PATTERN (NB-1.5)

Definition

Beliefs, attitudes, thoughts, and behaviors related to food, eating, and weight management, including classic eating disorders as well as less severe, similar conditions that negatively impact health.

Etiology (Cause/Contributing Risk Factors)

Factors gathered during the nutrition assessment process that contribute to the existence or the maintenance of pathophysiological, psychosocial, situational, developmental, cultural, and/or environmental problems:

- Familial, societal, biological/genetic, and/or environmental related obsessive desire to be thin
- Weight regulation/preoccupation significantly influences self-esteem

Signs/Symptoms (Defining Characteristics)

A typical cluster of subjective and objective signs and symptoms gathered during the nutrition assessment process that provide evidence that a problem exists; quantify the problem and describe its severity.

Nutrition Assessment Category	Potential Indicators of this Nutrition Diagnosis (one or more must be present)
Biochemical Data, Medical Tests and Procedures	• Decreased cholesterol, abnormal lipid profiles, hypoglycemia, hypokalemia [anorexia nervosa (AN)] • Hypokalemia and hypochloremic alkalosis [bulimia nervosa (BN)] • Hyponatremia, hypothyroid, leukopenia, elevated BUN (AN) • Urine positive for ketones (AN)
Anthropometric Measurements	• BMI < 17.5, arrested growth and development, failure to gain weight during period of expected growth, weight less than 85% of expected (AN) • BMI > 29 [eating disorder not otherwise specified (EDNOS)] • Significant weight fluctuation (BN)

Edition: 2007

DISORDERED EATING PATTERN (NB-1.5)

Physical Exam Findings	• Severely depleted adipose and somatic protein stores (AN)
	• Lanugo hair formation on face and trunk, brittle listless hair, cyanosis of hands and feet, and dry skin (AN)
	• Normal or excess adipose and normal somatic protein stores (BN, EDNOS)
	• Damaged tooth enamel (BN)
	• Enlarged parotid glands (BN)
	• Peripheral edema (BN)
	• Skeletal muscle loss (AN)
	• Cardiac arrhythmias, bradycardia (AN, BN)
	• Hypotension, low body temperature
	• Inability to concentrate (AN)
	• Positive Russell's Sign (BN) callous on back of hand from self-induced vomiting
	• Bradycardia (heart rate < 60 beats/min), hypotension (systolic < 90 mm HG), and orthostatic hypotension (AN)

Edition: 2007

BEHAVIORAL-ENVIRONMENTAL DOMAIN - Knowledge and Beliefs

DISORDERED EATING PATTERN (NB-1.5)

Food/Nutrition History	Reports or observations of:
	• Avoidance of food or calorie-containing beverages (AN, BN)
	• Fear of foods or dysfunctional thoughts regarding food or food experiences (AN, BN)
	• Denial of hunger (AN)
	• Food and weight preoccupation (AN, BN)
	• Knowledgeable about current diet fad (AN, BN, EDNOS)
	• Fasting (AN, BN)
	• Intake of larger quantity of food in a defined time period, a sense of lack of control over eating (BN, EDNOS)
	• Excessive physical activity (AN, BN, EDNOS)
	• Eating much more rapidly than normal, until feeling uncomfortably full, consuming large amounts of food when not feeling physically hungry; eating alone because of embarrassment, feeling very guilty after overeating (EDNOS)
	• Eats in private (AN, BN)
	• Irrational thoughts about food's affect on the body (AN, BN, EDNOS)
	• Pattern of chronic dieting
	• Excessive reliance on nutrition terming and preoccupation with nutrient content of foods
	• Inflexibility with food selection
Client History	• Self-induced vomiting, diarrhea, bloating, constipation, and flatulence (BN); always cold (AN)
	• Misuse of laxatives, enemas, diuretics, stimulants, and/or metabolic enhancers (AN,BN)
	• Muscle weakness, fatigue, cardiac arrhythmias, dehydration, and electrolyte imbalance (AN, BN)
	• Diagnosis, e.g., anorexia nervosa, bulimia nervosa, binge eating, eating disorder not otherwise specified, amenorrhea,
	• History of mood and anxiety disorders (e.g., depression, obsessive/compulsive disorder [OCD]), personality disorders, substance abuse disorders
	• Family history of ED, depression, OCD, anxiety disorders (AN, BN)
	• Irritability, depression (AN, BN)
	• Anemia
	• Avoidance of social events at which food is served

Edition: 2007

164

DISORDERED EATING PATTERN (NB-1.5)

References:

1. Anderson GH, Kennedy SH, eds. *The Biology of Feast and Famine*. New York: Academic Press; 1992.
2. American Psychiatric Association. *Diagnostic and statistical manual for mental disorders (fourth edition, text revision)*. APA Press: Washington DC; 2000.
3. American Psychiatric Association. Practice guidelines for the treatment of patients with eating disorders. *Am J Psychiatry*. 2000;157 (suppl):1-39.
4. Cooke RA, Chambers JB. Anorexia nervosa and the heart. *Br J Hosp Med*. 1995;54:313-317.
5. Fisher M. Medical complications of anorexia and bulimia nervosa. *Adol Med Stat of the Art Reviews*. 1992;3:481-502.
6. Gralen SJ, Levin MP, Smolak L, Murnen SK. Dieting and disordered eating during early and middle adolescents: Do the influences remain the same? *Int J Eating Disorder*. 1990;9:501-512.
7. Harris JP, Kriepe RE, Rossback CN. QT prolongation by isoproterenol in anorexia nervosa. *J Adol Health*. 1993;14:390-393.
8. Kaplan AS, Garfunkel PE, eds. *Medical Issues and the Eating Disorders: The Interface*. New York: Brunner/Manzel Publishers; 1993.
9. Keys A, Brozek J, Henschel A, Mickelson O, Taylor HL. *The Biology of Human Starvation, 2nd vol*. Minneapolis, MN: University of Minnesota Press; 1950.
10. Kirkley BG. Bulimia: clinical characteristics, development, and etiology. *J Am Diet Assoc*. 1986;86:468-475.
11. Kreipe RE, Uphoff M. Treatment and outcome of adolescents with anorexia nervosa. *Adolesc Med*.1992;16:519-540.
12. Kreipe RE, Birndorf DO. Eating disorders in adolescents and young adults. *Medical Clinics of North America*. 2000;84:1027-1049.
13. Mordasini R, Klose G, Greter H. Secondary type II hyperlipoproteinemia in patients with anorexia nervosa. *Metabolism*. 1978;27:71-79.
14. Position of the American Dietetic Association: Nutrition intervention in the treatment of anorexia nervosa, bulimia nervosa, and eating disorder not otherwise specified (EDNOS). *J Am Diet Assoc*. 2001;101:810-819.
15. Position of the American Dietetic Association: Nutrition intervention in the treatment of anorexia nervosa, bulimia nervosa, and eating disorder not otherwise specified (EDNOS). *J Am Diet Assoc*. 2001;101:810-819.
16. Rock C, Yager J. Nutrition and eating disorders: a primer for clinicians. *Int J Eat Disord*. 1987;6:267-280.
17. Rock, CL. Nutritional and medical assessment and management of eating disorders. *Nutr Clin Care*. 1999;2:332-343.
18. Schebendach J, Reichert-Anderson P. Nutrition in Eating Disorders. In: *Kraus's Nutrition and Diet Therapy*. Mahan K, Escott-Stump S (eds). McGraw- Hill: New York, NY; 2000.
19. Silber T. Anorexia nervosa: Morbidity and mortality. *Pediar Ann*. 1984; 13:851-859.
20. Swenne I. Heart risk associated with weight loss in anorexia nervosa and eating disorders: electrocardiographic changes during the early phase of refeeding. *Acta Paediatr*. 2000;89:447-452.
21. Turner JM, Bulsara MK, McDermott BM, Byrne GC, Prince RL, Forbes DA. Predictors of low bone density in young adolescent females with anorexia nervosa and other dieting disorders. *Int J Eat Disord*. 2001;30:245-251.

LIMITED ADHERENCE TO NUTRITION-RELATED RECOMMENDATIONS (NB-1.6)

Definition

Lack of nutrition-related changes as per intervention agreed on by client or population.

Etiology (*Cause/Contributing Risk Factors*)

Factors gathered during the nutrition assessment process that contribute to the existence or the maintenance of pathophysiological, psychosocial, situational, developmental, cultural, and/or environmental problems:

- Lack of social support for implementing changes
- Lack of value for behavior change or competing values
- Perception that time or financial constraints prevent changes
- Previous lack of success in making health-related changes
- Poor understanding of how and why to make the changes
- Unwilling or uninterested in applying information

Signs/Symptoms (*Defining Characteristics*)

A typical cluster of subjective and objective signs and symptoms gathered during the nutrition assessment process that provide evidence that a problem exists; quantify the problem and describe its severity.

Nutrition Assessment Category	Potential Indicators of this Nutrition Diagnosis (one or more must be present)
Biochemical Data, Medical Tests and Procedures	• Expected laboratory outcomes are not achieved
Anthropometric Measurements	• Expected anthropometric outcomes are not achieved
Physical Exam Findings	• Negative body language, e.g., frowning, lack of eye contact, fidgeting (Note: body language varies by culture)

Edition: 2007

BEHAVIORAL-ENVIRONMENTAL DOMAIN • Knowledge and Beliefs

LIMITED ADHERENCE TO NUTRITION-RELATED RECOMMENDATIONS (NB-1.6)

Food/Nutrition History
Reports or observations of: • Expected food/nutrition-related outcomes are not achieved • Inability to recall agreed on changes • Failure to complete any agreed on homework • Lack of compliance or inconsistent compliance with plan • Failure to keep appointments or schedule follow-up appointments • Lack of appreciation of the importance of making recommended nutrition-related changes • Uncertainty as to how to consistently apply food/nutrition information

Client History

References:
1. Crawford S. Promoting dietary change. *Can J Cardiol.* 1995;11(suppl A):14A-15A.
2. Kumanyika SK, Van Horn L, Bowen D, Perri MG, Rolls BJ, Czajkowski SM, Schron E. Maintenance of dietary behavior change. *Health Psychol.* 2000;19(1 suppl):S42-S56.
3. Position of the American Dietetic Association: Total diet approach to communicating food and nutrition information. *J Am Diet Assoc.* 2002;102:100-108.
4. Shepherd R. Resistance to changes in diet. *Proc Nutr Soc.* 2002;61:267-272.
5. U.S. Preventive Services Task Force. Behavioral counseling in primary care to promote a healthy diet. *Am J Prev Med.* 2003;24:93-100.

167

Edition: 2007

UNDESIRABLE FOOD CHOICES (NB-1.7)

Definition

Food and/or beverage choices that are inconsistent with US Recommended Dietary Intake, *US Dietary Guidelines*, or the Food Guide Pyramid, or with targets defined in the nutrition prescription or nutrition care process.

Etiology (*Cause/Contributing Risk Factors*)

Factors gathered during the nutrition assessment process that contribute to the existence or the maintenance of pathophysiological, psychosocial, situational, developmental, cultural, and/or environmental problems:

- Lack of prior exposure to or misunderstanding of information
- Language, religious, or cultural barrier impacting ability to apply information
- Learning disabilities, neurological or sensory impairment
- High level of fatigue or other side effect of medical, surgical or radiological therapy
- Inadequate access to recommended foods
- Perception that financial constraints prevent selection of food choices consistent with recommendations
- Food allergies and aversions impeding food choices consistent with guidelines
- Lacks motivation and or readiness to apply or support systems change
- Unwilling or uninterested in learning information
- Psychological limitations

Signs/Symptoms (*Defining Characteristics*)

A typical cluster of subjective and objective signs and symptoms gathered during the nutrition assessment process that provide evidence that a problem exists; quantify the problem and describe its severity.

Nutrition Assessment Category	Potential Indicators of this Nutrition Diagnosis (one or more must be present)
Biochemical Data, Medical Tests and Procedures	• Elevated lipid panel
Anthropometric Measurements	
Physical Exam Findings	• Findings consistent with vitamin/mineral deficiency or excess

Edition: 2007

BEHAVIORAL-ENVIRONMENTAL DOMAIN - Knowledge and Beliefs

UNDESIRABLE FOOD CHOICES (NB-1.7)

Food/Nutrition History	Reports or observations of:
	• Intake inconsistent with *US Dietary Guidelines* or Food Guide Pyramid (e.g., omission of entire nutrient groups, disproportionate intake [e.g., juice for young children])
	• Inaccurate or incomplete understanding of the guidelines
	• Inability to apply guideline information
	• Inability to select (e.g., access), or unwillingness, or disinterest in selecting, food consistent with the guidelines
Client History	• Conditions associated with a diagnosis or treatment, e.g., mental illness

References:
1. Birch LL, Fisher JA. Appetite and eating behavior in children. *Pediatr Clin North Am.*1995;42:931-953.
2. Butte N, Cobb K, Dwyer J, Graney L, Heird W, Richard K. The start healthy feeding guidelines for infants and toddlers. *J Am Diet Assoc.* 2004:104:3:442-454.
3. Position of the American Dietetic Association: Weight management. *J Am Diet Assoc.* 2002;102:1145-1155.
4. Dolecek TA, Stamlee J, Caggiula AW, Tillotson JL, Buzzard IM. Methods of dietary and nutritional assessment and intervention and other methods in the multiple risk factor intervention trial. *Am J Clin Nutr.* 1997;65(suppl):196S-210S.
5. Epstein LH, Gordy CC, Raynor HA, Beddome M, Kilanowski CK, Paluch R. Increasing fruit and vegetable intake and decreasing fat and sugar intake in families at risk for childhood obesity. *Obesity Res.* 2001:9:171-178.
6. Freeland-Graves J, Nitzke S. Total diet approach to communicating food and nutrition information. *J Am Diet Assoc.* 2002;102:100-108.
7. French SA. Pricing effects on food choices. *J Nutr.* 2003;133:S841-S843.
8. Glens K, Basil M, Mariachi E, Goldberg J, Snyder D. Why Americans eat what they do: taste, nutrition, cost, convenience and weight control concerns as influences on food consumption. *J Am Diet Assoc.* 1998;98:1118-1126.
9. Hampl JS, Anderson JV, Mullis R. The role of dietetics professionals in health promotion and disease prevention. *J Am Diet Assoc.* 2002;102:1680-1687.
10. Lin SH, Guthrie J, Frazao E. American children's' diets are not making the grade. *Food Review.* 2001;24: 8-17.
11. Satter E. Feeding dynamics: helping children to eat well. *J Pediatr Healthcare.* 1995:9:178-184.
12. Story M, Holt K, Sofka D, eds. *Bright futures in practice: Nutrition, 2ⁿᵈ Ed.* Arlington, VA: National Center for Education in Maternal Child Health; 2002.
13. Pelto GH, Levitt E, Thairu L. Improving feeding practices, current patterns, common constraints and the design of interventions. *Food Nutr Bull.* 2003;24:45-82.

Edition: 2007

169

PHYSICAL INACTIVITY (NB-2.1)

Definition

Low level of activity/sedentary behavior to the extent that it reduces energy expenditure and impacts health.

Etiology (Cause/Contributing Risk Factors)

Factors gathered during the nutrition assessment process that contribute to the existence or the maintenance of pathophysiological, psychosocial, situational, developmental, cultural, and/or environmental problems:

- Financial constraints that may prevent sufficient level of activity
- Harmful beliefs/attitudes about physical activity
- Injury or lifestyle change that reduces physical activity or activities of daily living
- Lack of prior exposure regarding need for physical activity or how to incorporate exercise, e.g., physical disability, arthritis
- Lack of role models, e.g., for children
- Lack of social support and/or environmental space or equipment
- Lack of safe environment for physical activity
- Lack of value for behavior change or competing values
- Time constraints

Signs/Symptoms (Defining Characteristics)

A typical cluster of subjective and objective signs and symptoms gathered during the nutrition assessment process that provide evidence that a problem exists; quantify the problem and describe its severity.

Nutrition Assessment Category	Potential Indicators of this Nutrition Diagnosis (one or more must be present)
Biochemical Data, Medical Tests and Procedures	
Anthropometric Measurements	
Physical Exam Findings	

Edition: 2007

PHYSICAL INACTIVITY (NB-2.1)

Food/Nutrition History	Reports or observations of: • Infrequent, low duration and/or low intensity physical activity • Large amounts of sedentary activities, e.g., TV watching, reading, computer use in both leisure and work/school • Barriers to physical activity, e.g., time constraints, availability of a safe environment for exercise
Client History	• Low cardiorespiratory fitness and/or low muscle strength • Medical diagnoses that may be associated with or result in decreased activity, e.g., arthritis, chronic fatigue syndrome, morbid obesity, knee surgery • Medications that cause somnolence and decreased cognition • Psychological diagnosis, e.g., depression, anxiety disorders

References:

1. Position of the American Dietetic Association: Weight management. *J Am Diet Assoc.* 2002;102:1145-1155.
2. Position of the American Dietetic Association: Total diet approach to communicating food and nutrition information. *J Am Diet Assoc* 2002;102:100-108.
3. Position of the American Dietetic Association: The role of dietetics professionals in health promotion and disease prevention. *J Am Diet Assoc.* 2002;102:1680-1687.

Edition: 2007

EXCESSIVE EXERCISE (NB-2.2)

Definition

An amount of exercise that exceeds that which is necessary to improve health and/or athletic performance.

Etiology (*Cause/Contributing Risk Factors*)

Factors gathered during the nutrition assessment process that contribute to the existence or the maintenance of pathophysiological, psychosocial, situational, developmental, cultural, and/or environmental problems:

- Disordered eating
- Irrational beliefs/attitudes about food, nutrition, and fitness
- "Addictive" behaviors/personality

Signs/Symptoms (*Defining Characteristics*)

A typical cluster of subjective and objective signs and symptoms gathered during the nutrition assessment process that provide evidence that a problem exists; quantify the problem and describe its severity.

Nutrition Assessment Category	Potential Indicators of this Nutrition Diagnosis (one or more must be present)
Biochemical Data, Medical Tests and Procedures	• Elevated liver enzymes, e.g., LDH, AST • Altered micronutrient status, e.g., decreased serum ferritin, zinc, and insulin-like growth factor-binding protein • Increased hematocrit • Suppressed immune function • Possibly elevated cortisol levels
Anthropometric Measurements	• Weight loss, arrested growth and development, failure to gain weight during period of expected growth (related usually to disordered eating)
Physical Exam Findings	• Depleted adipose and somatic protein stores (related usually to disordered eating) • Frequent and/or prolonged injuries and/or illnesses • Chronic muscle soreness

BEHAVIORAL-ENVIRONMENTAL DOMAIN ▪ Physical Activity and Function

EXCESSIVE EXERCISE (NB-2.2)

Food/Nutrition History	Reports or observations of:
	• Continued/repeated high levels of exercise exceeding levels necessary to improve health and/or athletic performance
	• Exercise daily without rest/rehabilitation days
	• Exercise while injured/sick
	• Forsaking family, job, social responsibilities to exercise
Client History	• Conditions associated with a diagnosis or treatment, e.g., anorexia nervosa, bulimia nervosa, binge eating, eating disorder not otherwise specified, amenorrhea
	• Chronic fatigue
	• Evidence of addictive, obsessive, or compulsive tendencies

Reference:
1. Aissa-Benhaddad A, Bouix D, Khaled S, Micallef JP, Mercier J, Bringer J, Brun JF. Early hemorheologic aspects of overtraining in elite athletes. *Clin Hemorheol Microcirc.* 1999;20:117-125.
2. American Psychiatric Association. *Diagnostic and Statistical Manual of Mental Disorders. 4th Ed.* Washington, DC: American Psychiatric Association; 1994.
3. Davis C, Brewer H, Ratusny D. Behavioral frequency and psychological commitment: necessary concepts in the study of excessive exercising. *J Behav Med.* 1993;16:611-628.
4. Davis C, Claridge G. The eating disorder as addiction: a psychobiological perspective. *Addict Behav.* 1998;23:463-475.
5. Davis C, Kennedy SH, Ravelski E, Dionne M. The role of physical activity in the development and maintenance of eating disorders. *Psychol Med.* 1994;24:957-967.
6. Klein DA, Bennett AS, Schebendach J, Foltin RW, Devlin MJ, Walsh BT. Exercise "addiction" in anorexia nervosa: model development and pilot data. *CNS Spectr.* 2004;9:531-537.
7. Lakier-Smith L. Overtraining, excessive exercise, and altered immunity: is this a helper-1 vs helper-2 lymphocyte response? *Sports Med.* 2003;33:347-364.
8. Position of the American Dietetic Association: Nutrition intervention in the treatment of anorexia nervosa, bulimia nervosa, and eating disorder not otherwise specified (EDNOS). *J Am Diet Assoc.* 2001;101:810-819.
9. Shephard RJ, Shek PN. Acute and chronic over-exertion: do depressed immune responses provide useful markers? *Int J Sports Med.* 1998;19:159-171.
10. Smith LL. Tissue trauma: the underlying cause of overtraining syndrome? *J Strength Cond Res.* 2004;18:185-193.
11. Urhausen A, Kindermann W. Diagnosis of overtraining: what tools do we have. *Sports Med.* 2002;32:95-102.

INABILITY OR LACK OF DESIRE TO MANAGE SELF-CARE (NB-2.3)

Definition

Lack of capacity or unwillingness to implement methods to support healthful Food- and nutrition-related behavior.

Etiology (Cause/Contributing Risk Factors)

Factors gathered during the nutrition assessment process that contribute to the existence or the maintenance of pathophysiological, psychosocial, situational, developmental, cultural, and/or environmental problems:

- Food- and nutrition-related knowledge deficit
- Lack of caretaker or social support for implementing changes
- Lack of developmental readiness to perform self-management tasks, e.g., pediatrics
- Lack of value for behavior change or competing values
- Perception that lack of resources (time, financial, support persons) prevent self-care
- Cultural beliefs and practices
- Learning disability, neurological or sensory impairment
- Prior exposure to incompatible information
- Not ready for diet/lifestyle change
- Unwilling or uninterested in learning/applying information
- No self-management tools or decision guides

Signs/Symptoms (Defining Characteristics)

A typical cluster of subjective and objective signs and symptoms gathered during the nutrition assessment process that provide evidence that a problem exists; quantify the problem and describe its severity.

Nutrition Assessment Category	Potential Indicators of this Nutrition Diagnosis (one or more must be present)
Biochemical Data, Medical Tests and Procedures	
Anthropometric Measurements	
Physical Exam Findings	

Edition: 2007

INABILITY OR LACK OF DESIRE TO MANAGE SELF-CARE (NB-2.3)

Food/Nutrition History	Reports or observations of: • Inability to interpret data or self-management tools • Embarrassment or anger regarding need for self-monitoring • Uncertainty regarding changes could/should be made in response to data in self-monitoring records
Client History	• Diagnoses that are associated with self-management, e.g., diabetes mellitus, obesity, cardiovascular disease, renal or liver disease • Conditions associated with a diagnosis or treatment, e.g., cognitive or emotional impairment • New medical diagnosis or change in existing diagnosis or condition

References:
1. Position of the American Dietetic Association: Providing nutrition services for infants, children, and adults with developmental disabilities and special health care needs. *J Am Diet Assoc.* 2004;104:97-107.
2. Crawford S. Promoting dietary change. *Can J Cardiol.* 1995;11(suppl A):14A-15A.
3. Falk LW, Bisogni CA, Sobal J. Diet change processes of participants in an intensive heart program. *J Nutr Educ.* 2000;32:240-250.
4. Glasgow RE, Hampson SE, Strycker LA, Ruggiero L. Personal-model beliefs and social-environmental barriers related to diabetes self-management. *Diabetes Care.* 1997;20:556-561.
5. Keenan DP, AbuSabha R, Sigman-Grant M, Achterberg C, Ruffing J. Factors perceived to influence dietary fat reduction behaviors. *J Nutr Educ.*1999;31:134-144.
6. Kumanyika SK, Van Horn L, Bowen D, Perri MG, Rolls BJ, Czajkowski SM, Schron E. Maintenance of dietary behavior change. *Health Psychol.* 2000;19(1 suppl):S42-S56.
7. Sporny, LA, Contento, Isobel R. Stages of change in dietary fat reduction: Social psychological correlates. *J Nutr Educ.* 1995;27:191.

Edition: 2007

175

IMPAIRED ABILITY TO PREPARE FOODS/MEALS (NB-2.4)

Definition

Cognitive or physical impairment that prevents preparation of foods/meals.

Etiology (*Cause/Contributing Risk Factors*)

Factors gathered during the nutrition assessment process that contribute to the existence or the maintenance of pathophysiological, psychosocial, situational, developmental, cultural, and/or environmental problems:

- Learning disability, neurological or sensory impairment
- Loss of mental or cognitive ability, e.g., dementia
- Physical disability
- High level of fatigue or other side effect of therapy

Signs/Symptoms (*Defining Characteristics*)

A typical cluster of subjective and objective signs and symptoms gathered during the nutrition assessment process that provide evidence that a problem exists; quantify the problem and describe its severity.

Nutrition Assessment Category	Potential Indicators of this Nutrition Diagnosis (one or more must be present)
Biochemical Data, Medical Tests and Procedures	
Anthropometric Measurements	
Physical Exam Findings	
Food/Nutrition History	Reports or observations of: • Decreased overall intake • Excessive consumption of convenience foods, preprepared meals, and foods prepared away from home resulting in an inability to adhere to nutrition prescription • Uncertainty regarding appropriate foods to prepare based on nutrition prescription • Inability to purchase and transport foods to one's home
Client History	• Conditions associated with a diagnosis or treatment, e.g., cognitive impairment, cerebral palsy, paraplegia, sight impairment, rigorous therapy regimen, recent surgery

Edition: 2007

BEHAVIORAL-ENVIRONMENTAL DOMAIN - Physical Activity and Function

IMPAIRED ABILITY TO PREPARE FOODS/MEALS (NB-2.4)

References:

1. Andren E, Grimby G. Activity limitations in personal, domestic and vocational tasks: a study of adults with inborn and early acquired mobility disorders. *Disabil Rehabil.* 2004;26:262-271.
2. Andren E, Grimby G. Dependence in daily activities and life satisfaction in adult subjects with cerebral palsy or spina bifida: a follow-up study. *Disabil Rehabil.* 2004;26:528-536.
3. Fortin S, Godbout L, Braun CM. Cognitive structure of executive deficits in frontally lesioned head trauma patients performing activities of daily living. *Cortex.* 2003;39:273-291.
4. Godbout L, Doucet C, Fiola M. The scripting of activities of daily living in normal aging: anticipation and shifting deficits with preservation of sequencing. *Brain Cogn.* 2000;43:220-224.
5. Position of the American Dietetic Association: Providing nutrition services for infants, children, and adults with developmental disabilities and special health care needs. *J Am Diet Assoc.* 2004;104:97-107.
6. Position of the American Dietetic Association: Domestic food and nutrition security. *J Am Diet Assoc.* 2002;102:1840-1847.
7. Position of the American Dietetic Association: Addressing world hunger, malnutrition, and food insecurity. *J Am Diet Assoc.* 2003;103:1046-1057.
8. Sandstrom K, Alinder J, Oberg B. Descriptions of functioning and health and relations to a gross motor classification in adults with cerebral palsy. *Disabil Rehabil.* 2004;26:1023-1031.

177

POOR NUTRITION QUALITY OF LIFE (NQOL) (NB-2.5)

Definition

Diminished NQOL scores related to food impact, self image, psychological factors social/interpersonal, physical, or self efficacy.

Etiology (*Cause/Contributing Risk Factors*)

Factors gathered during the nutrition assessment process that contribute to the existence or the maintenance of pathophysiological, psychosocial, situational, developmental, cultural, and/or environmental problems:

- Food and nutrition knowledge–related deficit
- Not ready for diet/lifestyle change
- Negative impact of current or previous medical nutrition therapy (MNT)
- Food or activity behavior-related difficulty
- Poor self-efficacy
- Altered body image
- Food insecurity
- Lack of social support for implementing changes

Signs/Symptoms (*Defining Characteristics*)

A typical cluster of subjective and objective signs and symptoms gathered during the nutrition assessment process that provide evidence that a problem exists; quantify the problem and describe its severity.

Nutrition Assessment Category	Potential Indicators of this Nutrition Diagnosis (one or more must be present)
Biochemical Data, Medical Tests and Procedures	
Anthropometric Measurements	
Physical Exam Findings	

POOR NUTRITION QUALITY OF LIFE (NQOL) (NB-2.5)

Food/Nutrition History	Reports or observations of: • Unfavorable NQOL rating • Frustration or dissatisfaction with MNT recommendations • Inaccurate or incomplete information related to MNT recommendations • Inability to change food- or activity-related behavior • Concerns about previous attempts to learn information • Unwillingness or disinterest in learning information
Client History	• New medical diagnosis or change in existing diagnosis or condition • Recent other lifestyle or life changes, e.g., quit smoking, initiated exercise, work change, home relocation

References:

1. Barr JT, Schumacher GE. The need for a nutrition-related quality-of-life measure. *J Am Diet Assoc.* 2003;103:177-180.
2. Barr JT, Schumacher GE. Using focus groups to determine what constitutes quality of life in clients receiving medical nutrition therapy: First steps in the development of a nutrition quality-of-life survey. *J Am Diet Assoc.* 2003;103:844-851.

SELF-FEEDING DIFFICULTY (NB-2.6)

Definition

Impaired actions to place food or beverages in mouth.

Etiology (Cause/Contributing Risk Factors)

Factors gathered during the nutrition assessment process that contribute to the existence or the maintenance of pathophysiological, psychosocial, situational, developmental, cultural, and/or environmental problems:

- Inability to grasp cups and utensils for self-feeding
- Inability to support and/or control head and neck
- Lack of coordination of hand to mouth
- Limited physical strength or range of motion
- Inability to bend elbow or wrist
- Inability to sit with hips square and back straight
- Limited access to foods conducive for self-feeding
- Limited vision
- Reluctance or avoidance of self-feeding

Signs/Symptoms (Defining Characteristics)

A typical cluster of subjective and objective signs and symptoms gathered during the nutrition assessment process that provide evidence that a problem exists; quantify the problem and describe its severity.

Nutrition Assessment Category	Potential Indicators of this Nutrition Diagnosis (one or more must be present)
Biochemical Data, Medical Tests and Procedures	
Anthropometric Measurements	• Weight loss
Physical Exam Findings	• Dry mucous membranes, hoarse or wet voice, tongue extrusion

Edition: 2007

SELF-FEEDING DIFFICULTY (NB-2.6)

Food/Nutrition History	Reports or observations of:
	• Being provided with foods that may not be conducive to self-feeding, e.g., peas, broth-type soups
	• Poor lip closure, drooling
	• Dropping of cups, utensils
	• Emotional distress, anxiety, or frustration surrounding mealtimes
	• Failure to recognize foods
	• Forgets to eat
	• Inappropriate use of food
	• Refusal to eat or chew
	• Dropping of food from utensil (splashing and spilling of food) on repeated attempts to feed
	• Utensil biting
Client History	• Conditions associated with a diagnosis or treatment of, e.g., neurological disorders, Parkinson's, Alzheimer's, Tardive dyskinesia, multiple sclerosis, stroke, paralysis, developmental delay
	• Physical limitations, e.g., fractured arms, traction, contractures
	• Surgery requiring recumbent position
	• Dementia/organic brain syndrome
	• Dysphagia
	• Shortness of breath
	• Tremors

References:

1. Consultant Dietitians in Healthcare Facilities. *Dining Skills Supplement: Practical Interventions for Caregivers of Eating Disabled Older Adults.* Pensacola, FL: American Dietetic Association; 1992.
2. Morley JE. Anorexia of aging: physiological and pathologic. *Am J Clin Nutr.* 1997; 66:760-773.
3. Position of the American Dietetic Association: Providing nutrition services for infants, children, and adults with developmental disabilities and special health care needs. *J Am Diet Assoc.* 2004;104:97-107.
4. Sandman P, Norberg A, Adolfsson R, Eriksson S, Nystrom L. Prevalence and characteristics of persons with dependency on feeding at institutions. *Scand J Caring Sci.* 1990;4:121-127.
5. Siebens H, Trupe E, Siebens A, Cooke F, Anshen S, Hanauer R, Oster G. Correlates and consequences of feeding dependency. *J Am Geriatr Soc.* 1986;34:192-198.
6. Vellas B, Fitten LJ, eds. *Research and Practice in Alzheimer's Disease.* New York, NY: Springer Publishing Company; 1998.

INTAKE OF UNSAFE FOOD (NB-3.1)

Definition

Intake of food and/or fluids intentionally or unintentionally contaminated with toxins, poisonous products, infectious agents, microbial agents, additives, allergens, and/or agents of bioterrorism.

Etiology (*Cause/Contributing Risk Factors*)

Factors gathered during the nutrition assessment process that contribute to the existence or the maintenance of pathophysiological, psychosocial, situational, developmental, cultural, and/or environmental problems:

- Lack of knowledge about potentially unsafe food
- Lack of knowledge about proper food/feeding, (infant and enteral formula, breast milk) storage and preparation
- Exposure to contaminated water or food, e.g., community outbreak of illness documented by surveillance and/or response agency
- Mental illness, confusion, or altered awareness
- Inadequate food storage equipment/facilities, e.g., refrigerator
- Inadequate safe food supply, e.g., inadequate markets with safe, uncontaminated food

Signs/Symptoms (*Defining Characteristics*)

A typical cluster of subjective and objective signs and symptoms gathered during the nutrition assessment process that provide evidence that a problem exists; quantify the problem and describe its severity.

Nutrition Assessment Category	Potential Indicators of this Nutrition Diagnosis (one or more must be present)
Biochemical Data, Medical Tests and Procedures	• Positive stool culture for infectious causes, such as listeria, salmonella, hepatitis A, *E. coli, Cyclospora* • Toxicology reports for drugs, medicinals, poisons in blood or food samples
Anthropometric Measurements	
Physical Examination Findings	• Evidence of dehydration, e.g., dry mucous membranes, damaged tissues

182

INTAKE OF UNSAFE FOOD (NB-3.1)

Food/Nutrition History	Reports or observations of intake of potential unsafe foods: • Mercury content of fish, non-food items (pregnant and lactating women) • Raw eggs, unpasteurized milk products, soft cheeses, undercooked meats (infants, children, immunocompromised persons, pregnant and lactating women, and elderly) • Wild plants, berries, mushrooms • Unsafe food/feeding storage and preparation practices (enteral and infant formula, breast milk)
Client History	• Conditions associated with a diagnosis or treatment, e.g., foodborne illness, such as, bacterial, viral, and parasitic infection, mental illness, dementia • Poisoning by drugs, medicinals, and biological substances • Poisoning from poisonous food stuffs and poisonous plants • Diarrhea, cramping, bloating, fever, nausea, vomiting, vision problems, chills, dizziness, headache • Cardiac, neurologic, respiratory changes

References:

1. Centers for Disease Control and Prevention. Diagnosis and Management of Foodborne Illnesses: A Primer for Physicians and Other Health Care Professionals. Available at: www.cdc.gov/mmwr/preview/mmwrhtml/rr5304a1.htm. Accessed July 2, 2004.
2. Food Safety and Inspection Service. The Fight BAC Survey Tool and Data Entry Tool. Available at: www.fsis.usda.gov/OA/fses/bac_datatool.htm. Accessed July 2, 2004.
3. Gerald BL, Perkin JE. Food and water safety. *J Am Diet Assoc.* 2003;103:1203-1218.
4. Partnership for Food Safety Education. Four steps. Available at: http://www.fightbac.org/foursteps.cfm?section=4. Accessed July 2, 2004.

LIMITED ACCESS TO FOOD (NB-3.2)

Definition

Diminished ability to acquire food from sources (e.g., shopping, gardening, meal delivery), due to financial constraints, physical impairment, caregiver support, or unsafe living conditions (e.g., crime hinders travel to grocery store). Limitation to food because of concerns about weight or aging.

Etiology (*Cause/Contributing Risk Factors*)

Factors gathered during the nutrition assessment process that contribute to the existence or the maintenance of pathophysiological, psychosocial, situational, developmental, cultural, and/or environmental problems:

- Caregiver intentionally or unintentionally not providing access to food, e.g., unmet needs for food or eating assistance, abuse/neglect
- Community and geographical constraints for shopping and transportation
- Lack of financial resources or lack of access to financial resources to purchase sufficient food
- Limited or absent community supplemental food programs, e.g., food pantry, shelter
- Failure to participate in food programs such as WIC, National School Lunch Program, food stamps
- Physical or psychological limitations that diminish ability to shop, e.g., walking, sight, mental/emotional health

Signs/Symptoms (*Defining Characteristics*)

A typical cluster of subjective and objective signs and symptoms gathered during the nutrition assessment process that provide evidence that a problem exists; quantify the problem and describe its severity.

Nutrition Assessment Category	Potential Indicators of this Nutrition Diagnosis (one or more must be present)
Biochemical Data, Medical Tests and Procedures	• Indicators of macronutrient or vitamin/mineral status as indicated by physical findings, food/nutrition, and client history
Anthropometric Measurements	• Growth failure, based on National Center for Health Statistics (NCHS) growth standards • Underweight (BMI <18.5)
Physical Exam Findings	• Findings consistent with vitamin/mineral deficiency

LIMITED ACCESS TO FOOD (NB-3.2)

Food/Nutrition History	Reports or observations of: • Food faddism • Belief that aging can be slowed by dietary limitations and extreme exercise • Hunger • Inadequate intake of food and/or specific nutrients • Limited supply of food in home • Limited variety of foods
Client History	• Malnutrition, vitamin/mineral deficiency • Illness or physical disability • Conditions associated with a diagnosis or treatment, e.g., mental illness, dementia • Lack of suitable support systems

References:
1. Position of the American Dietetic Association: Domestic food and nutrition security. *J Am Diet Assoc.* 2002;102:1840-1847.
2. Position of the American Dietetic Association: Addressing world hunger, malnutrition, and food insecurity. *J Am Diet Assoc.* 2003;103:1046-1057.

185

Nutrition Care Process Step 3. Nutrition Intervention

INTRODUCTION

Nutrition intervention is the third step in the Nutrition Care Process, preceded by nutrition assessment and nutrition diagnosis. Nutrition intervention is defined as purposefully planned actions designed with the intent of changing a nutrition-related behavior, risk factor, environmental condition, or aspect of health status for an individual (and his/her family or caregivers), target group, or the community at large. A dietetics professional works in conjunction with the patient/client(s) and other health care providers, programs, or agencies during the nutrition intervention phase.

While nutrition intervention is one step in the process, it consists of two interrelated components—planning and implementation. Planning involves prioritizing the nutrition diagnoses, conferring with the patient/client and/or others, reviewing practice guides and policies, and setting goals and defining the specific nutrition intervention strategy. Implementation of the nutrition intervention is the action phase that includes carrying out and communicating the plan of care, continuing data collection, and revising the nutrition intervention strategy, as warranted, based on the patient/client response.

When drafting the specific nutrition intervention terms, the Standardized Language Task Force endeavored to include the type of information necessary for medical record documentation, billing, and the description of nutrition interventions for research. Further, it is intentional that the nutrition intervention terminology distinguishes between two distinct nutrition interventions, such as nutrition education and nutrition counseling. The plan can include more that one nutrition intervention that may be implemented simultaneously during the actual interaction with the patient/client.

The nutrition intervention terminology is organized into four classes—Food and/or Nutrient Delivery, Nutrition Education, Nutrition Counseling, and Coordination of Nutrition Care. Each class is defined with subclasses of nutrition interventions. Reference sheets for each nutrition intervention term define the nutrition intervention, list typical details for the nutrition intervention, and illustrate the potential connection to the nutrition diagnoses.

The nature of a single nutrition intervention encounter with a patient/client can be described in many ways. It could include face-to-face contact with the patient/client or an encounter via electronic mail (e-mail) or telephone. The encounter may involve an individual or group and may be described in varying increments of contact time. Throughout the course of nutrition care, the practitioner and patient/client might engage in several encounters (i.e., interactions, visits, contacts) aimed at helping the patient/client implement the nutrition intervention(s). Nutrition interventions in the Food and/or Nutrient Delivery class and Coordination of Nutrition Care class may occur without direct patient/client contact.

At all levels of practice, practitioners are competent to provide many types of nutrition interventions. However, practitioner roles and responsibilities vary with experience, education, training, practice setting, employer expectations, and local standards of care. Responsible dietetics professionals assure that they are competent to practice by participating in continuing education activities and obtaining necessary education, training, and credentials related to their area of practice. The Scope of Dietetics Practice and Framework documents (available at www.eatright.org/cps/rde/xchg/ada/hs.xsl/career_7225_ENU_HTML.htm) provide guidance to the practitioner in identifying activities within and outside the Scope of Practice. The ADA Code of Ethics, Dietetic Practice Groups, and specialty groups also have documents that help identify appropriate practitioner roles and responsibilities.

Individualized nutrition interventions, based on a patient's/client's needs identified through nutrition assessment and nutrition diagnosis is the product of this step of the nutrition care process. Using a standardized terminology for describing the nutrition interventions extends the ability of the dietetics professional to document, communicate, and research the impact of nutrition care on health and disease.

NUTRITION INTERVENTION COMPONENTS

Planning and implementation are the two components of nutrition intervention. These components are interrelated, and a dietetics professional will make decisions about the nutrition intervention when both planning and implementation are feasible.

Planning the Nutrition Intervention

As a practitioner plans the nutrition intervention, he/she prioritizes the nutrition diagnoses, based on the severity of the problem, safety, patient/client need, likelihood that the nutrition intervention will impact the problem, and the patient/client perception of importance.

To determine which nutrition diagnosis can be positively impacted, a practitioner needs to examine the relationship between the pieces of the nutrition diagnosis and the nutrition intervention. It has been previously established that the nutrition diagnosis defines the problem, etiology, and the signs and symptoms based on data from the nutrition assessment.

Relationships

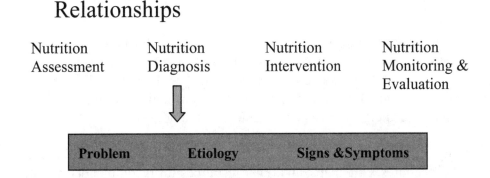

Nutrition Assessment   Nutrition Diagnosis   Nutrition Intervention   Nutrition Monitoring & Evaluation

| Problem | Etiology | Signs &Symptoms |

The nutrition intervention is directed, whenever possible, at the etiology or cause of the problem identified in the PES (i.e., problem, etiology, and signs/symptoms) statements.

Relationships

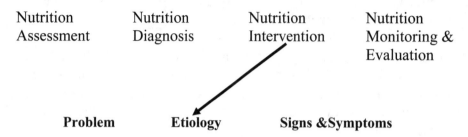

Follow-up monitoring of the signs and symptoms is used to determine the impact of the nutrition intervention on the etiology of the problem.

Relationships

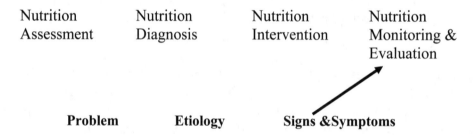

There is an exception to these relationships in the nutrition care process. In some cases, it is not possible to direct the nutrition intervention at the etiology if the etiology cannot be changed by a dietetics professional. For example, if Excessive Energy Intake (NI-1.5) is caused by depression the nutrition intervention is aimed at reducing the impact of the signs and symptoms of the problem, e.g., weight gain due to energy intake more than estimated needs.

Another aspect of planning the nutrition intervention is referring to evidence-based guidelines, institutional policies and procedures, care maps, and other resources for recommended nutrition interventions, medical nutrition therapy goals, behavior changes, and/or expected outcomes. *ADA's MNT Evidence-Based Guides for Practice* provides science-based recommendations for nutrition interventions. Dietetics practitioners should carefully examine resources to determine if the recommendations are evidence-based.

An essential part of planning the nutrition intervention is detailing the Nutrition Prescription. The nutrition prescription concisely states the patient/client's individualized recommended dietary intake of energy and/or selected foods or nutrients based on current reference standards and dietary guidelines and the patient's/client's health condition and nutrition diagnosis. It is determined using the assessment data, the nutrition diagnostic statement (PES), current evidence, policies and procedures, and patient/client values and preferences. The nutrition prescription either drives the nutrition intervention selection or is the context within which the nutrition intervention should be implemented. With the nutrition prescription defined, the dietetics practitioner identifies the specific nutrition intervention strategies and establishes the patient/client-focused goals to be accomplished.

Goal Setting

This is the time to establish clear patient/client goals that are measurable, achievable, and time-defined. In many cases, the goals are jointly set with the patient/client; however, this is not always possible in the case of patients/clients receiving enteral or parenteral nutrition, for example. In goal setting, the individual(s) responsible for the associated actions to achieve the goals is/are clearly identified.

These steps are essential because it is impossible to assess the impact of the nutrition intervention without quantifying or qualifying the goals so they can be measured. If the goals are not achievable even the most appropriate nutrition intervention could be judged as unsuccessful. Additionally, the time for achieving the individual goals should be delineated into short-term (next visit) and long-term goals (over the course of the nutrition intervention).

The parties responsible for establishing the goals and the associated actions—such as joint development with patient/client and/or family or solely provider-directed (e.g., patient/client unable to participate in interaction and family/other not available)—needs to be documented.

> Planning Summary:
> - Prioritize the nutrition diagnoses, based on problem severity, safety, patient/client need, likelihood that the nutrition intervention will impact the problem, and patient/client perception of importance
> - Consult *ADA's MNT Evidence-Based Guides for Practice* and other practice guides/policies
> - Confer with patient/client and other caregivers, or refer to policies throughout planning step
> - Detail the nutrition prescription and identify the specific nutrition intervention strategies
> - Determine patient/client-focused goals/expected outcomes
> - Define time and frequency of care

Implementing the Nutrition Intervention

Implementation is the action portion of the nutrition intervention in which professionals carry out and communicate the plan of care to all relevant parties, continue the data collection that was initiated with the nutrition assessment, and revise the nutrition intervention based on the patient/client response.

Once a practitioner has verified that the nutrition intervention is occurring, the data collected will also provide evidence of the response(s) and potentially lead to revision of the nutrition intervention.

Implementation Summary:
- Action phase
  - Communicate the plan of care
  - Carry out the plan
  - Continue data collection
- Other aspects
  - Individualize nutrition intervention
  - Collaborate with other colleagues
  - Follow-up and verify that nutrition intervention is occurring
  - Adjust intervention strategies, if needed, as response occurs

NUTRITION INTERVENTION TERMS

The Standardized Language Task Force identified four classes of nutrition interventions—Food and/or Nutrient Delivery, Nutrition Education, Nutrition Counseling, and Coordination of Care—and defined subclasses within them. These terms are intended to be used by all dietetics professionals in all nutrition intervention settings (e.g., community, public health, home care, long-term care, private practice, and pediatric and adult acute care). Currently, the nutrition intervention terms are being tested for usability and validity in clinical settings. The specific nutrition intervention terms are:

Food and/or Nutrient Delivery (ND) refers to an individualized approach for food/nutrient provision.

Meal and Snacks (ND-1)— meals are regular eating events that include a variety of foods consisting of grains and/or starches, meat and/or meat alternatives, fruits and vegetables, and milk or milk products. A snack is defined as food served between regular meals.

Enteral and Parenteral Nutrition (ND-2)—nutrition provided through the gastrointestinal tract via tube, catheter, or stoma that delivers nutrients distal to the oral cavity (enteral) or the administration of nutrients intravenously (centrally or peripherally) (parenteral).

Supplements (ND-3)—foods or nutrients that are not intended as a sole item or a meal or diet, but that are intended to provide additional nutrients.

Medical Food Supplement (ND-3.1)—commercial or prepared foods or beverages intended to supplement the nutrient intake in energy, protein, carbohydrate, fiber, and/or fat, which may also contribute to vitamin and mineral intake.
Vitamin and Mineral Supplement (ND-3.2)— a product that is intended to supplement vitamin or mineral intake.
Bioactive Substance Supplement (ND-3.3)—a product that is intended to supplement bioactive substances (e.g., plant stanol and sterol esters, psyllium).

Feeding Assistance (ND-4)—accommodation or assistance in eating designed to restore the patient's/client's ability to eat independently, support adequate nutrient intake, and reduce the incidence of unplanned weight loss and dehydration.

Feeding Environment (ND-5)—adjustment of the physical environment, temperature, convenience, and attractiveness of the location where food is served that impacts food consumption.

Nutrition-Related Medication Management (ND-6)—modification of a drug or herbal to optimize patient/client nutritional or health status.

Nutrition Education (E) is a formal process to instruct or train a patient/client in a skill or to impart knowledge to help patients/clients voluntarily manage or modify food choices and eating behavior to maintain or improve health.

> *Initial/Brief Nutrition Education (E-1)*—instruction or training intended to build or reinforce basic nutrition-related knowledge, or to provide essential nutrition-related information until patient/client returns.

> *Comprehensive Nutrition Education (E-2)*—instruction or training intended to lead to in-depth nutrition-related knowledge and/or skills in given topics.

Nutrition Counseling (C-1) is a supportive process, characterized by a collaborative counselor-patient/client relationship, to set priorities, establish goals, and create individualized action plans that acknowledge and foster responsibility for self-care to treat an existing condition and promote health.

Coordination of Nutrition Care (RC) is consultation with, referral to, or coordination of nutrition care with other health care providers, institutions, or agencies that can assist in treating or managing nutrition-related problems.

> *Coordination of Other Care During Nutrition Care (RC-1)*—facilitating services or interventions with other professionals, institutions, or agencies on behalf of the patient/client prior to discharge from nutrition care.

> *Discharge and Transfer of Nutrition Care to New Setting or Provider (RC-2)*—discharge planning and transfer of nutrition care from one level or location of care to another.

Nutrition Education vs Nutrition Counseling

As mentioned earlier, it is intentional to *separate* nutrition education and nutrition counseling despite the fact that a practitioner may use both of these nutrition interventions at one time.

Nutrition education involves the transfer of knowledge, tailored to the specific knowledge deficit identified in the PES statement. *Nutrition counseling* involves behavior and attitude change, focused on the underlying behavioral and environmental etiologies identified in the nutrition assessment and documented in the PES statement. The etiologies leading to the two interventions differ. Knowledge deficit or no previous exposure to information would lead to nutrition education. Etiologies reflecting attitudinal issues (e.g., readiness to change, lack of willingness to change) would lead to counseling. In these cases the patient/client knows what to do but has been unable to make or sustain a behavioral change. Therefore, these nutrition interventions are *separated* to highlight the difference between them and to show the true nature of the interaction(s) between professional and patient/client. This will assist a practitioner in thinking about providing distinct education and counseling approaches, while moving seamlessly between these two activities.

Use of Nutrition Interventions Based on Practice Setting

The typical use of the nutrition interventions may vary by practice setting, but are not limited based upon the practice setting.

- Food and/or Nutrient Delivery nutrition interventions will commonly be used by practitioners in institutional settings (e.g., hospitals, long-term care) and home care.
- Nutrition Education interventions—Initial/Brief Education (E-1) and Comprehensive Education (E-2)—Initial/Brief Education will be utilized more often in institutionalized settings and Comprehensive Education will be utilized more often in outpatient/noninstitutionalized settings (e.g., outpatient offices, private practice, community).
- Nutrition Counseling will likely be used more by professionals in outpatient/noninstitutionalized settings (e.g., outpatient offices, private practice, community) due to the nature of the nutrition intervention and the practice setting.
- Coordination of Nutrition Care interventions will be used by practitioners from a variety of practice settings.

It is important to reiterate that these are *typical* uses of specific nutrition interventions. Dietetics professionals in any practice setting can use the complete array of nutrition interventions as needed.

NUTRITION INTERVENTION REFERENCE SHEETS

A reference sheet for each nutrition intervention has been developed that includes: the nutrition intervention label and its definition, descriptive details of the nutrition intervention, and the nutrition diagnoses with which the nutrition intervention might typically be used. Additional considerations pertinent to the nutrition intervention are also included. A partial example of a nutrition intervention reference sheet follows here:

> *Example*
> **Feeding Assistance (ND-4)**
> **Defined as** accommodation or assistance in eating designed to restore the patient's/client's ability to eat independently, support adequate nutrient intake, and reduce the incidence of unplanned weight loss and dehydration.
> **Details of Nutrition Intervention**: A typical nutrition intervention might be further described with the following details:
> - Recommends, implements, or orders adaptive equipment, feeding position, feeding cues, meal set-up, or mouth care to facilitate eating
> - Recommends, designs, or implements a restorative dining program
> - Recommends, designs, or implements a feeding assistance training program
> - Recommends, designs, or implements menu selections that foster, promote, and maintain independent eating

These reference sheets are designed to assist practitioners with consistent and correct utilization of the nutrition interventions and are available beginning on page 201.

ENCOUNTER DETAILS

A single nutrition intervention encounter (i.e., interactions, visits, contacts, sessions) includes time spent reviewing the medical record or patient/client information and direct (i.e., face-to-face) or indirect (e.g., electronic, phone) contact with the patient/client and his/her family or caregiver. With the expanded use of electronic communication has come the growth of nutrition interventions via methods like e-mail and webinars (seminars on the Internet), along with phone and teleconference encounters.

Encounters may involve an individual or group where:

- An individual is one person with his/her family or caregiver
- A group is intended to meet more than one individual's needs

A typical method to indicate contact time in ambulatory care is in increments of 15 minutes (one unit = 15 minutes). Naturally, throughout a course of nutrition care, the practitioner and patient/client might engage in several encounters.

Roles and Responsibilities

Dietetics practice is such that practitioners differ in their need, desire, opportunity, experience, or credentials to perform various nutrition interventions. Generalist professionals may maintain competence in a wide variety of nutrition interventions, while specialty practitioners may develop in-depth expertise with a few nutrition interventions. Some of the nutrition interventions described in the reference sheets (e.g., nutrition counseling, enteral and parenteral nutrition, or nutrition-related medication management) may require specialty or advanced education and/or training.

Practice roles and responsibilities may vary according to employer expectations or institutional tradition. Regulations, in certain practice settings, may be interpreted as restricting intervention to that authorized by order of a physician or others. Protocols may be used to allow interventions to be implemented or modified. Clinical privileges allow practitioners to autonomously intervene according to a specified scope of practice. Obtaining clinical privileges or being granted authority to make independent changes to a patient/client's nutrition prescription or nutrition intervention may be needed. In some situations, such as private practice or community settings, a dietetics practitioner may have complete autonomy. Further, depending on the setting, the practitioner may assume various levels of autonomy for different nutrition interventions. Examples are provided below:

- *Implements the specified nutrition intervention; recommends initiating, modifying, or discontinuing a nutrition intervention as appropriate.* On completion of a nutrition assessment, the practitioner may recommend (verbally or by writing) refinements, modifications, or alternative nutrition interventions that require affirmation before they can be implemented.

> *Example*: The practitioner assesses a patient/client on a general diet and notices elevated serum cholesterol and triglyceride levels. The practitioner recommends a modification of the nutrition prescription to the physician or nurse practitioner, and modifies the nutrition prescription on affirmation of the recommendation.

• *Implements, within the parameters of an approved protocol or algorithm, initiation, modification, or discontinuance of a nutrition intervention.* On completion of a nutrition assessment, the practitioner modifies the original nutrition intervention within preapproved parameters.

> *Example*: The practitioner assesses a patient/client with a general nutrition prescription and notices elevated serum cholesterol, triglyceride, and blood glucose levels. According to an approved treatment algorithm, the practitioner can implement a "heart healthy" nutrition prescription for any patient/client with a serum cholesterol level more than 200 mg/dL. The practitioner changes the nutrition prescription to "heart healthy", initiates patient/client nutrition education, and documents the change and other details of the nutrition intervention in the medical record. Because the algorithm does not specify the nutrition intervention for hyperglycemia, the practitioner must provide (verbally or in writing) recommendations for an additional carbohydrate restriction or management in the nutrition prescription, then await affirmation for implementation.

• *Independently orders initiation, modification, or discontinuance of a nutrition intervention based on a scope of practice. Authority may be specified in an approved clinical privileging document or inherent in the setting.* On completion of the nutrition assessment the practitioner is able to initiate, modify, or discontinue a nutrition intervention based on independent clinical judgment.

> *Example*: The practitioner assesses a patient/client with a general nutrition prescription, and notices elevated serum cholesterol, triglyceride levels, and blood glucose levels. In this setting, a practitioner has the autonomy to order, change, and implement nutrition prescriptions designed to manage disorders of lipid, carbohydrate, protein, and energy metabolism. The practitioner changes the nutrition prescription to "heart healthy" with consistent carbohydrate intake and initiates patient/client nutrition education and other details of the nutrition intervention as appropriate.

The table provides examples of the common level of autonomy in a few practice settings:

Setting	Common Triggers	Common Levels of Autonomy
Inpatient	Physician or advanced practice nurse **orders** a diet or **requests** a consultation or the patient is **identified** at risk by screening criteria	• Implements the specified nutrition intervention; recommends initiating, modifying, or discontinuing a nutrition intervention. • Implements, within the parameters of an approved protocol or algorithm, initiation, modification, or discontinuance of a nutrition intervention. • Independently orders initiation, modification, or discontinuance of a nutrition intervention based on a scope of practice. Authority is usually specified in an approved clinical privileging document.
Outpatient	Physician or advanced practice nurse **refers** the patient/client or the patient/client is **self-referred**	• Implements the specified nutrition intervention; recommends initiating, modifying, or discontinuing a nutrition intervention. • Implements, within the parameters of an approved protocol or algorithm, initiation, modification, or discontinuance of a nutrition intervention. • Independently orders initiation, modification, or discontinuance of a nutrition intervention based on a scope of practice. Authority may be specified in an approved clinical privileging document or inherent in practice setting.
Private Practice	Physician or advanced practice nurse **refers** the patient/client or the patient/client is **self-referred**	• Independently orders initiation, modification, or discontinuance of a nutrition intervention based on scope of practice.
Community	Client is **self-referred** or is identified at risk by screening criteria	• Independently orders initiation, modification, or discontinuance of a nutrition intervention based on scope of practice.

As mentioned earlier, the Scope of Dietetics Practice and Framework documents provide guidance to the practitioner in identifying activities within and outside the Dietetics Scope of Practice. The entire Scope of Dietetics Practice documents are available on ADA's web site at www.eatright.org/cps/rde/xchg/ada/hs.xsl/career_7225_ENU_HTML.htm. Dietetic Practice Groups and specialty organizations have documents that help identify appropriate practitioner roles and responsibilities and practitioners should refer to these reports for guidance.

SUMMARY

Using a defined nutrition intervention terminology will assist the profession in communicating within and among a variety of providers. It will also be instrumental in documenting and researching the impact the profession has on specific diagnoses and/or etiologies in all patient/client populations. The nutrition intervention reference sheets are a tool that professionals can use to select strategies and implement this aspect of the nutrition care process. Finally, evaluation of the nutrition intervention terminology is planned and will guide possible future modifications.

REFERENCES

1. Davis AM, Baker SS, Leary RA. Advancing clinical privileges for support practitioners: the dietitian as a model. *Nutr Clin Pract.* 1995;10:98-103.
2. Hager M. Hospital therapeutic diet orders and the Centers for Medicare & Medicaid Services: Steering through regulations to provide quality nutrition care and avoid survey citations. *J Am Diet Assoc.* 2006;106:198-204.
3. Kieselhorst KJ, Skates J, Pritchett E. American Dietetic Association: Standards of practice in nutrition care and updated standards of professional performance. *J Am Diet Assoc.* 2005;105:641-645.
4. Kulkarhi K, Boucher J, Daly A, Shwide-Slavin C, Silvers B, Maillet JO, Pritchett E. American Dietetic Association: Standards of practice and standards of professional performance for registered dietitians (generalist, specialty, and advanced) in diabetes care. *J Am Diet Assoc.* 2005;105:819-824.
5. Lacey K, Pritchett E. Nutrition care process and model: ADA adopts road map to quality care and outcomes management. *J Am Diet Assoc.* 2003;103:1061-1072.
6. Mahan L, Escott-Stump S. *Krause's Food, Nutrition, & Diet Therapy. 11th ed.* Philadelphia, PA: Saunders; 2000.
7. Miller R, Rollnick S. *Motivational Interviewing: Preparing People for Change, 2nd ed.* New York, NY: Guilford Press; 2002.
8. Moreland K, Gotfried M, Vaughn L. Development and implementation of the clinical privileges for dietitian nutrition order writing program at a long-term acute-care hospital. *J Am Diet Assoc.* 2002;102:72-74.
9. Myers EF, Barnhill G, Bryk J. Clinical privileges: missing piece of the puzzle for clinical standards that elevate responsibilities and salaries for registered dietitians. *J Am Diet Assoc.* 2002;102:123-132.
10. O'Sullivan Maillet J, Skates J, Pritchett E. American Dietetic Association: Scope of dietetics practice framework. *J Am Diet Assoc.* 2005;105:634-640.
11. Silver H, Wellman N. Nutrition diagnosing and order writing: value for practitioners, quality for clients. *J Am Diet Assoc.* 2003;103:1470-1472.

Problem _____

Etiology _____

Signs/Symptoms _____

Nutrition Prescription
The patient's/client's individualized recommended dietary intake of energy and/or selected foods or nutrients based on current reference standards and dietary guidelines and the patient's/client's health condition and nutrition diagnosis. (specify)

_____

_____

Intervention #1_____

Goal (s) _____

_____

Intervention #2 _____

Goal (s) _____

_____

Intervention #3_____

Goal (s) _____

_____

FOOD AND/OR NUTRIENT DELIVERY   ND

Meal and Snacks   ND-1
Regular eating event (meal); food served between regular meals (snack).
- ❏ General/healthful diet
- ❏ Modify distribution, type, or amount of food and nutrients within meals or at specified time
- ❏ Specific foods/beverages or groups
- ❏ Other *(specify)* _____

Enteral and Parenteral Nutrition   ND-2
Nutrition provided through the GI tract via tube, catheter, or stoma (enteral) or intravenously (centrally or peripherally) (parenteral).
- ❏ Initiate enteral or parenteral nutrition
- ❏ Modify rate, concentration, composition or schedule
- ❏ Discontinue enteral or parenteral nutrition
- ❏ Insert enteral feeding tube
- ❏ Site care
- ❏ Other *(specify)* _____

SUPPLEMENTS   ND-3

Medical Food Supplements   ND-3.1
Commercial or prepared foods or beverages that supplement energy, protein, carbohydrate, fiber, or intake.
Type
- ❏ Commercial beverage
- ❏ Commercial food
- ❏ Modified beverage
- ❏ Modified food
Purpose
(specify)_____

Vitamin and Mineral Supplements   ND-3.2
Supplemental vitamins or minerals.
- ❏ Multivitamin/mineral
- ❏ Vitamin
  - ❏ A   ❏ C
  - ❏ Thiamin   ❏ D
  - ❏ Riboflavin   ❏ E
  - ❏ Niacin   ❏ K
  - ❏ Folate   ❏ Multivitamin
  - ❏ Other *(specify)*_____
- ❏ Mineral
  - ❏ Calcium   ❏ Iron
  - ❏ Potassium   ❏ Zinc
  - ❏ Phosphorus   ❏ Magnesium
  - ❏ Multi-trace elements
  - ❏ Other *(specify)*_____

Bioactive Substance Supplement   ND-3.3
Supplemental bioactive substances.
- ❏ Initiate
- ❏ Dose change
- ❏ Form change
- ❏ Route change
- ❏ Administration schedule
- ❏ Discontinue
(specify) _____

Feeding Assistance   ND-4
Accommodation or assistance in eating.
- ❏ Adaptive equipment
- ❏ Feeding position
- ❏ Meal set-up
- ❏ Mouth care
- ❏ Other *(specify)* _____

Feeding Environment   ND-5
Adjustment of the factors where food is served that impact food consumption.
- ❏ Lighting
- ❏ Odors
- ❏ Distractions
- ❏ Table height
- ❏ Table service/set up
- ❏ Room temperature
- ❏ Other *(specify)* _____

Nutrition-Related Medication Management   ND-6
Modification of a drug or herbal to optimize patient/client nutritional or health status.
- ❏ Initiate
- ❏ Dose change
- ❏ Form change
- ❏ Route change
- ❏ Administration schedule
- ❏ Discontinue
(specify) _____

NUTRITION EDUCATION   E

Initial/Brief Nutrition Education   E-1
Build or reinforce basic or essential nutrition-related knowledge.
- ❏ Purpose of the nutrition education
- ❏ Priority modifications
- ❏ Survival information
- ❏ Other *(specify)* _____

Comprehensive Nutrition Education   E-2
Instruction or training leading to in-depth nutrition-related knowledge or skills.
- ❏ Purpose of the nutrition education
- ❏ Recommended modifications
- ❏ Advanced or related topics
- ❏ Result interpretation
- ❏ Other *(specify)* _____

NUTRITION COUNSELING   C

Nutrition Counseling   C-1
A supportive process to set priorities, establish goals, and create individualized action plans that acknowledge and foster responsibility for self-care.
- ❏ Theory or approach
  - ☐ Behavior modification
  - ☐ Cognitive-behavioral theory
  - ☐ Social learning theory
  - ☐ Transtheoretical
  - ☐ Other *(specify)* _____
- ❏ Strategies
  - ☐ Cognitive restructuring
  - ☐ Goal setting
  - ☐ Motivational interviewing
  - ☐ Problem solving
  - ☐ Rewards/reinforcement
  - ☐ Self-monitoring
  - ☐ Social support
  - ☐ Stimulus control/contingency management
  - ☐ Stress management
  - ☐ Other *(specify)*_____
- ❏ Phase
  - ☐ Involving
  - ☐ Exploring
  - ☐ Resolving
  - ☐ Closing

COORDINATION OF NUTRITION CARE   RC

Coordination of Other Care During Nutrition Care   RC-1
Facilitating services with other professionals, institutions, or agencies during nutrition care.
- ❏ Team meeting
- ❏ Referral to RD with different expertise
- ❏ Collaboration/referral to other providers
- ❏ Referral to community agencies/programs
(specify) _____

Discharge and Transfer of Nutrition Care to New Setting or Provider   RC-2
Discharge planning and transfer of nutrition care from one level or location of care to another.
- ❏ Collaboration/referral to other providers
- ❏ Referral to community agencies/programs
(specify) _____

NUTRITION INTERVENTION TERMS AND DEFINITIONS

Nutrition Intervention Term	Term Number	Definition	Reference Sheet Page Numbers
DOMAIN: FOOD AND/OR NUTRIENT DELIVERY	ND	**Individualized approach for food/nutrient provision.**	
Meals and Snacks	ND-1	Meals are defined as regular eating events that include a variety of foods consisting of grains and/or starches, meat and/or meat alternatives, fruits and vegetables, and milk or milk products. A snack is defined as food served between regular meals.	201-202
Enteral and Parenteral Nutrition	ND-2	Enteral nutrition is defined as nutrition provided through the gastrointestinal (GI) tract via tube, catheter, or stoma that delivers nutrients distal to the oral cavity. Parenteral nutrition is defined as the administration of nutrients intravenously, centrally (delivered into a large-diameter vein, usually the superior vena cava adjacent to the right atrium) or peripherally (delivered into a peripheral vein, usually of the hand or forearm).	203-204
Supplements	ND-3	Foods or nutrients that are not intended as a sole item or a meal or diet, but that are intended to provide additional nutrients.	
Medical Food Supplements	ND-3.1	Commercial or prepared foods or beverages intended to supplement energy, protein, carbohydrate, fiber, and/or fat intake that may also contribute to vitamin and mineral intake.	205-206
Vitamin and Mineral Supplements	ND-3.2	A product that is intended to supplement vitamin or mineral intake.	207-208

Edition: 2007

NUTRITION INTERVENTION TERMS AND DEFINITIONS

Nutrition Intervention Term	Term Number	Definition	Reference Sheet Page Numbers
Bioactive Substance Supplement	ND-3.3	A product that is intended to supplement bioactive substances (e.g., plant stanol and sterol esters, psyllium).	209
Feeding Assistance	ND-4	Accommodation or assistance in eating designed to restore the patient's/client's ability to eat independently, support nutrient intake, and reduce the incidence of unplanned weight loss and dehydration.	210-211
Feeding Environment	ND-5	Adjustment of the physical environment, temperature, convenience, and attractiveness of the location where food is served that impacts food consumption.	212-213
Nutrition-Related Medication Management	ND-6	Modification of a drug or herbal to optimize patient/client nutritional or health status.	214-215
DOMAIN: NUTRITION EDUCATION	**E**	**Formal process to instruct or train a patient/client in a skill or to impart knowledge to help patients/clients voluntarily manage or modify food choices and eating behavior to maintain or improve health.**	
Initial/Brief Nutrition Education	E-1	Instruction or training intended to build or reinforce basic nutrition-related knowledge, or to provide essential nutrition-related information until patient/client returns.	216-217
Comprehensive Nutrition Education	E-2	Instruction or training intended to lead to in-depth nutrition-related knowledge and/or skills in given topics.	218-219

199

Edition: 2007

NUTRITION INTERVENTION TERMS AND DEFINITIONS

Nutrition Intervention Term	Term Number	Definition	Reference Sheet Page Numbers
DOMAIN: NUTRITION COUNSELING	C	**A supportive process, characterized by a collaborative counselor-patient/client relationship, to set priorities, establish goals, and create individualized action plans that acknowledge and foster responsibility for self-care to treat an existing condition and promote health.**	
Nutrition Counseling	C-1	A supportive process, characterized by a collaborative counselor-patient/client relationship, to set priorities, establish goals, and create individualized action plans that acknowledge and foster responsibility for self-care to treat an existing condition and promote health.	220-221
DOMAIN: COORDINATION OF NUTRITION CARE	RC	**Consultation with, referral to, or coordination of nutrition care with other providers, institutions, or agencies that can assist in treating or managing nutrition-related problems.**	
Coordination of Other Care During Nutrition Care	RC-1	Facilitating services or interventions with other professionals, institutions, or agencies on behalf of the patient/client prior to discharge from nutrition care.	222-224
Discharge and Transfer of Nutrition Care to New Setting or Provider	RC-2	Discharge planning and transfer of nutrition care from one level or location of care to another.	225-226

MEALS AND SNACKS (ND-1)

Definition: Meals are defined as regular eating events that include a variety of foods consisting of grains and/or starches, meat and/or meat alternatives, fruits and vegetables, and milk or milk products. A snack is defined as food served between regular meals.

Details of Intervention:

A typical intervention might be further described with the following details:

- Recommend, implement, or order an appropriate distribution of type or quantity of food and nutrients within meals or at specified times
- Identify specific food/beverage(s) or groups for meals and snacks

Typically used with the following:

Nutrition Diagnostic Terminology Used in PES Statements	Common Examples (Not intended to be inclusive)
Nutrition Diagnoses	• Increased energy expenditure (NI-1.2) • Excessive fat intake (NI-51.2) • Excessive carbohydrate intake (NI-53.2) • Inconsistent carbohydrate intake (NI-53.4)
Etiology	• Lack of access to healthful food choices, e.g., food provided by caregiver • Physiologic causes, e.g., increased energy needs due to increased activity level or metabolic change, malabsorption • Psychological causes, e.g., disordered eating • Difficulty chewing, swallowing, extreme weakness

201

MEALS AND SNACKS (ND-1)

Signs and Symptoms
Biochemical Data, Medical Tests and Procedures
• Serum cholesterol level > 200 mg/dL
• Hemoglobin A1C > 6%
Physical Assessment
• Weight change
• Dental caries
• Diarrhea in response to carbohydrate feeding
Food/Nutrition History
• Cultural or religious practices that do not support modified food/nutrition intake
• Changes in physical activity
• Intake of inappropriate foods
Client History
• Conditions associated with diagnosis or treatment, e.g., surgery, trauma, sepsis, diabetes mellitus, inborn errors of metabolism, digestive enzyme deficiency, obesity
• Chronic use of medications that increase or decrease nutrient requirements or impair nutrient metabolism

Other considerations *(e.g., patient/client negotiation, patient/client needs and desires, and readiness to change)*

- Compliance skills and abilities
- Economic concerns with purchasing special food items
- Willingness/ability to change behavior to comply with diet
- Availability/access to a qualified practitioner for follow-up and monitoring

References:

1. Lacey K, Pritchett E. Nutrition Care Process and Model: ADA adopts road map to quality care and outcomes management. *J Am Diet Assoc.* 2003;103:1061-1071.

Edition: 2007

ENTERAL AND PARENTERAL NUTRITION (ND-2)

Definition: Enteral nutrition is defined as nutrition provided through the gastrointestinal (GI) tract via tube, catheter, or stoma that delivers nutrients distal to the oral cavity. Parenteral nutrition is defined as the administration of nutrients intravenously, centrally (delivered into a large-diameter vein, usually the superior vena cava adjacent to the right atrium) or peripherally (delivered into a peripheral vein, usually of the hand or forearm).

Details of Intervention:

A typical intervention might be further described with the following details:

- Recommend, implement, or order changes in the rate, composition, schedule, and/or duration of feeding
- Recommend, implement, or order the initiation, route, and discontinuation of enteral nutrition
- Insert the feeding tube, provide tube site care; administer feedings
- Change dressings and provide line care
- Review changes in the intervention with the patient/client(s) and/or caregivers

Typically used with the following:

Nutrition Diagnostic Terminology Used in PES Statements	Common Examples (Not intended to be inclusive)
Nutrition Diagnoses	• Swallowing difficulties (NC-1.1) • Altered GI function (NC-1.4) • Inadequate oral food/beverage intake (NI-2.1) • Inadequate intake from enteral/parenteral nutrition infusion (NI-2.3) • Excessive intake from parenteral nutrition infusion (NI-2.4)
Etiology	• Altered gastrointestinal tract function, inability to absorb nutrients • Inability to chew/swallow

203

Edition: 2007

ENTERAL AND PARENTERAL NUTRITION (ND-2)

Signs and Symptoms	Physical Assessment
	• Weight loss > 10% in 6 months, > 5% in 1 month
	• Obvious muscle wasting
	• Skin turgor (tenting, edema)
	• Growth failure
	• Insufficient maternal weight gain
	• BMI < 18.5
	Food/Nutrition History
	• Intake < 75% of requirements (insufficient intake)
	• Existing or expected inadequate intake for 7-14 days
	Client History
	• Malabsorption, maldigestion
	• Emesis
	• Diffuse peritonitis, intestinal obstruction, paralytic ileus, intractable diarrhea or emesis, gastrointestinal ischemia, or perforated viscus, short-bowel syndrome

Other considerations *(e.g., patient/client negotiation, patient/client needs and desires, and readiness to change)*

• End-of-life issues, ethical considerations, patient/client rights and family/caregiver issues.
• Other nutrient intake (oral, parenteral, or enteral nutrition)
• Enteral formulary composition and product availability
• Availability/access to a qualified practitioner for follow-up and monitoring
• Economic constraints that limit availability of food/enteral/parenteral products

References:

1. A.S.P.E.N. Board of Directors and Standards Committee. Definition of terms, style, and conventions used in A.S.P.E.N. guidelines and standards. *Nutr Clin Pract.* 2005;20:281-285.
2. A.S.P.E.N. Board of Directors and the Clinical Guidelines Task Force. Guidelines for the use of parenteral and enteral nutrition in adult and pediatric patients. *JPEN J Parenter Enteral Nutr.* 2002;26:1SA-138SA.
3. McClave SA, Lowen CC, Kleber MJ, Nicholson JF, Jimmerson SC, McConnell JW, Jung LY. Are patients fed appropriately according to their caloric requirements? *JPEN J Parenter Enteral Nutr.* 1998;22:375-381.
4. Mirtallo J, Canada T, Johnson D, Kumpf V, Petersen C, Sacks G, Seres D, Guenter P. Task force for the revision of safe practices for parenteral nutrition. *JPEN J Parenter Enteral Nutr.* 2004;28:S39-S70.

Edition: 2007

MEDICAL FOOD SUPPLEMENTS (ND-3.1)

Definition: Commercial or prepared foods or beverages intended to supplement energy, protein, carbohydrate, fiber, and/or fat intake that may also contribute to vitamin and mineral intake.

Details of Intervention:

A typical intervention might be further described with the following details:

- Recommend, implement, or order changes in an individualized feeding plan including the initiation, composition, type, frequency, timing, and discontinuation of oral supplements
- Describe the purpose of the supplement (e.g., to supplement energy, protein, carbohydrate, fiber, and/or fat intake)

Typically used with the following:

Nutrition Diagnostic Terminology Used in PES Statements	Common Examples (Not intended to be all inclusive)
Nutrition Diagnoses	- Inadequate oral food/beverage intake (NI-2.1) - Inadequate fluid intake (NI-3.1) - Increased nutrient needs (NI-5.1)
Etiology	- Neurologic deficit (stroke) - Difficulty chewing or swallowing - Food allergies or intolerance - Altered GI function - Partial GI obstruction
Signs and Symptoms	Physical Examination Findings - Weight loss > 10% in 6 months or > 5% in 1 month - Obvious muscle wasting - Poor skin turgor (tenting or edema) Food/Nutrition History - Insufficient usual food/beverage intake Client History - Diagnosis consistent with elevated nutrient needs - Potential for repletion of nutritional status - Ability to feed self - Choking on foods, oral/facial trauma - Insufficient vitamin-mineral intake

205

MEDICAL FOOD SUPPLEMENTS (ND-3.1)

Other considerations *(e.g., patient/client negotiation, patient/client needs and desires, and readiness to change)*

- Appetite sufficient to take medical food supplements
- System constraints that prevent meeting the client's preferences for specific flavors, textures, foods and the timing of feedings
- Availability of feeding assistance
- Economic concerns and product/food availability

References:
1. Milne AC, Avenell A, Potter J. Meta-analysis: Protein and energy supplementation in older people. *Ann Intern Med.* 2006;144:37-48.

VITAMIN OR MINERAL SUPPLEMENTS (ND-3.2)

Definition: A product that is intended to supplement vitamin or mineral intake.

Details of Intervention:

A typical intervention might be further described with the following details:

- Recommend, implement, or order initiation, change in administration schedule and dose/form/route, or discontinuation of a vitamin and/or mineral supplement

Typically used with the following:

Nutrition Diagnostic Terminology Used in PES Statements	Common Examples (Not intended to be inclusive)
Nutrition Diagnoses	• Inadequate vitamin intake (NI-54.1) • Excessive vitamin intake (NI-54.2) • Inadequate mineral intake (NI-55.1) • Excessive mineral intake (NI-55.2) • Food–medication interaction (NC-2.3) • Food- and nutrition-related knowledge deficit (NB-1.1) • Undesirable food choices (NB-1.7)
Etiology	• Poor intake of nutrient dense foods that contain vitamins and minerals • Excessive use of vitamin and mineral supplements • Medical diagnosis consistent with altered vitamin and mineral requirements • Malabsorption of vitamins and minerals
Signs and Symptoms	Physical Examination Findings • Cutaneous abnormalities consistent with vitamin and mineral deficiency of excess Food/Nutrition History • Nutrient intake analysis reveals vitamin and mineral intake more or less than recommended • Laboratory or radiologic indexes of vitamin-mineral depletion

207

FOOD AND/OR NUTRIENT DELIVERY DOMAIN

VITAMIN OR MINERAL SUPPLEMENTS (ND-3.2)

Other considerations (e.g., patient/client negotiation, patient/client needs and desires, and readiness to change)

- Emerging scientific evidence to support the use of vitamin and mineral supplements in specific populations
- Availability of a qualified practitioner with additional education/training in the use of vitamin and mineral supplements in practice
- Economic considerations and product availability

References:

1. Federal Food, Drug and Cosmetic Act. US Code, Title 21, Chapter 9, Subchapter II, Section 321 (ff). 2000 Edition. Available at: http://frwebgate.access.gpo.gov/cgi-bin/getdoc.cgi?dbname=browse_usc&docid=Cite:+21USC321. Accessed April 26, 2005.
2. Position of the American Dietetic Association: Fortification and nutritional supplements. *J Am Diet Assoc.* 2005;105:1300-1311.

BIOACTIVE SUBSTANCE SUPPLEMENT (ND-3.3)

Definition: A product that is intended to supplement bioactive substances (e.g., plant stanol and sterol esters, psyllium).

Details of Intervention:

A typical intervention might be further described with the following details:

- Recommend, implement, or order initiation, changed in administration schedule or dose/form/route, or discontinuation of a bioactive substances (e.g., soluble fiber, soy protein, fish oils, plant sterol and stanol esters)

Typically used with the following:

Nutrition Diagnostic Terminology Used in PES Statements	Common Examples (Not intended to be inclusive)
Nutrition Diagnoses	• Inadequate bioactive substance intake (NI-4.1) • Excessive bioactive substance intake (NI-4.2) • Excessive alcohol intake (NI-4.3) • Food–medication interaction (NC-2.3) • Food- and nutrition-related knowledge deficit (NB-1.1) • Undesirable food choices (NB-1.7)
Etiology	• Poor intake of bioactive substance–containing foods • Excessive use of bioactive substance supplements
Signs and Symptoms	Food/Nutrition History • Nutrient intake analysis reveals bioactive substance intake more or less than recommended Client History • Medical diagnosis associated with increased bioactive substance need

Other considerations *(e.g., patient/client negotiation, patient/client needs and desires, and readiness to change)*

- Emerging scientific evidence to support the use of bioactive supplements in specific populations
- Availability of a qualified practitioner with additional education/training in the use of bioactive supplements in practice

References

1. Position of the American Dietetic Association: Functional foods. *J Am Diet Assoc.* 2004;104:814-826.

Edition: 2007

FEEDING ASSISTANCE (ND-4)

Definition: Accommodation or assistance in eating designed to restore the patient's/client's ability to eat independently, support adequate nutrient intake, and reduce the incidence of unplanned weight loss and dehydration.

Details of Intervention:

A typical intervention might be further described with the following details:

- Recommend, implement, or order adaptive equipment, feeding position, feeding cues, meal set-up, or mouth care to facilitate eating
- Recommend, design, or implement a restorative dining program
- Recommend, design, or implement a feeding assistance training program
- Recommends, designs, or implements menu selections that foster, promote, and maintain independent eating

Typically used with the following:

Nutrition Diagnostic Terminology Used in PES Statements	Common Examples (Not intended to be inclusive)
Nutrition Diagnoses	• Inadequate energy intake (NI-1.4) • Inadequate oral/food beverage intake (NI-2.1) • Involuntary weight loss (NC-3.2)
Etiology	• Physical disability • Poor food/nutrient intake • Decreased memory/concentration problems
Signs and Symptoms	Physical Examination Findings • Dropping the utensils or food • Weight loss Client History • Cerebral palsy, stroke, dementia • Refusal to use prescribed adaptive eating devices, or follow prescribed positioning techniques

Other considerations *(e.g., patient/client negotiation, patient/client needs and desires, and readiness to change)*

- Acceptance of feeding assistance/feeding devices
- Poor environment to foster adequate intake
- Lack of individual to provide assistance at meal time

Edition: 2007

FOOD AND/OR NUTRIENT DELIVERY DOMAIN

FEEDING ASSISTANCE (ND-4)

- Lack of training in methods of feeding assistance
- Lack of available physical therapy, occupational therapy, or speech therapy evaluations
- Ability to understand the reasoning behind the recommendations and then want to make personal changes

References:
1. Consultant Dietitians in Health Care Facilities. *Eating Matters: A training Manual for Feeding Assistants.* Chicago, IL: Consultant Dietitians in Health Care Facilities, American Dietetic Association; 2003.
2. Niedert K, Dorner B, eds. *Nutrition Care of the Older Adult, 2nd edition.* Chicago, IL: Consultant Dietitians in Health Care Facilities, American Dietetic Association; 2004.
3. Position of the American Dietetic Association: Liberalization of the diet prescription improves quality of life for older adults in long-term care. *J Am Diet Assoc.* 2005;105:1955-1965.
4. Position of the American Dietetic Association: Providing nutrition services for infants, children, and adults with developmental disabilities and special health care needs. *J Am Diet Assoc.* 2004;104:97-107.
5. Robinson GE, Leif B, eds. *Nutrition Management and Restorative Dining for Older Adults: Practical Interventions for Caregivers.* Chicago, IL: Consultant Dietitians in Health Care Facilities, American Dietetic Association; 2001.
6. Russell C, ed. *Dining Skills: Practical Interventions for the Caregivers of Older Adults with Eating Problems.* Consultant Dietitians in Health Care Facilities. Chicago, IL: American Dietetic Association; 2001.
7. Simmons SF, Osterweil D, and Schnelle JF. Improving food intake in nursing home residents with feeding assistance: A staffing analysis. *J Gerontol A Biol Sci Med Sci.* 2001;56:M790-M794.
8. Simmons SF, Schnelle JF. Individualized feeding assistance care for nursing home residents: Staffing requirements to implement two interventions. *J Gerontol A Biol Sci Med Sci.* 2004;59:M966-M973.

FEEDING ENVIRONMENT (ND-5)

Definition: Adjustment of the physical environment, temperature, convenience, and attractiveness of the location where food is served that impacts food consumption.

Details of Intervention:

A typical intervention might be further described with the following details:

- Recommend, implement, or order changes in table service/colors/set up/height, room temperature and lighting, meal schedule, menu choice, appetite enhancers, proper positioning, and minimize distractions and odors
- Recommend, implement, or order seating arrangements considering groupings that inspire social interactions

Typically used with the following:

Nutrition Diagnostic Terminology Used in PES Statements	Common Examples (Not intended to be inclusive)
Nutrition Diagnoses	• Inadequate oral food/beverage intake (NI-2.1) • Disordered eating pattern (NB-1.5) • Self-feeding difficulty (NB-2.6)
Etiology	• Dementia • Inability to stick to task/easily distracted by others
Signs and Symptoms	Food/Nutrition History • Changes in appetite attributed to mealtime surroundings • Easily distracted from eating • Food sanitation and safety issues • Available foods not of the patient's choosing • Decline in patient/client ability to eat independently Client History • Pacing, wandering, changes in affect

Other considerations *(e.g., patient/client negotiation, patient/client needs and desires, and readiness to change)*

- Resources available to improve/modify the feeding environment

212

FOOD AND/OR NUTRIENT DELIVERY DOMAIN

FEEDING ENVIRONMENT (ND-5)

References:
1. Niedert K, Dorner B, eds. *Nutrition Care of the Older Adult, 2nd edition*. Chicago, IL: Consultant Dietitians in Health Care Facilities, American Dietetic Association; 2004.
2. Position of the American Dietetic Association: Liberalization of the diet prescription improves quality of life for older adults in long-term care. *J Am Diet Assoc.* 2005;105:1955-1965.
3. Position of the American Dietetic Association: Providing nutrition services for infants, children, and adults with developmental disabilities and special health care needs. *J Am Diet Assoc.* 2004;104:97-107.
4. Robinson GE, Leif B, eds. *Nutrition Management and Restorative Dining for Older Adults: Practical Interventions for Caregivers*. Chicago, IL: Consultant Dietitians in Health Care Facilities, American Dietetic Association; 2001.
5. Russell C, ed. *Dining Skills: Practical Interventions for the Caregivers of Older Adults with Eating Problems*. Consultant Dietitians in Health Care Facilities. Chicago, IL: American Dietetic Association; 2001.

213

Edition: 2007

NUTRITION-RELATED MEDICATION MANAGEMENT (ND-6)

Definition: Modification of a drug or herbal to optimize patient/client nutritional or health status.

Details of Intervention:

A typical intervention might be further described with the following details:

- Recommend, implement, order initiation, changes in dose/form/route, change in administration schedule, or discontinuance of medications or herbals including insulin, appetite stimulants, digestive enzymes, or probiotics

Typically used with the following:

Nutrition Diagnostic Terminology Used in PES Statements	Common Examples (Not intended to be inclusive)
Nutrition Diagnoses	• Altered GI function (NC-1.4) • Impaired nutrient utilization (NC-2.1) • Food–medication interaction (NC-2.3)
Etiology	• Appetite insufficient resulting in adequate nutrient intake • Frequent hypo- or hyperglycemia • Pancreatic insufficiency • Malabsorption of fat, protein, lactose, or other carbohydrates • Polypharmacy and medication abuse • Drug toxicity
Signs and Symptoms	Physical Examination Findings • Thin, wasted appearance Food/Nutrition History • Sufficient oral intake • Report of herbal use Client History • Diabetes with poorly controlled blood sugar

Edition: 2007

NUTRITION-RELATED MEDICATION MANAGEMENT (ND-6)

Other considerations *(e.g., patient/client negotiation, patient/client needs and desires, and readiness to change)*

- Availability/access to a clinical pharmacist
- Availability of a qualified practitioner with appropriate pharmacology training and/or education

References:

1. Position of the American Dietetic Association: Integration of medical nutrition therapy and pharmacotherapy. *J Am Diet Assoc.* 2003;103:1363-1370.
2. Kris-Etherton P, Pearson T. Over-the-counter statin medications: Emerging opportunities for RDs. *J Am Diet Assoc.* 2000;100:1126-1130.
3. Moyers B. Medications as adjunct therapy for weight loss: Approved and off-label agents in use. *J Am Diet Assoc.* 2005;105:948-959.

215

Edition: 2007

INITIAL/BRIEF NUTRITION EDUCATION (E-1)

Definition: Instruction or training intended to build or reinforce basic nutrition-related knowledge, or to provide essential nutrition-related information until patient/client returns.

Details of Intervention:

A typical intervention might be further described related the following details:

- Discuss the purpose of the nutrition education intervention
- Communicate relationship between nutrition and specific disease/health issue
- Begin instruction of nutrition issue of most concern to patient/client's health and well-being
- Provide basic nutrition-related educational information until client is able to return for comprehensive education

Typically used with the following:

Nutrition Diagnostic Terminology Used in PES Statements	Common Examples (Not intended to be inclusive)
Nutrition Diagnoses	• Food–medication interaction (NC-2.3) • Food- and nutrition-related knowledge deficit (NB-1.1) • Harmful beliefs/attitudes about food- or nutrition-related topics (NB-1.2) • Self-monitoring deficit (NB-1.4) • Other: Any diagnoses related to inadequate, excessive, inappropriate, or inconsistent intake
Etiology	• Capacity for learning • Knowledge deficit related to newly diagnosed medical condition • Interest and/or motivation • Medical or surgical procedure requiring modified diet • Unable to distinguish legitimate from false information
Signs and Symptoms	Food/Nutrition History • Unable to explain purpose of the nutrition prescription or rationale for nutrition prescription in relationship to disease/health • Expresses need for additional information or clarification of education or additional time to learn information • Unable to select appropriate foods or supplements • Unable to choose appropriate timing, volume, or preparation/handling of foods

216

NUTRITION EDUCATION DOMAIN

INITIAL/BRIEF NUTRITION EDUCATION (E-1)

Other considerations *(e.g., patient/client negotiation, patient/client needs and desires, and readiness to change)*

- Met with several providers in one day and is unable or unwilling to receive more nutrition education at this time
- Profile reflects complicated situation warranting additional education/instruction
- Being discharged from the hospital
- Caregiver unavailable at time of nutrition education
- Baseline knowledge
- Learning style
- Other education and learning needs, e.g., new medication or other treatment administration

References:

1. Position of the American Dietetic Association: Total diet approach to communicating food and nutrition information. *J Am Diet Assoc* 2002;102:100-108.
2. Holli BB, Calabrese RJ, O'Sullivan-Maillet J. *Communication and education skills for dietetics professionals*. 4th ed. New York, NY: Lipincott Williams and Wilkins; 2003.
3. Sahyoun NR, Pratt CA, Anderson A. Evaluation of nutrition education interventions for older adults: A proposed framework. *J Am Diet Assoc*. 2004;104:58-69.
4. Contento I. The effectiveness of nutrition education and implications for nutrition education policy, programs, and research: a review of research. *J Nutr Ed*. 1995;27: 279-283.
5. Medeiros LC, Butkus SN, Chipman H, Cox RH, Jones L, Little D. A logic model framework for community nutrition education. *J Nutr Educ Behav*. 2002;37: 197-202.

Edition: 2007

COMPREHENSIVE NUTRITION EDUCATION (E-2)

Definition: Instruction or training intended to lead to in-depth nutrition-related knowledge and/or skills in given topics.

Details of Intervention:

A typical intervention might be further described with the following details:

- Provide information related to purpose of the nutrition prescription
- Initiate thorough instruction of relationship between nutrition and disease/health
- Explain detailed or multiple nutrition prescription modifications recommended given patient/client situation
- Introduce more advanced nutrition topics related to patient/condition (e.g., saturated and *trans* fatty acid intake vs. total fat intake, glucometer use, home tube feeding and feeding pump training, menu planning, food purchasing and preparation)
- Commence training on interpreting medical or other results to modify nutrition prescription (e.g., distribution of carbohydrates throughout the day based on blood glucose monitoring results)

Typically used with the following:

Nutrition Diagnostic Terminology Used in PES Statements	Common Examples (Not intended to be inclusive)
Nutrition Diagnoses	• Food–medication interaction (NC-2.3) • Food- and nutrition-related knowledge deficit (NB-1.1) • Harmful beliefs/attitudes about food- or nutrition-related topics (NB-1.2) • Self-monitoring deficit (NB-1.4) • Other: Any diagnoses related to inadequate or excessive, inappropriate, or inconsistent intake
Etiology	• Deficient understanding of relevant nutrition-related topics • Exposure to incorrect food and nutrition information • Lack of skill in self management techniques
Signs and Symptoms	Food/Nutrition History • Expresses desire for knowledge/information • Food and nutrient intake assessment indicates food choice incompatible with recommendations

218

NUTRITION EDUCATION DOMAIN

COMPREHENSIVE NUTRITION EDUCATION (E-2)

Other considerations *(e.g., patient/client negotiation, patient/client needs and desires, and readiness to change)*

- Profile reflects complicated situation warranting additional education/instruction
- Increased capacity and willingness to learn information
- Quality of life may be enhanced with in-depth nutrition education and understanding
- Baseline knowledge
- Lifestyle factors
- Education approaches that enhance knowledge/skill transfer

References:

1. Position of the American Dietetic Association: Total diet approach to communicating food and nutrition information. *J Am Diet Assoc.* 2002;102:100-108.
2. Carmona RH. Improving Health Literacy: Preventing Obesity with education. *J Am Diet Assoc.* 2005;105:S9-S10.
3. Contento I. The effectiveness of nutrition education and implications for nutrition education policy, programs, and research: a review of research. *J Nutr Educ.* 1995;27: 279-283.
4. Holli BB, Calabrese RJ, O'Sullivan-Maillet J. *Communication and education skills for dietetics professionals.* 4th ed. New York, NY: Lipincott Williams and Wilkins; 2003.
5. Holmes AL, Sanderson B, Maisiak R, Brown R, Bittner V. Dietitian services are associated with improved patient outcomes and the MEDFICTS dietary assessment questionnaire is a suitable outcome measure in cardiac rehabilitation. *J Am Diet Assoc.* 2005;105:1533-1540.
6. Medeiros LC, Butkus SN, Chipman H, Cox RH, Jones L, Little D. A logic model framework for community nutrition education. *J Nutr Educ Behav.* 2005;37:197-202.
7. Sahyoun NR, Pratt CA, Anderson A. Evaluation of nutrition education interventions for older adults: A proposed framework. *J Am Diet Assoc.* 2004;104:58-69.

Edition: 2007

219

NUTRITION COUNSELING (C-1)

Definition: A supportive process, characterized by a collaborative counselor-patient/client relationship, to set priorities, establish goals, and create individualized action plans that acknowledge and foster responsibility for self-care to treat an existing condition and promote health.

Details of Intervention:

A typical intervention might be further described with the following details:

- Theory or approach
  - ○ Behavior modification
  - ○ Cognitive-behavioral
  - ○ Social learning theory
  - ○ Transtheoretical model
  - ○ Other

- Strategies
  - ○ Cognitive restructuring
    - > identify thought that intervenes between stimulus and response
  - ○ Goal setting
  - ○ Motivational interviewing, including eliciting change talk and using:
    - > open-ended questions
    - > affirmation
    - > reflection
    - > summarization
  - ○ Problem solving
    - > brainstorm several solutions
    - > discuss pros and cons
    - > techniques to decrease resistance
  - ○ Rewards/reinforcement
  - ○ Self-monitoring
    - > food intake, e.g., amount, time
    - > exercise, e.g., activity, duration, intensity
    - > other, e.g., weight, glucose
  - ○ Social support
  - ○ Stimulus control/contingency management
    - > antecedents to response
    - > consequences of behavior
    - > environmental change
    - > accountability for change
  - ○ Stress management
  - ○ Other

- Phase
  - ○ Involving
  - ○ Exploration-education
  - ○ Resolving
  - ○ Closing

220

NUTRITION COUNSELING DOMAIN

NUTRITION COUNSELING (C-1)

Typically used with the following:

Nutrition Diagnostic Terminology Used in PES Statements	Common Examples (Not intended to be inclusive)
Nutrition Diagnoses	• Harmful beliefs/attitudes about food- or nutrition-related topics (NB-1.2) • Self-monitoring deficit (NB-1.4) • Disordered eating pattern (NB-1.5) • Undesirable food choices (NB-1.7) • Physical inactivity (NB-2.1) • Other: Any diagnoses related to inadequate, excessive, inappropriate, or inconsistent intake
Etiology	• Denial of need for change • Any behavior that is inconsistent with healthy habits, e.g., eating fast food at lunch when other restaurant options are readily available • Perception that change will be hard • Pattern of negative thoughts
Signs and Symptoms(Defining Characteristics)	Food/Nutrition History • Absent or incomplete self-monitoring records • Unable to describe strategies or recognize need for relapse prevention • Inability to problem-solve • Disbelief in ability to accomplish nutrition recommendations • Negative self-talk • Evidence of excessive, inadequate, inappropriate, or inconsistent intake related to needs

Other considerations *(e.g., patient/client negotiation, patient/client needs and desires, and readiness to change)*

• Lifestyle factors

References:
1. Position of the American Dietetic Association: Weight management. *J Am Diet Assoc.* 2002;102:1145-1155.
2. Berkel LA, Carlow Poston WS, Reeves RS, Foreyt JP. Behavioral interventions for obesity. *J Am Diet Assoc.* 2005;105;S35-S43.
3. Cooper Z, Fairburn CG. A new cognitive behavioural approach to the treatment of obesity. *Behav Res Ther.* 2001;39:499-511.
4. Emmons KM, Rollnick S. Motivational interviewing in health care settings. Opportunities and limitations. *Am J Prev Med.* 2001;20:68-74.
5. Harris-Davis E, Haughton B. Model for multicultural nutrition counseling competencies. *J Am Diet Assoc.* 2000;100:1178-1185.
6. Kirk S, Scott BJ, Daniels SR. Pediatric obesity epidemic: Treatment options. *J Am Diet Assoc.* 2005;105:S44-S51.
7. Mahan L, Escott-Stump S. *Krause's Food, Nutrition, & Diet Therapy.* 11th ed. Philadelphia, PA: Saunders; 2000.
8. Miller R, Rollnick S. *Motivational Interviewing: Preparing People for Change, 2nd ed.* New York, NY: Guilford Press; 2002.
9. Resnicow K, Yaroch AL, Davis A, Wang DT, Carter S, Slaughter L, Coleman D, Baranowski T. Go Girls!: Results from a nutrition and physical activity program for low-income, overweight African-American adolescent females. *Health Educ Behav.* 2000;27:616-631.
10. Resnicow K, Taylor R, Baskin M, McCarty F. Results of Go Girls!: A weight control program for overweight African-American adolescent females. *Obes Res.* 2005;13:1739-1748.
11. Snetselaar L. *Nutrition Counseling in Lifestyle Change.* New York, NY: CRC Press; 2006.

Edition: 2007

221

COORDINATION OF OTHER CARE DURING NUTRITION CARE (RC-1)

Definition: Facilitating services or interventions with other professionals, institutions, or agencies on behalf of the patient/client prior to discharge from nutrition care.

Details of Intervention:

A typical intervention might be further described with the following details:

- Holding a team meeting to develop a comprehensive plan of care
- A formal referral for care by other dietetics professionals who provide different expertise
- Collaboration with or referral to others such as the physician, dentist, physical therapist, social worker, occupational therapist, speech therapist, nurse, pharmacist, or other specialist dietitian
- Referral to an appropriate agency/program (e.g., home delivered meals, WIC, food pantry, soup kitchen, food stamps, housing assistance, shelters, rehabilitation, physical and mental disability programs, education training, and employment programs)

Typically used with the following:

Nutrition Diagnostic Terminology Used in PES Statements	Common Examples (Not intended to be inclusive)
Nutrition Diagnoses	• Inadequate oral food and beverage intake (NI 2.1) • Involuntary weight loss (NC-3.2) • Excessive alcohol intake (NI-4.3) • Inappropriate intake of food fats (NI-51.3) • Overweight/obesity (NC-3.3) • Physical inactivity (NB-2.1) • Food–medication interaction (NC-2.3) • Self-feeding difficulty (NB-2.6) • Limited access to food (NB-3.2)

Edition: 2007

COORDINATION OF OTHER CARE DURING NUTRITION CARE (RC-1)

Etiology	**Physical Examination Findings** • Physical disability with impaired feeding ability, other impairments related to activities of daily living • Growth and development issues **Food/Nutrition History** • Inadequate intake • Nutrient drug interactions **Psychological/Social History** • Transportation issues • Food acceptance issues • Developmental issues • Economic considerations impacting food/nutrient intake
Signs and Symptoms	**Physical Examination Findings** • Weight loss • Unacceptable growth rates compared to standard growth charts **Food/Nutrition History** • More than 10% weight loss in 6 months • Hyperglycemia and weight loss • Poor wound healing **Client History** • Inability to procure food • Anorexia nervosa • Lack of access to food sources • Lack of food preparation skills

Other considerations *(e.g., patient/client negotiation, patient/client needs and desires, and readiness to change)*

• Availability of services related to patient/client need (specialty dietitians, clinical pharmacists, speech pathologists, nurse practitioners, etc.)
• Anticipated duration of health care encounter/hospital or long-term care discharge
• Resources available for care
• Medicare/Medicaid/insurance guidelines and restrictions
• Food assistance program (e.g., food stamp program) guidelines and regulations

223

Edition: 2007

COORDINATION OF NUTRITION CARE DOMAIN

COORDINATION OF OTHER CARE DURING NUTRITION CARE (RC-1)

References:

1. Position of the American Dietetic Association. Nutrition, aging, and the continuum of care. *J Am Diet Assoc.* 2000;100:580-595.
2. Mclaughlin C, Tarasuk V, Kreiger N. An examination of at-home food preparation activity among low-income, food insecure women. *J Am Diet Assoc.* 2003;103:1506-1512.
3. Greger JL, Maly A, Jensen N, Kuhn J, Monson K, Stocks A. Food pantries can provide nutritionally adequate food packets but need help to become effective referral units for public assistance programs. *J Am Diet Assoc.* 2002;102:1125-1128.
4. Olson CM, Holben DH. Position of the American Dietetic Association: Domestic food and nutrition security. *J Am Diet Assoc.* 2002;102:1840-1847.
5. Millen BE, Ohls JC, Ponza M, McCool AC. The elderly nutrition program: An effective national framework for preventive nutrition interventions. *J Am Diet Assoc.* 2002;102:234-240.

224

Edition: 2007

DISCHARGE AND TRANSFER OF NUTRITION CARE TO A NEW SETTING OR PROVIDER (RC-2)

Definition: Discharge planning and transfer of nutrition care from one level or location of care to another.

Details of Intervention:

A typical intervention might be further described with the following details:

- Change in the nutrition prescription with consideration for changes in patient/client schedule, activity level, and food/nutrient availability in the new setting
- Collaboration with or referral to others such as the physician, dentist, physical therapist, social worker, occupational therapist, speech therapist, nurse, pharmacist, or other specialist dietitian
- Referral to an appropriate agency/program (e.g., home delivered meals, WIC, food pantry, soup kitchen, food stamps, housing assistance, shelters, rehabilitation, physical and mental disability programs, education, training and employment programs)

Typically used with the following:

Nutrition Diagnostic Terminology Used in PES Statements	Common Examples (Not intended to be inclusive)
Nutrition Diagnoses	• Inadequate oral food/beverage intake (NI-2.1) • Imbalance of nutrients (NI-5.5) • Inappropriate intake of food fats (NI-51.3) • Food–medication interaction (NC-2.3) • Underweight (NC-3.1) • Overweight/obesity (NC-3.3) • Impaired ability to prepare foods/meals (NB-2.4) • Self-feeding difficulty (NB-2.6)
Etiology	Food/Nutrition History • Long-term insufficient intake mandating home enteral or parenteral nutrition • Growth and development considerations requiring intervention in a new setting

225

Edition: 2007

DISCHARGE AND TRANSFER OF NUTRITION CARE TO A NEW SETTING OR PROVIDER (RC-2)

Signs and Symptoms

Biochemical Data, Medical Tests and Procedures
- Abnormal lab values

Anthropometric Measurements
- Inappropriate weight status
- Continuing weight gain or loss

Food/Nutrition History
- Inappropriate dietary practices
- Harmful beliefs and attitudes

Client History
- Treatment failure
- Readmission

Other considerations *(e.g., patient/client negotiation, patient/client needs and desires, and readiness to change)*

- Availability of discharge planning services, options for care
- Preferences for the level and location of care
- Resources available for care
- Medicare/Medicaid/insurance guidelines and restrictions
- Health literacy
- Ability to implement treatment at home
- Food assistance program (e.g., food stamp program) guidelines and regulations

References:

1. Baker EB, Wellman NS. Nutrition concerns for discharge planning for older adults: A need for multidisciplinary collaboration. *J Am Diet Assoc.* 2005;105:603-607.
2. Position of the American Dietetic Association. Nutrition, aging, and the continuum of care. *J Am Diet Assoc.* 2000;100:580-595.

Nutrition Care Process: Case Study A
Examples of Charting in Various Formats

It is recommended that practitioners document each step of the Nutrition Care Process. Typically, documentation is entered in writing or electronically into the medical record. The Nutrition Care Process describes documentation of Assessment, Diagnosis, Intervention, Monitoring, and Evaluation (ADIME) steps (1). In a pilot study, this format was shortened to the Assessment, Diagnosis, and Intervention (ADI) with monitoring and evaluation incorporated into the nutrition intervention step (2). Implementation of the Nutrition Care Process is not dependent upon a specific format for documentation. The diagnostic and nutrition intervention terminology can be incorporated into existing documentation formats such as narrative and SOAP notes. The example below illustrates how the Nutrition Diagnosis, PES Statement, and nutrition intervention terminology can be incorporated into narrative and SOAP notes and also illustrates the ADIME format.

Case:
HO is a 47-year-old man who is married with three children ages 13, 15, and 17 years. HO is 5'11" tall and weighs 235 pounds (BMI 32.8). While playing college baseball, HO weighed about 185 pounds, but when he stopped playing and began coaching, his weight drifted up to 200 pounds. About 3 years ago, he took a job as a junior high school principal. The principal's job requires much more desk work, and, despite walking the halls regularly between periods at the large urban school, HO doesn't get much exercise. He has verbalized the need to "get back in shape."

HO's family history is a concern. Both of his parents have type 2 diabetes. HO's father was forced into retirement a year after his foot was amputated because of complications from the diabetes. Two of HO's older brothers have been told to lose weight in order to reduce their risk of developing type 2 diabetes. His younger sister recently gave birth to her third child and was diagnosed with gestational diabetes during the pregnancy.

Because his first son will enter college next year, HO is thinking about the future. He is thinking about how he will prepare for his children's college education and, eventually, their weddings. He would like to be healthy enough to play baseball with his grandchildren when they arrive. He is becoming concerned about his health and realizes that he needs to do something about his weight. A recent visit to his physician was a great relief because no problems other than obesity were identified. The physician emphasized the importance of weight loss and referred HO to an RD for a weight reduction program.

The RD interviewed HO and found:
HO was born in Mexico, but emigrated to the United States at age 4 with his parents. His family owned a restaurant, and he learned to cook at an early age. He often prepares traditional foods from Mexico and fries these foods in lard. His North American-born wife does some of the cooking and prepares meals with meat, potatoes, fruits and vegetables, and gravy.

HO does not eat breakfast, stating that with five people in the house getting ready for work and school each morning, there is too much of a rush to stop for a meal. When he arrives at school, HO usually stops by the school cafeteria to purchase cookies or a large muffin, which he eats with butter. He drinks several cups of coffee with sugar and cream at his desk during the morning. He eats lunch in the school cafeteria, often requesting large portions of meats and other foods he likes. After lunch, he usually drinks at least one sweetened soda. He is usually at school until late afternoon, and may return for evening activities. On these evenings, he enjoys the "all you can eat buffet" at a family restaurant near his home. He eats a variety of foods, including fruits, vegetables and salads. His weakness is flour tortillas slathered with butter or sour cream, and he eats several with each evening meal taken at home. HO eats dessert only on special occasions. Because the family is busy, there are plenty of "snack foods" available, and he usually has an "after dinner snack" when he returns home from evening activities.

HO's alcohol intake is moderate, limited to 2 or 3 cans of beer on a Friday or Saturday night if he and his wife go out with friends. Analysis of a 24-hour diet recall combined with a food frequency questionnaire reveals that HO's typical intake is approximately 4,200 calories with about 200 grams/day of total fat, about 100 grams of saturated fat, and about 20% of calories from sugar or other concentrated sweets.

Because his job and family require so much of his time, HO does not regularly exercise.

Nutrition Diagnosis:
Excessive Oral Food/Beverage Intake NI-2.2 (P) related to a knowledge deficit of portion sizes and meal planning (E), as evidenced by weight gain of 35lbs during the last 3 years and estimated oral intake of 2,200 kcal/day more than estimated needs (S).

Nutrition Intervention:
Nutrition Prescription: Reduction of food intake to approximately 2,550 calories per day with approximately 30% of calories from fat and < 10% of intake from saturated fat. **Initial/Brief Education (E-1)** on portion sizes of food and survival skills. **Coordination of Other Health Care During Nutrition Care (RC-1)** with referral to a 6-week weight-loss program.

Narrative Format	SOAP Format	ADIME Format*
HO is a 47-year-old male referred for a 35# weight gain (from 200 to 235 #) over the last 3 years since taking a sedentary job. His family history includes diabetes, but he has no medical problems (BMI ~33). Diet history reveals a intake of 4,200 kcal with 200 grams of fat, 100 grams of saturated fat, and a high consumption of high-calorie beverages. He eats two meals and snacks throughout the day. He does not exercise regularly. He likes most foods.	**S** (subjective): Pt. states that he is 47 years old. He has gained 35# (from 200 to 235#) over the last 3 years since taking a sedentary job. His family history includes diabetes, but he has no medical problems. He reports no breakfast, frequent snacking, high-calorie beverage intake throughout the day, and large portions at lunch and dinner. His alcohol intake is limited to social occasions. He rarely finds time for exercise due to a busy work and family schedule. He likes most foods.	
	O (objective): Ht. 5'11"; Current weight 235#; BMI 32.8; no medical problems.	
HO has a nutrition diagnosis of **Excessive Oral Food/Beverage Intake NI-2.2** related to knowledge deficit of portion size and meal planning as evidenced by weight gain of 35# over the last 3 years and estimated oral intake of 1,650 kcal/day more than estimated needs of 2,550 kcal/day. His **Nutrition Prescription (ND-1)** is 2,550 calories per day with approximately 30% of calories from fat and < 10% of intake from saturated fat. After **Initial/Brief Education (E-1)** on portion sizes of food and survival skills as described in the *ADA Nutrition Care Manual.* **Coordination of Other Health Care During Nutrition Care (RC-1)** with referral to a 6-week weight-loss program and follow-up in 6 weeks.	**A** (assessment): Analysis reveals intake of approximately 4,200 calories, 200 grams/day of total fat, 100 grams of saturated fat, and 20% of calories from sugar or other concentrated sweets. Pt. is about 45# above the upper limit for ideal weight of 189#. Calorie intake is 1,650 kcal/day more than estimated needs of 2,550 kcal. Nutrition Diagnosis: **Excessive Oral Food/Beverage Intake (NI-2.2)** related to knowledge deficit of portion size and meal planning as evidenced by weight gain of 35# over the last 3 years and oral intake of 1,650 kcal/day more than estimated needs of 2,550 kcal/day.	**A** (assessment): Analysis reveals intake of approximately 4,200 calories, 200 grams/day of total fat, 100 grams of saturated fat, and 20% of calories from sugar or other concentrated sweets. Pt. is about 45# above the upper limit for his ideal weight range. Calorie intake is 1,650 kcal/day more than estimated needs of 2,550 kcal.

Edition: 2007

Case Study A: Examples Incorporating the Nutrition Diagnosis, PES statement, and Nutrition Intervention into Various Styles of Charting

Narrative Format	SOAP Format	ADIME Format*
		D (diagnosis): **Excessive Oral Food/Beverage Intake (NI-2.2)** related to knowledge deficit of portion size and meal planning as evidenced by weight gain of 35# over the last 3 years and estimated oral intake of 1,650 kcal/day more than estimated needs of 2,550 kcal/day.
	P (plan) **Nutrition Prescription (ND-1)** 2,550 calories per day with approximately 30% of calories from fat and < 10% of intake from saturated fat. **Initial/Brief Education (E-1)** on portion sizes of food and survival skills as described in the ADA Nutrition Care Manual. **Coordination of Other Health Care During Nutrition Care (RC-1)** with referral to a 6-week weight-loss program, and return for follow-up in 6 weeks.	**I** (intervention): **Nutrition Prescription (ND-1)** 2,550 calories per day with approximately 30% of calories from fat and < 10% of intake from saturated fat. **Initial/Brief Education (E-1)** on portion sizes of food and survival skills as described in the ADA Nutrition Care Manual. **Coordination of Other Health Care During Nutrition Care (RC-1)** with referral to a 6-week weight-loss program.
		M (monitor): Monitor understanding of weight reduction principles and caloric intake. Monitor weight in 6 weeks.
		E (evaluation): Weight change over time.

* In some settings, the ADIME format has been abbreviated to the ADI format.

diagnosis might change over time.

Session	Topic	Session Details	Follow-up Notes
Session 1	Diet and lifestyle modifications	Review food records and agree on goals for intake modification. Educate on portion sizes.	Review of food records and discussion with HO suggest that he is unaware of the amount of food appropriate to maintain his desirable weight. His nutrition diagnosis continues to be **Excessive Oral Food/Beverage Intake NI-2.2** related to knowledge deficit of portion size and meal planning as evidenced by weight gain of 35# over the last 3 years and estimated oral intake of 1,650 kcal/day more than estimated needs of 2,550 kcal/day.
Session 2	Meal planning and nutrient-dense foods	Review food records and goals for intake modification. Review portion sizes and educate on appropriate substitutions for high-calorie, high-fat foods.	Review of food records and discussion with HO suggest that he has made some progress, and has lost 2-3 pounds. However, he continues to eat large portions of food at school and at restaurant meals. **Excessive Oral Food/Beverage Intake NI-2.2** related to knowledge deficit of portion size and meal planning as evidenced by weight gain of 35# over the last 3 years and estimated oral intake of 1,650 kcal/day more than estimated needs of 2,550 kcal/day.
Session 3	Meal planning and eating out	Review food records and goals for intake modification. Review substitutions for high-calorie, high-fat foods, and educate on strategies when eating out.	Review of food records and discussion with HO suggest that he lost another pound this week, but he needs more information on how to avoid eating too much when eating out. **Excessive Oral Food/Beverage Intake NI-2.2** related to knowledge deficit of portion size and meal planning as evidenced by weight gain of 35# over the last 3 years and estimated oral intake of 1,650 kcal/day more than estimated needs of 2,550 kcal/day.

231

Edition: 2007

Case Study A: This table demonstrates how the weight loss program addresses HO's nutrition diagnosis, and how that nutrition diagnosis might change over time.

Session	Topic	Session Details	Follow-up Notes
Session 4	Meal planning and preparation	Review food records and goals for intake modification. Review strategies for eating out and educate on lower calorie, lower fat cooking techniques	Review of food records suggests that HO has reduced his oral food and beverage intake to about 2,500 kcal/day on most days. However, he has not yet increased his activity level. Therefore the nutrition diagnosis of **Excessive Oral Food/Beverage Intake NI-2.2** is resolved, and the nutrition diagnosis of **Physical inactivity NB-2.1** related to lack of understanding of the caloric equivalents of exercise as evidenced by report of large amounts of sedentary activities including desk work and computer use.
Session 5	Exercise and physical activity	Review food records and goals for intake. Review cooking techniques and develop a physical activity plan.	Review of food records suggests that HO has continued to comply with his diet, loosing 1 or 2 pounds per week, but he has not initiated a physical activity program. **Physical inactivity NB-2.1** related to lack of understanding of the caloric equivalents of exercise as evidenced by report of large amounts of sedentary activities including desk work and computer use
Session 6	Weight maintenance	Develop long-term goals. Review weight-reduction strategies, and discuss a long-term weight maintenance plan.	

References

1. Lacey K, Pritchett E. Nutrition Care Process and Model: ADA adopts road map to quality care and outcomes management. *J Am Diet Assoc.* 2003;103:1061-1071.

2. Mathieu J, Foust M, Ouellette P. Implementing nutrition diagnosis, step two in the nutrition care process and model: challenges and lessons learned in two health care facilities. *J Am Diet Assoc.* 2005;105:1636-1640.

Nutrition Care Process: Case Study B
Examples of Charting in Various Formats

Case:
JG is a 68-year-old woman with a history of type 2 diabetes, chronic renal failure (which is treated with hemodialysis three times weekly), and peripheral vascular disease. She has been noncompliant with her insulin regimen, routinely experiencing blood glucose levels in the 250-300mg/dL range when tested at the dialysis center. Over the last 3 months, she developed a venous stasis ulcer just above her ankle. Despite aggressive care at a wound center, she developed gangrene and was admitted to the hospital for a below the knee amputation. For 2 days after surgery, she did well, but then she developed a rapid heart rate and increased respiratory rate, and her temperature spiked to 102° Fahrenheit. The intensive care team was consulted, and JG was transferred to the intensive care unit.

The RD reviewed the medical record and found:
JG was transferred to the intensive care unit for management of sepsis and respiratory failure 3 nights ago. She is being mechanically ventilated intermittently at 16 breaths per minute (IMV of 16). The fraction of inspired oxygen (FiO_2) is 60%, and positive end expiratory pressure (PEEP) is 6 cm H_2O. Her mean arterial pressure is 70. Renal replacement therapy consists of hemodialysis, which is still being done three times a week; most recently on the previous afternoon (Day –1). There is no notation of any vomiting or diarrhea, and her last bowel movement was two days ago (Day –2).

Blood cultures were positive for *Staphylococcus epidermis*. Antibiotics were started, and empiric coverage of a suspected fungemia was begun. She received fluid boluses of 500 mL of 0.45 saline twice on ICU admission, and is now receiving 0.45 saline at 40 mL/hour. She receives no other fluids except what is needed to administer her medication.

Physical Exam Findings:
JG is 5'5" tall and before surgery weighed 147 pounds (approximately 67 kg). She appears overweight and has edema in her remaining ankle and foot. There is a nasogastric tube in place. Her abdomen is soft, and she has occasional hypoactive bowel sounds.

Food/Nutrition History:
As JG is unable to communicate, her family provided a history. They state that she is noncompliant with her diabetic diet, but she limits high-potassium fruits. They also state that her appetite was good prior to hospital admission. A conversation with the RD at the dialysis center reveals that her weight was stable over the last 6 months. Presently, she is receiving 20 mL/hour of a 1 calorie per mL enteral formula through the nasogastric (NG) tube.

JG Biochemical Data:

	Day -3	Day - 2	Day -1	Day 0 (today)
Sodium (mEq/L)	135	134	132	132
Potassium (mEq/L)	3.4	4.6	4.8	3.2
Chloride (mEq/L)	109	111	113	109
CO_2 (mEq/L)	19	17	17	19
BUN (mg/dL)	87	93	97	85
Creatinine (mg/dL)	5.7	6.1	5.8	5.6
Blood Glucose (mg/dL)	341	184	136	129
Magnesium (mEq/L)	1.9	2.1	2.4	1.8
Phosphorus (mg/dL)	6.3	7.1	6.9	6.4
Calcium (mg/dL)	8.1	7.9	8.0	7.8
Albumin (mg/dL)	2.4	2.3	2.5	2.3
Weight (kg)	61	61	63	67
Intake in liters (all sources)	1.6	3.4	5.1	
Output in liters (includes dialysis)	1.1	0.1	1.1	

Intravenous (IV) Medications:
Vancomycin 1 g q12 h — IV
Theophylline 200 mg q8 h — per nasogastric tube (NGT)
Captopril 25 mg tid — per NGT
Furosemide 40 mg each day — per NGT
Potassium Chloride 20 mEq each day — per NGT
Insulin drip at 2 units per hour — IV
Propofol at 5 mcg/kg/min — IV
Amphotericin 50 mg each day — IV
Multiple vitamin liquid, 10 mL each day — per NGT

Narrative Format	SOAP Format	ADIME Format*
This 68-year-old female was transferred to the ICU with sepsis and respiratory failure following a BKA five days ago. Her history includes diabetes mellitus (DM) treated with insulin. She receives hemodialysis three times weekly for chronic renal failure and is noncompliant with her diet at home, but does avoid high-potassium foods. The RD at the dialysis center states her weight has been stable. Currently, she is mechanically ventilated and is being treated for a staph infection and suspected fungemia. She receives potassium supplementation and has had normal serum potassium levels over the last 3 days. Phosphate binders have not been restarted since surgery. Her blood glucose level is being controlled with an insulin drip. Propofol is to be discontinued this afternoon. Her fluid status is 5 L positive over the last 3 days and the medical team wants to limit her fluid intake. She is receiving a 1 kcal/mL enteral feeding at 20 mL/hour providing 480 kcal/20 grams of protein/56 grams of carbohydrate and 21 grams of fat, which she appears to be tolerating without difficulty. **Nutrition Prescription** is 1,675 calories and 100 grams of protein (25 kcal/kg and 1.5 grams of protein) with low phosphorus intake in minimal volume.	**S** (subjective): Deferred as patient is receiving mechanical ventilation. Family states that her appetite/intake was good prior to admission. The RD at the dialysis center states her weight has been stable. **O** (objective): Ht. 5'5''; current weight 67 kg; medical problems include sepsis, poorly controlled DM now treated effectively with an insulin drip, chronic renal failure treated with hemodialysis 3 times weekly. Patient underwent BKA for gangrenous ulcer 5 days ago. She is now receiving a 1 kcal/mL enteral formula at 20 mL/hr. Medications and laboratory data reviewed. **A** (assessment): **Nutrition Prescription** is 1,675 calories and 90 grams of protein (25 kcal/kg and 1.5 grams of protein) with low phosphorus intake in minimal volume. **Nutrition Diagnosis** is **Inadequate intake from enteral nutrition infusion (NI-2.3)** related to need to concentrate and advance enteral formula as evidenced by comparison of nutrient intake with estimated needs.	**A** (assessment): Review of the medical record and conversations with family and dialysis center RD reveal a 68-year-old female transferred to the ICU with sepsis and respiratory failure following a BKA five days ago. Her history included diabetes mellitus treated with insulin. She receives hemodialysis 3 times weekly for chronic renal failure and is noncompliant with her diet at home, but she does avoid high-potassium foods. The RD at the dialysis center states her weight has been stable.

Case Study B: Examples Incorporating the Nutrition Diagnosis, PES statement, and Nutrition Intervention into Various Styles of Charting an Initial Assessment

Narrative Format	SOAP Format	ADIME Format*
Nutrition Diagnosis is **Inadequate Intake from Enteral Nutrition Infusion (NI-2.3)** related to need to concentrate and advance enteral formula as evidenced by comparison of nutrient intake with estimated needs. **Nutrition Intervention** is **Enteral or Parenteral Nutrition (ND -3)** to change the composition of the enteral feeding to 2 kcal/mL thus increasing the caloric intake to 960 kcal/day with 42 g protein in a minimal volume. A second nutrition intervention is **Coordination of Other Health Care During Nutrition Care (RC-1).** Discussed reordering phosphate binders with the medical team. Discussed maximally concentrating IV medication with the pharmacist so that enteral feeding can be advanced to goal as tolerated.		Currently, she is mechanically ventilated and is being treated for a staph infection and suspected fungemia. She receives potassium supplementation with normal serum potassium levels over the last 3 days. Phosphate binders have not been restarted since surgery. Her blood glucose levels are being controlled with an insulin drip. Her fluid status is 5 L positive over the last 3 days and the medical team wants to limit her fluid intake. She is receiving a 1 kcal/mL enteral feeding at 20 mL/hour providing 480 kcal/20 grams of protein/ 56 grams of carbohydrate and 21 grams of fat which she appears to be tolerating without difficulty. Her height is 5'5" and she weighed 147# (67 kg) on admission. Her current weight is 67 kg. Her labs are as expected for her diagnosis, including hypoalbuminemia reflective of positive fluid status. Medications noted and her blood sugars are coming under control with an insulin drip.

D (diagnosis): Inadequate Intake from Enteral Nutrition Infusion (NI-2.3) related to fluid restriction as evidenced by comparison of nutrient intake with estimated needs. |

Case Study B: Examples incorporating the Nutrition Diagnosis, PES statement, and Nutrition Intervention like Values By Age 31

Charting an Initial Assessment

Narrative Format	SOAP Format	ADIME Format*
	P (plan): Coordination of Other Health Care During Nutrition Care (RC-1) Discussed reordering phosphate binders with the medical team. Discussed maximally concentrating IV medication with the pharmacist so that enteral feeding can be advanced to goal as tolerated.	**I (intervention): Nutrition Prescription Enteral or Parenteral Nutrition (ND -3)** Recommend changing the composition of the enteral feeding to 2 kcal/mL formula providing 960 kcal/day with 42 g protein in a minimal volume. **Coordination of Other Health Care During Nutrition Care (RC-1)** Discussed reordering phosphate binders with the medical team. Discussed maximally concentrating IV medication with the pharmacist so that enteral feeding can be advanced to goal as tolerated.
		M (monitor): Tolerance to enteral feedings and fluid status; serum phosphorus, magnesium, and potassium levels and ongoing need for potassium supplementation.
		E (evaluation): Comparison of intake to estimated needs.

* In some settings, the ADIME format has been abbreviated to the ADI format.

237

Case Study B: Follow-up Documentation (Day +1)

JG's tube feeding was changed overnight to the goal rate of 35 mL/hr of 2 kcal/mL feeding. The propofol was discontinued as planned but other medications continue unchanged. JG is scheduled for dialysis today.

Biochemical Data

	Day +1
Sodium (mEq/L)	130
Potassium (mEq/L)	3.0
Chloride (mEq/L)	117
CO_2 (mEq/L)	16
BUN (mg/dL)	93
Creatinine (mg/dL)	5.9
Blood Glucose (mg/dL)	121
Magnesium (mEq/L)	1.6
Phosphorus (mg/dL)	6.8
Calcium (mg/dL)	7.8
Albumin (mg/dL)	2.1
Weight (kg)	69

Case Study B: Examples Incorporating the Nutrition Diagnosis, PES statement, and Nutrition Intervention into Various Styles of Charting a Follow-up Note

Narrative Format	SOAP Format	ADIME Format*
Phosphate binders have not been restarted since surgery. Her blood glucose levels are being controlled with an insulin drip. Her fluid status is 8 L positive over the last 3 days and the medical team continues to limit her fluid intake. She is receiving a 2 kcal/mL enteral feeding at 32 mL/hour providing 1,536 kcal/ 58 grams of protein/ 76 grams of carbohydrate and 77 grams of fat, which she appears to be tolerating. **Nutrition Prescription** is 1,675 calories and 100 grams of protein (25 kcal/kg and 1.5 grams of protein), low phosphorus intake in minimal volume. **Nutrition Diagnosis** is **Inadequate Intake from Enteral Nutrition Infusion (NI-2.3)** related to need to supplement protein intake as evidenced by comparison of protein intake with estimated needs. **Nutrition Intervention** is **Enteral or Parenteral Nutrition (ND-3)** to change the composition of the enteral feeding by adding 20 grams of protein to it. A second Nutrition Intervention is **Coordination of Other Health Care During Nutrition Care (RC-1).** Discussed reordering phosphate binders with the medical team.	**S (subjective):**

O (Objective): Propofol d/c'd yesterday. Labs reviewed. Feedings running at goal rate of 32 mL/hour.

A (Assessment): Patient tolerating feedings without difficulty. **Nutrition Prescription** is 1,675 calories and 100 grams of protein (25 kcal/kg and 1.5 grams of protein) with low phosphorus intake in minimal volume. **Nutrition Diagnosis** is **Inadequate Intake from Enteral Nutrition Infusion (NI-2.3)** related to need to supplement protein intake as evidenced by comparison of protein intake with estimated needs.

P (Plan): Nutrition Intervention is **Enteral or Parenteral Nutrition (ND-3)** to change the composition of the enteral feeding by adding 20 grams of protein to it. A second nutrition intervention is **Coordination of Other Health Care During Nutrition Care (RC-1) Discussed** reordering phosphate binders with the medical team. | **A (Assessment):** Feeding increased to goal rate this AM. Patient tolerating feedings without difficulty. **Nutrition Prescription** is 1,675 calories and 100 grams of protein (25 kcal/kg and 1.5 grams of protein) with low phosphorus intake in minimal volume.

D (Diagnosis): Inadequate Intake from Enteral Nutrition Infusion (NI-2.3) related to need to supplement protein intake as evidenced by comparison of protein intake with estimated needs.

I (Intervention): Enteral or Parenteral Nutrition (ND-3) to change the composition of the enteral feeding by adding 20 grams of protein to it. **Coordination of Other Health Care During Nutrition Care (RC-1).** Discussed reordering phosphate binders with the medical team. |

239

Edition: 2007

References

1. Lacey K, Pritchett E. Nutrition Care Process and Model: ADA adopts road map to quality care and outcomes management. *J Am Diet Assoc.* 2003;103:1061-1071.

2. Mathieu J, Foust M, Ouellette P. Implementing nutrition diagnosis, step two in the nutrition care process and model: challenges and lessons learned in two health care facilities. *J Am Diet Assoc.* 2005;105:1636-1640.

Implementing Nutrition Diagnosis, Step Two in the Nutrition Care Process and Model: Challenges and Lessons Learned in Two Health Care Facilities

Jennifer Mathieu; Mandy Foust, RD; Patricia Ouellette, RD

In adherence to the American Dietetic Association's (ADA) Strategic Plan goal of establishing and implementing a standardized Nutrition Care Process (NCP) in the hopes of "increasing demand and utilization of services provided by members" (1), dietetics professionals in two health care facilities established an NCP pilot program in 2005, in collaboration with ADA. The pilot sites were the Virginia Hospital Center in Arlington and the Veterans Affairs Medical Center in San Diego, CA.

This article gives a background on the NCP and Model, the standardized language used in the nutrition diagnosis step, medical record documentation, and an explanation of how the two sites came to participate in the pilot program. It also provides a timeline for each site's implementation of the NCP, including challenges faced and lessons learned. Similarities and differences in approaches will also be discussed. Managers from both facilities will offer advice to facilities who are contemplating implementation of the NCP and nutrition diagnoses in the future.

J. Mathieu is a freelance writer, Houston, TX. M. Foust is clinical nutrition manager, Virginia Hospital Center, Arlington. P. Ouellette is deputy director of nutrition and food services, Veterans Affairs Medical Center, San Diego, CA.

Address correspondence to: Jennifer Mathieu, 5639 Berry Creek Dr, Houston, TX 77017. E-mail: jenmathieu27@yahoo.com
0002-8223/05/10510-0019$30.00/0
doi: 10.1016/j.jada.2005.07.015

BACKGROUND

ADA developed a four-step NCP and Model that appeared in the August 2003 issue of the *Journal*. The NCP consists of four "distinct but interrelated and connected steps"—Nutrition Assessment, Nutrition Diagnosis, Nutrition Intervention, and Nutrition Monitoring and Evaluation (2). The NCP and Model were developed by the Quality Management Committee Work Group with input from the House of Delegates.

This new model calls for dietetics professionals to incorporate a new step—making a nutrition diagnosis—which involves working with defined terminology. It also asks dietetics professionals to chart their diagnosis in the form of a statement that establishes the patient's Problem (diagnostic label), Etiology (cause/contributing risk factors), and Signs and Symptoms (defining characteristics). This is known as a PESS statement, and makes up the heart of the NCP's second step—nutrition diagnosis.

"The second step is the culture shift," says Susan Ramsey, MS, RD, senior manager of medical nutrition services for Sodexho and a member of ADA's Research Committee. "The second step forces us to make a one-line statement. It brings the whole assessment into one clear vision."

According to the article by Lacey and Pritchett, using the new model provides many benefits. The model defines a common language that allows nutrition practice to be more measurable, creates a format that enables the process to generate quantitative and qualitative data that can then be analyzed and interpreted, serves as the structure to validate nutrition care, and shows how the care

that was provided does what it intends to do (2). It also gives the profession a greater sense of autonomy, says Ramsey: "It's given us responsibility for our work instead of looking for permission from others."

The nutrition diagnostic labels and reference sheets were developed by the Standardized Language Task Force, chaired by Sylvia Escott-Stump, MA, RD. It is from this list that dietetics professionals utilizing the NCP list the P (problem) part of the PESS statement. According to Escott-Stump, this Standardized Language will help bring dietetics professionals a new focus and the ability to target their interventions into more effective results that will match the patient nutrition diagnosis (problem).

It is Escott-Stump's belief that documenting nutrition diagnoses, interventions, and outcomes will allow dietetics professionals to better track diagnoses over several clients, allowing the profession to be more likely to track the types of nutrition diagnoses that clients have, and be able to state that the profession affects certain types of acute and chronic diseases more than others.

"For example, now we believe that our impact on cardiovascular, endocrine, and renal diseases is strong, but we may find that our professionals impact gastrointestinal disorders the most," says Escott-Stump. "By having standardized language, we will be able to validate or correct our suspicions."

This pilot implementation of the nutrition care model also tested a new method of charting that differs from the traditional Subjective Objective Assessment Plan format (SOAP). The new ADI template stands for Assessment, Diagnosis, and Intervention (including Monitoring and Evaluation).

According to Dr Esther Myers, PhD, RD, FADA, ADA's Research and Scientific Affairs director, ADA plans to expand these two pilot tests through the Peer Network for Nutrition Diagnosis in the next 2 years. This group of dietetics professionals will receive additional training and networking opportunities to assist them as they implement this new model within their facility and then share their knowledge with other dietetics professionals in their geographical region.

Their experience will be used to determine what additional implementation tools are needed. In addition, a formal research project will be conducted through the Dietetics Practice Based Research Network in early 2006.

IMPLEMENTATION OF THE PROGRAM
Virginia Hospital Center

Mandy Foust, RD and Clinical Nutrition Manager of the Virginia Hospital Center, is contracted through Sodexho to oversee patient services at the 400-bed facility. In December 2004, Foust, who had learned about PESS statements while in school, decided to have her college dietetic intern Anne Avery research current changes and updates in charting for dietetics professionals.

Avery spoke with Dr Myers and discussed the possibility of the Virginia Hospital Center serving as a pilot site for the new model. Foust was excited about the idea for several reasons. "To me, the nutrition care model is a clinically based, concise way of charting that sets goals and is more standardized with other disciplines," she says. Until the implementation of the pilot project, the RDs on staff at the Virginia Hospital Center used the SOAP format of charting.

A conference call took place between Foust, Dr Myers, Avery, and Avery's internship director at Virginia Tech. Foust selected one of her five inpatient registered dietitians (RDs) to serve as the first RD to use the new method. It was decided Avery would present an in-service on the nutrition care model to the dietetics professionals on staff. This in-service provided the RDs with introductory information, the four steps of the NCP, PESS statements, diagnostic labeling, and an explanation of why the changes would be beneficial.

Foust says there were concerns from her staff about the new method. These included that the new ADI charting format would not allow them to be thorough enough and that it seemed "too cookie cutter." Staff also expressed concern that it would be difficult to sum up two or more serious problems in one PESS statement. They also worried that physicians would be wary of the term "nutrition diagnosis."

Over several days in mid-December, Foust arranged meetings with several hospital administrators, including the vice president of the hospital, the chief nursing officer, the medical staff president, and the chief of the nutrition committee to get their feedback on the pilot project. She also kept her supervisor at Sodexho abreast of the situation. "Because I am a contractor, I want to make sure I'm covering my bases," says Foust. She says the Virginia Hospital Center is "very interdisciplinary" and that she wanted there to be an awareness of the upcoming changes.

Administrators initially had questions about how the new method would benefit patients, but Foust says after she met with them and presented them with information on the nutrition care model, they were receptive to the changes. The physician who served as chief of the hospital's nutrition committee had concerns about the idea of a nutrition diagnosis. Foust says she reassured him that the new method did not ask RDs to make a medical diagnosis or interfere with a physician's orders.

After the nutrition committee approved the project in early January 2005, Foust was asked to inform several other hospital staff members about the new format, including the chief of surgery and the chief of surgical education. Because the first RD to participate in the pilot project worked in the intensive care unit (ICU), Foust was also asked to notify the medical director of the ICU, two ICU nurse educators, and the ICU patient care director via formal letters. Responses to these letters encouraged Foust to seek approval for the project from the hospital's patient-monitoring committee.

During the end of January, while waiting for a response from the patient-monitoring committee, Foust met for about an hour each week with

the RD who would be the first to use the new method. The RD used actual patients from her daily census to begin practicing PESS statements and ADI charting. Foust shared the results with Dr Myers and the Standardized Language Task Force often. Through early to mid-February, the RD submitted her notes in both the SOAP format and the new format as a way of practicing the new method.

At the end of January, the patient monitoring committee gave the project its approval. Before implementation officially occurred, Foust requested permission and modified the Hakel-Smith Coding Instrument as an auditing tool to evaluate the charts. She also developed a questionnaire for allied health professionals to give feedback on the new system of charting.

On February 16, 2005, the ICU RD, Korinne Umbaugh, officially began submitting all of her notes using the ADI template. Foust audited two to three charts each day. In late February, a second RD began using the new method of charting. On March 28, a third RD began the process. By the middle of April, all five RDs were using the ADI template, with the fifth RD beginning the process on the second week of the month.

Throughout the entire transition, Foust met formally and informally with staff RDs both individually and in groups. Foust says at least 20 minutes of each weekly hour-long staff meeting continues to be spent discussing the new method of charting and reviewing PESS statements. At this time Foust is editing about 10% of the charts.

Unfortunately, Foust did not receive as many completed questionnaires as she hoped for from allied health professionals. However, her initial chart audits showed that by the end of April the staff had become much more comfortable with the process. Audits revealed notes that steadily became more direct and concise, as well as more outcome-oriented. Extraneous information was not included as often.

Veterans Affairs Medical Center, San Diego

Patricia Ouellette, RD, is the deputy director of nutrition and food services for the Veterans Affairs (VA) Medical

Center in San Diego, CA. The Medical Center is a 238-bed facility. There are three RDs who focus on the inpatient areas of the facility.

In January 2004, the facility's director of nutrition and food service, Ginger Hughes, MS, RD, distributed the August 2003 article by Karen Lacey, MS, RD and Ellen Pritchett, RD, about the NCP that appeared in the *Journal*. The staff was advised to read the article and become familiar with it. In the fall of 2004, internship program director Tere Bush-Zurn and outpatient dietitian Teresa Hilleary received a scholarship to attend the Nutrition Diagnosis Roundtable for Educators workshop at ADA's 2004 Food & Nutrition Conference & Expo. Bush-Zurn and Hilleary relayed what they learned with the rest of their staff when they returned to California.

In November 2004, a staff meeting was held to discuss questions and concerns surrounding the NCP and PESS statements. The staff agreed to start using the PESS statements as soon as possible. After a December 2004 workshop presented by a visiting Lacey, the staff agreed that they wanted to work toward transitioning to the nutrition care model and would serve as a pilot site.

"It evolved after a year of looking at the process and after a lot of discussions with the staff," says Ouellette. "We are a teaching institution and we wanted to challenge ourselves in terms of our practice. We also have a dietetic internship program and feel responsible for providing the interns with the most progressive concepts in our field of practice."

As with the Virginia Hospital Center RDs, the RDs at the VA Medical Center had been using the SOAP format for many years and they had similar concerns over whether the new method would be deemed thorough enough. They were also concerned that one PESS statement would not be enough if the patient had several complicated problems.

Based on staff consensus, in February 2005 the staff started devoting time at the weekly staff meeting to discussing issues related to the new method. The staff practiced writing PESS statements and shared the results with each other during this time. They also discussed questions and concerns related to the new method.

At the same time, several staff members, including the staff's performance improvement/information technology dietitian, worked separately to develop a point-and-click computer version of the inpatient initial nutrition assessment ADI template that could be used by the inpatient RDs on staff when writing their notes.

During the last week in March, the inpatient RDs spent 1 week writing their notes using both the old SOAP method and the new template. On April 4, the staff officially implemented the new version of charting for the inpatient initial nutrition assessments and stopped using the SOAP method completely. For the first month after the official implementation, Ouellette checked every inpatient initial nutrition assessment chart note and provided weekly feedback to the staff.

In May, the auditing components were incorporated into the NFS Periodic Performance Review plan implemented as part of the Joint Commission on Accreditation of Healthcare Organizations' continuous readiness philosophy. Although not required, they believed this was a good way to continue to audit and document the process.

Ouellette continued to meet with RDs individually as problems and questions developed about the change. Her initial audits revealed that the majority of the staff used the same five to six diagnostic labels. She also assessed that after 2 weeks of using the new ADI template exclusively, PESS statements markedly improved and chart notes became more focused and concise. After 3 weeks, the amount of time spent on the notes shortened, suggesting that the staff was becoming more comfortable with the process.

In regard to diagnostic labels, Ouellette's staff began the practice of utilizing two diagnostic labels and combining them into one PESS statement if the two conditions were closely related (eg, difficulty swallowing and chewing difficulty).

The monitoring component of the process still needs to be observed carefully, as many of Ouellette's staff members are not yet in the habit of stating which specific laboratory tests need to be performed.

SIMILARITIES AND DIFFERENCES

The biggest difference between the two sites was the time spent seeking approval for the project before proceeding. As a contractor, Foust believed she needed to secure approval from several different administrators before beginning implementation. Ouellette's approval process occurred much more informally. Ouellette says this is because the VA allows flexibility in how Nutrition and Food Service processes are carried out.

Another difference centered on the way staff RDs began participating in the implementation. Ouellette's staff discussed the process for about a year before they all began the new method of charting at the same time. Ouellette and her staff wanted to work with only one inpatient charting template at a time, and this allowed them to do so. Also, Ouellette believed that if the SOAP method template was available, RDs might be tempted to go back to the old format that they felt most comfortable using.

After the staff in-service, Foust started one of her RDs on the new method and others followed over a period of months. As the implementation was occurring, the staff had several meetings to discuss the new changes. Foust believed this gradual method of implementation allowed time for RDs who were having trouble with the new method to learn from RDs who were actively working with it.

The similarities between both sites included the increased amount of administrative time spent on the change (especially at the manager level) as well as the decision to focus the change on inpatient areas only. Foust and Ouellette both said this decision was made because inpatient cases tend to be more complex, and if these cases could be dealt with successfully it would be even easier to make the transition with outpatient cases. The sites shared another similarity in that the types of concerns held by the staffs were nearly identical, as were the challenges they faced and the lessons they learned.

CHALLENGES AND LESSONS LEARNED

According to Foust and Ouellette, the biggest challenge for both sites was assisting their RDs in completely changing the way they think about their chart notes. "It's a brand new language," says Foust. "My RDs are already seeing 14, 16 patients a day, and it's a long process when you're starting something new."

Both managers say their RDs had a hard time excluding extraneous language. In the SOAP format, for example, RDs were used to including information about everything from decades-old surgeries, the patient's general mood, and other aspects of the patient's condition that are not relevant to a nutrition diagnosis. With the nutrition care model, the charting must be much more exact. "This new method requires us to focus on establishing a nutrition label and forces us to restrict our charting to what is relevant to that nutritional diagnosis," says Ouellette.

Also challenging for the RDs was the creation of the PESS statements. "They initially roadblock with the PESS," says Foust. "It is a completely different way of formatting your thoughts. It's moving from a very conversational way of charting to a more clinical-sounding, concise note. This results in a struggle when first charting."

Staff members at both sites had concerns over what to do when there seemed to be two separate but equally important problems. After discussions with Dr Myers, it was decided that, on occasion, two PESS statements can be used.

Ouellette adds that another challenge comes from the fact that the nutrition care model means a different way of approaching formatting the chart note. "The chart note really has to be decided after determining the PESS statement," says Ouellette. "The statement can only be determined after a thorough nutritional assessment. The chart review and patient consultation method are the same, but the structuring of the chart note is quite different. We no longer do this in a linear fashion. We start from the middle with the PESS statement and complete both ends—assessment and goals—from there."

RDs also struggled with how to write PESS statements for patients that simply had no nutrition risk. Foust says she urged her staff to recognize that if they were experts in making a nutrition diagnosis, they could say that at certain times there is no nutrition diagnosis. Ouellette

adds that it might be a good idea to create a category of "potential" diagnostic labels that could be used for patients who are basically stable with tube feedings or dialysis, but who still need to be monitored.

While the PESS statement proved to be the most difficult hurdle, RDs also had to learn to be more specific when it came time to express how they would monitor and evaluate their patients. It wasn't enough to write "monitor labs," says Foust. "You need to give specific labs and then follow with an explanation and expected outcomes."

For managers, keeping morale of staff up was a challenge. This was especially true for RDs who spoke of feeling stifled by the new method and who constantly feared they were making a mistake. Managers learned they needed to spend extra time encouraging their RDs and reminding them that they were working on a cutting-edge project.

"All of my RDs are competent and brilliant," says Foust. "Changing the way they chart and implementing new techniques can cause doubt. This can potentially alter their clinical self-confidence, and you want to maintain a positive outlook to avoid this."

Both Foust and Ouellette say it was beneficial to work in groups on PESS statements and learn from each other, being sure to highlight well-written charts as well as the ones that that needed attention. Foust and Ouellette also learned that not every RD would learn at the same pace. While RDs who had been in the profession for a shorter amount of time were often able to grasp the concept faster, Ouellette adds that, in general, the RDs who had the easiest time were the ones with personality types that adjusted well to change, regardless of experience level.

ADVICE TO SITES READY FOR IMPLEMENTATION

Both Foust and Ouellette offer similar advice to sites seeking to implement the NCP and model. Both suggest an in-service for the staff and the distribution of materials well ahead of implementation. Ouellette also suggests providing training from a knowledgeable source, as was the case with Karen Lacey speaking to

her staff using ADA slides describing the NCP.

Both managers suggest setting aside a generous portion of the weekly staff meeting time to discuss the model, review PESS statements, answer questions, and motivate the staff with positive feedback.

While Foust and Ouellette had different experiences in terms of seeking approval from the administration to implement the program, both suggest allowing time to meet with the necessary people in the facility, as the approval needed will differ from facility to facility.

Most of all, Ouellette and Foust suggest that future managers and staffs remind themselves that transitioning to the nutrition care model is a beneficial but time-consuming process that requires patience. Both say they have seen marked improvements among their staff over time, and many of the initial challenges have been overcome with patience and practice.

"You're changing the way you're thinking, you're changing the way you're charting—it's a huge change," says Ouellette. "There are no shortcuts you can take, but my staff is excited about being on the forefront. It's certainly a worthwhile thing."

Adds Foust, "This continues to be an excellent, groundbreaking experience."

The authors would like to acknowledge the contributions of the following people in the preparation of this article: Susan Ramsey, MS, RD, senior manager of medical nutrition services for Sodexho who also serves on ADA's Research Committee; Sylvia Escott-Stump, MA, RD, Standardized Language Task Force Chair; and Esther Myers, PhD, RD, FADA, ADA's Research and Scientific Affairs director.

References
1. American Dietetic Association Strategic Plan. Available at: http://www.eatright.org (member-only section). Accessed April 17, 2005.
2. Lacey K, Pritchett E. Nutrition Care Process and Model: ADA adopts road map to quality care and outcomes management. *J Am Diet Assoc.* 2003;103:1061-1072.

TIMELINES OF IMPLEMENTATION

Virginia Hospital Center

December 2004
- Idea of participating in pilot project presented to facility.
- Staff in-service held to educate staff about the NCP, ADI charting, and PESS statements.
- Meetings between clinical nutrition manager and hospital administrators to discuss the NCP and seek approval for participation in the pilot project.

January 2005
- Hospital nutrition committee approves the pilot project.
- Other hospital administrators, including those on the unit where the first RD to participate in the project works, are informed of the pilot project.
- The hospital's patient-monitoring committee approves the pilot project.
- Throughout the month of January, the first RD to take part in the project meets regularly with clinical nutrition manager to practice ADI charting and PESS statements.
- Clinical nutrition manager obtains permission and modifies the Hakel-Smith Coding Instrument as a way of auditing charts.

February 2005
- From early to mid-February, the first RD to participate in the project charts using both the ADI and SOAP formats before formally transitioning to the ADI method alone on February 16.
- In late February, a second RD begins to exclusively use the ADI method of charting.

March 2005
- By the end of March, a third RD has transitioned to the ADI method of charting.
- Throughout the entire process, the clinical nutrition manager meets formally and informally with RDs both individually and in groups to discuss concerns and monitor progress.
- Throughout the process, at least 20 minutes of each weekly staff meeting are devoted to reviewing the ADI method of charting, PESS statements, questions, and concerns.

April 2005
- By the start of April, a fourth RD is exclusively using the ADI method of charting, with the fifth and final RD making the transition by mid-April.
- The clinical nutrition manager audits 10% of charts.

Veterans Affairs Medical Center, San Diego

January 2004
- Director of nutrition and food services distributes journal articles about the NCP to staff.

October 2004
- Two staff members attend the Nutrition Diagnosis Roundtable for Educators workshop at ADA's Food & Nutrition Conference & Expo and share what they learn with the rest of the staff upon their return.

November 2004
- A staff meeting is held to discuss questions and concerns surrounding the NCP and PESS statements.

December 2004
- ADA's Karen Lacey, Chair of ADA's Quality Management Working Group on the NCP, provides the staff with a workshop on the NCP.

February 2005
- The staff begins to devote time during each weekly staff meeting to practice using the new method and to share PESS statements.
- Several staff members, including the staff's performance improvement/information technology dietitian, develop a point-and-click computer version of the ADI template for the staff to use.

March 2005
- Toward the end of March, the staff spends 1 week using both the SOAP format and the new ADI template to chart notes.

April 2005
- On April 4, the staff officially implements the new method of charting exclusively.
- The deputy director of nutrition and food service checks each inpatient initial nutrition assessment chart note and provides feedback to individuals.

May 2005
- Ongoing auditing was accomplished by incorporating the auditing elements into the periodic performance review plan implemented to ensure continuous readiness for the Joint Commission on Accreditation of Healthcare Organization's review.

NUTRITION CARE PROCESS AND MODEL WORK GROUP

Karen Lacey, MS, RD, Chair
Elvira Johnson, MS, RD
Kessey Kieselhorst, MPA, RD
Mary Jane Oakland, PhD, RD, FADA
Carlene Russell, RD, FADA
Patricia Splett, PhD, RD, FADA
Staff Liaisons:
Harold Holler, RD
Esther Myers, PhD, RD, FADA
Ellen Pritchett, RD
Karri Looby, MS, RD

The work group would like to extend a special thank you to Marion Hammond, MS, and Naomi Trostler, PhD, RD, for their assistance in development of the NCP and Model.

STANDARDIZED LANGUAGE TASK FORCE

Sylvia Escott-Stump, MA, RD, Chair
Peter Beyer, MS, RD
Christina Biesemeier, MS, RD, FADA
Pam Charney, MS, RD
Marion Franz, MS, RD
Karen Lacey, MS, RD
Carrie LePeyre, RD
Kathleen Niedert, MBA, RD, FADA
Mary Jane Oakland, PhD, RD, FADA
Patricia Splett, PhD, MPH, RD
Frances Tyus, MS, RD

The task force would like to extend a special thank you to Naomi Trostler, PhD, RD, FADA.

American Dietetic Association: Scope of Dietetics Practice Framework

Julie O'Sullivan Maillet, PhD, RD, FADA; Janet Skates, MS, RD, FADA; Ellen Pritchett, RD

Dietetics practitioners, like most health care practitioners, are often faced with the difficult question of whether an activity is within their scope of practice. As your Association, the American Dietetics Association (ADA) is faced with providing guidance on the breadth and depth of dietetics practice.

With dietetics practitioners taking on shifting and more diverse roles, as well as specialty and advanced practice, the Association committed itself to equipping its members with new tools to operate in a diverse, highly changeable environment. The result is the Scope of Dietetics Practice Framework, which serves as a cornerstone for the profession. The framework is a flexible decision-making structure that empowers practitioners to provide safe, effective, and timely health care services.

J. O'Sullivan-Maillet is the associate dean for Academic Affairs and research chairman at the University of Medicine and Dentistry of New Jersey, Newark, the co-chair of the Practice Definitions Task Force, and a member of the ADA Ethics Committee. J. Skates is a consultant in private practice in Kingsport, TN, co-chair of the Practice Definitions Task Force, a member of the Quality Management Committee, and Tennessee delegate to the House of Delegates. E. Pritchett is the director of Quality and Outcomes at the American Dietetics Association, Chicago, IL.

Questions regarding the Scope of Dietetics Practice Framework may be addressed to Ellen Pritchett, RD, at epritchett@eatright.org.

0002-8223/05/10504-0014$30.00/0
doi: 10.1016/j.jada.2005.02.001

The framework was approved by the ADA House of Delegates on November 3, 2003. For more history behind its development and more detail about the Framework, consult the Web site at www.eatright.org. This site will continue to evolve as the members of the Association use it to help realize ADA's vision of its members as the most valued source of food and nutrition information.

THE BASIC FRAMEWORK

The Framework is an umbrella that encompasses the entire practice of dietetics. It is for use by practicing registered dietitians (RDs), dietetics technicians, registered (DTRs), and dietetics students as a career-development guide. It can also be used as an aid to organizations when making employment decisions.

The Framework covers three broad areas:

- Foundation knowledge—definition of dietetics as a profession, five characteristics of the profession, and educational resources. These are resources and information that every professional should know.
- Evaluation resources—code of ethics and standards of practice and professional performance outlined for RDs, DTRs, and specialty or advanced professionals. These are evaluation tools that practitioners and their managers can use to gauge and channel performance. For example, a DTR can apply the DTR Standards of Practice to ensure that he or she is following accepted practice in his or her day-to-day work, to determine whether a particular competency falls within the scope of his or her work, or to ensure that his or her role description is accurate and comprehensive.
- Decision aids—decision tree, deci-

sion analysis tool, definition of terms, and other resources that practitioners can apply to their situations to further define the scope of their practice. The first two aids can be used to determine whether a requested service, such as providing instruction on the use of an insulin pump for a patient with diabetes, falls within one's legitimate qualified scope of practice. These tools are especially helpful when state, federal, and ADA documents do not clearly delineate responsibility. The Definition of Terms sets a common vocabulary for practitioners to use when discussing professional matters.

There are four underlying assumptions in the design of this scope: (a) the assumption that level of experience, skills, and proficiency with respect to identified activities varies among individuals; (b) the assumption that dietetics practitioners may not be competent to practice in all aspects of the field; (c) the assumption that individual practitioners are expected to practice only in areas in which they are competent; and (d) the assumption that practitioners should pursue additional education and experience to expand the scope of their personal dietetics practice.

HOW THE FRAMEWORK IS STRUCTURED

The Framework consists of three building blocks that, when viewed together, describe the full range of roles, responsibilities, and activities that dietetics practitioners are educated and authorized to perform today. To facilitate the growth of the profession and the growth of individual practitioners into new roles and areas of responsibility, the blocks have been designed with flexible boundaries. Within the blocks, spe-

Block One: Foundation Knowledge			
Definition of Dietetics as a Profession: "The integration and application of principles derived from the sciences of food, nutrition, management, communication, and biological, physiological, behavioral, and social sciences to achieve and maintain optimal human health" within flexible scope of practice boundaries to capture the breadth of the profession.			
Five Characteristics of the Profession	**Professionals Who Demonstrate This Characteristic . . .**	**Core Professional Resources**	
Code of Ethics	Follow a Code of Ethics for practice	Code of Ethics	Ethics Opinions
Body of Knowledge	Possess a unique theoretical body of knowledge and science-based knowledge that leads to defined skills, abilities, and norms	Philosophy and Mission: ● Research Philosophy and Diagram	Research, Position Papers, Practice Papers, Published Literature
Education	Demonstrate competency at selected level by meeting set criteria and passing credentialing exams	CADE[a] Core Competencies and Emphasis Areas	CDR[b] Certification (RD[c], DTR[d])
Autonomy	● Are reasonably independent and self-governing in decision-making and practice ● Demonstrate critical thinking skills ● Take on roles that require greater responsibility and accountability both professionally and legally ● Stay abreast of new knowledge and technical skills	The CDR Professional Development Portfolio Process offers a framework for credentialed professionals to develop specific goals, identify learning needs, and pursue continuing education opportunities. This may encompass certificates (such as weight management), specialty certificates (such as CSR[e]), advanced practice certification, or advanced degrees.	
Service	Provide food and nutrition care services for individuals and population groups and other stakeholders. Additional functions may include: ● Managing food and other material resources ● Marketing services and products ● Teaching dietitians and other professionals or students ● Conducting research ● Managing human resources ● Managing facilities	Nutrition Care Process and Model *Nutrition Care Manual*	Nationally developed guidelines ADA Evidence-Based Guides for Practice
		Practice-Based Evidence ■ Dietetics Practice Outcomes Research ■ Dietetics Practice Audit	

Figure 1. Scope of Dietetics Practice Framework—Block One: Foundation Knowledge. [a]CADE=Commission on Accreditation for Dietetics Education. [b]CDR=Commission on Dietetic Registration. [c]RD=registered dietitian. [d]DTR=dietetics technician, registered. [e]CSR=board-certified specialist in renal nutrition.

Block Two: Evaluation Resources		
Code of Ethics	DTR[a] Standards of Practice in Nutrition Care RD[b] Standards of Practice in Nutrition Care ↓	Standards of Professional Performance for Dietetics Professionals ↓
	RD Specialty or RD Advanced Standards of Practice	RD Specialty or RD Advanced Standards of Professional Performance

Figure 2. Scope of Dietetics Practice Framework—Block Two: Evaluation Resources. [a]DTR=dietetics technician, registered. [b]RD=registered dietitian.

cific tools are provided to inform, enable, and support practitioners' career decisions.

Dietetics practitioners work in a variety of environments and serve many different functions. Because of the dynamic nature of our profession, a flexible algorithmic approach was adopted. An algorithm is a series of steps that can be followed to solve a problem or achieve a goal. In the ADA's case, there are a multitude of goals and pathways. For example, the needs of RDs who specialize in witness testimony or diabetes care are quite different from those of DTRs who have just entered the profession. Given this variance in applications and needs, the Framework should be viewed as an umbrella that describes, rather than defines, the safe, sanc-

Block Three: Decision Aids		
Decision Analysis Tool	Decision Tree	Definition of Terms
Supporting Documentation for use with Decision Tree and Decision Analysis Tool		

Licensure/Certification/Credentials Examples include: State Licensure, Commission on Dietetic Registration Credentials, Specialty Certificates, Advanced Practice Certification, or Advanced Degrees **Organizational Privileging** **Individual** Commission on Dietetic Registration **Professional Development Portfolio** Portfolio Learning Plan and Learning Activities Log	**Evidence-Based Practice** ● Existing Research and Literature ● ADA Position and Practice Papers, Ethics Opinions ● Nationally-Developed Guidelines and ADA Guides for Practice **Practice-Based Evidence** ● Dietetics Practice Outcomes Research

Figure 3. Scope of Professional Practice Framework—Block Three: Decision Aids.

tioned practice of dietetics, including its foundations, career progression, and tools for negotiating dietetics practice.

The Framework captures core responsibilities based on formal education and training at the entry level (Foundation Knowledge), then builds from there to encompass practice grounded in knowledge, skills, and experience, including additional certification or advanced degrees (Evaluation Resources). The Framework also provides tools for helping practitioners grow their practice in response to changing role or job needs (Decision Aids). This approach allows our profession to evolve as new research and practice trends emerge. Viewed in entirety, the Framework can be seen as a series of stepping stones that guide the profession into the future at the individual practitioner level and, through our combined efforts, at the collective level.

BLOCK ONE: FOUNDATION KNOWLEDGE

Every profession, from clergy to accounting to medicine, defines precisely what it is that the profession does and the specific behaviors that practitioners must carry out to engage in the profession. Generally, those characteristics include a code of ethics, a body of knowledge, education, a certain level of autonomy, and service.

Dietetics is a broad discipline incorporating many venues. The best definition of the profession says that dietetics "is the integration and application of principles derived from the sciences of food, nutrition, management, communication, and biolog-

ical, physiological, behavioral, and social services to achieve and maintain optimal human health" (1). This definition was reaffirmed by the ADA Board of Directors in September 2003. The definition of the profession and its key characteristics are the foundation of our profession—both the everyday, working knowledge of who we are and what we do as professionals, and why we are uniquely, distinctly dietetics professionals and not physicians or nurses. This clear understanding guides our practice along safe, acceptable lines; trains students for successful practice; ensures our certification process adequately measures competence; and holds us accountable for the services we render and methods we pursue to offer them to the public.

Core resources available to dietetics professionals align with each characteristic (Figure 1). To act within the scope of dietetics practice, we must consider its definition, our individual competency, and the core documents that lay the foundation for our profession: our Code of Ethics (2), our entry-level educational competencies (3), our process and model for nutrition care (4), and our standards of practice and professional performance (5). These, along with position papers, evidence-based guides for practice, and research, define the core of our profession.

BLOCK TWO: EVALUATION RESOURCES

The evaluation resources continue on from the Foundation knowledge and include the Code of Ethics, the Standards of Practice in Nutrition Care, and the Standards of Professional

Performance (Figure 2). Major expansion is anticipated in this area with the Standards of Practice and Standards of Professional Performance for Registered Dietitians (Generalist, Specialty, and Advanced) in Diabetes Care in next month's issue of the *Journal of the American Dietetic Association*, as well as several others anticipated within the year.

The new Standards of Practice in nutrition care, which are based on the Nutrition Care Process and Model, the Commission on Accreditation for Dietetics Education (CADE) educational core competencies; research impacting the profession; and the updated Standards of Professional Performance are presented in the article by Kieselhorst and colleagues (5) in this month's issue of the *Journal*, and are key resources in evaluating the scope of practice within the profession (5).

Together with relevant state, federal, and licensure laws, these resources serve as a guide for ensuring safe and effective dietetics practices. They may also be used to evaluate performance, to make hiring decisions, to determine whether a particular activity falls within an individual's legitimate scope of the practice or to initiate regulatory reform.

BLOCK THREE: DECISION AIDS

Dietetics practitioners must practice safely, ethically, and effectively when presented with new challenges within a health care environment that is highly diverse and evolving. Although the dietetics profession as a whole has flexible boundaries, individual practitioners must take responsibility for

Block One: Foundation Knowledge

Definition of Dietetics as a Profession: "The integration and application of principles derived from the sciences of food, nutrition, management, communication, and biological, physiological, behavioral, and social sciences to achieve and maintain optimal human health" within flexible scope of practice boundaries to capture the breadth of the profession.

Five Characteristics of the Profession	Professionals Who Demonstrate This Characteristic ...	Core Professional Resources	
Code of Ethics	Follow a Code of Ethics for practice	Code of Ethics	Ethics Opinions
Body of Knowledge	Possess a unique body of theoretical and science-based knowledge that leads to defined skills, abilities, and norms	Philosophy and Mission: • Research Philosophy and Diagram	Research, Position Papers, Practice Papers, Published Literature
Education	Demonstrate competency at selected level by meeting set criteria and passing credentialing exams	CADE[a] Core Competencies and Emphasis Areas	CDR[b] Certification (RD[c], DTR[d])
Autonomy	• Are reasonably independent and self-governing in decision-making and practice • Demonstrate critical thinking skills • Take on roles that require greater responsibility and accountability both professionally and legally • Stay abreast of new knowledge and technical skills	The CDR Professional Development Portfolio Process offers a framework for credentialed professionals to develop specific goals, identify learning needs, and pursue continuing education opportunities. This may encompass certificates (such as weight management), specialty certificates (such as CSR[e]), advanced practice certification, or advanced degrees.	
Service	Provide food and nutrition care services for individuals and population groups and other stakeholders. Additional functions may include: • Managing food and other material resources • Marketing services and products • Teaching dietitians and other professionals or students • Conducting research • Managing human resources • Managing facilities	Nutrition Care Process and Model	Nationally developed guidelines / ADA Evidence-Based Guides for Practice
		Practice-Based Evidence • Dietetics Practice Outcomes Research • Dietetics Practice Audit	

The Framework consists of three building blocks with flexible boundaries. The blocks describe the full range of responsibilities, roles, and activities that dietetics professionals are educated and authorized to perform. The flexible boundaries allow for new roles to emerge. Because of the complexity of our profession, it is impossible to present this information as a list of isolated activities that are parceled out at different levels. Rather, a stepped algorithmic approach is needed to capture the breadth of the profession, allow individual practitioners to draw from the full range of resources, and lend our scope of practice the flexibility it needs to evolve as new research in dietetics and practice emerge.

From an individual perspective, whether an activity is within your scope of practice is influenced by every level of the Framework— our Foundation Knowledge, Code of Ethics, Standards of Practice, and Standards of Professional Performance—as well as by licensure and certification laws, research, guides for practice and expert opinion, and new research.

Block Two: Evaluation Resources

The evaluation resources listed here are intended for use in conjunction with relevant state, federal and licensure laws. Together with the laws, they serve as a guide for ensuring safe and effective dietetics practice. Practitioners can use them **to evaluate performance, make hiring decisions, determine whether a particular activity falls within the legitimate scope of the practice, or to initiate regulatory reform.** The core standards are based on the Nutrition Care Process and Model (NCPM) and Commission on Accreditation for Dietetics Education (CADE) educational core competencies). Specialty and advanced standards can evolve for specific practice areas.

Code of Ethics	DTR Standards of Practice in Nutrition Care / RD Standards of Practice in Nutrition Care	Standards of Professional Performance for Dietetics Professionals
	↓	↓
	RD Specialty or RD Advanced Standards of Practice	RD Specialty or RD Advanced Standards of Professional Performance

Block Three: Decision Aids

The healthcare environment in which we work is highly diverse and always evolving. The resources listed here are intended to help dietetics professionals respond to new demands. By using the Decision Tree and Decision Analysis Tool, professionals can fully consider whether a new role or activity falls within the legitimate scope of their practices, and thereby grow their practices to encompass new areas. This is particularly helpful when state, federal, organizational and educational guidelines have not yet expanded to address a need. The other resources can be applied to seek guidance when making such decisions, or when effecting change at the local or national level to reflect emerging trends and needs.

Decision Analysis Tool	Decision Tree	Definition of Terms
Supporting Documentation for use with Decision Tree and Decision Analysis Tool		

Licensure/ Certification/Credentials Examples include: State Licensure, CDR Credentials, Specialty Certificates, Advanced Practice Certification, or Advanced Degrees. **Organizational Privileging** **Individual CDR Professional Development Portfolio** *Portfolio* Learning Plan and Learning Activities Log	**Evidence Based Practice** • Existing Research and Literature • ADA Position and Practice Papers, Ethics Opinions • Nationally-Developed Guidelines and ADA Guides for Practice **Practice Based Evidence** • Dietetics Practice Outcomes Research

The arrows reflect the flexible, dynamic nature of the Framework. At both the individual practitioner level and our collective professional level, developments in one area of the Framework influence others. For example, as new trends in dietetics practice emerge, education, certification, and standards of practice and professional performance will change to address them. Likewise, as a practitioner tailors his or her individual scope of practice through experience and training, this will influence the resources utilized at every level.

Figure 4. American Dietetic Association Scope of Dietetics Practice Framework. [a]CADE=Commission on Accreditation for Dietetics Education. [b]CDR=Commission on Dietetic Registration. [c]RD=registered dietitian. [d]DTR=dietetics technician, registered. [e]CSR=board-certified specialist in renal nutrition.

When to Use the Decision Analysis Tool: Use this tool to determine whether a specific requested service or act falls within your individualized scope of practice. This tool can be used in conjunction with the Decision Tree, or separate from it.

Instructions for Use: Complete each section, and then follow the instructions at the end of each section.

Part A: General Review

1. Describe the activity or service to be performed:

_____

_____

2. Review the practice expectations (job description, policies and procedures) and core competencies for your level (DTR, RD, or RD Specialty/Advanced Practice) to determine whether the service or act is permitted.
3. Review the Code of Ethics, Standards of Practice in Nutrition Care, and Standards of Professional Performance for your practice level to determine whether the service or act is permitted.
4. Review any licensure laws to determine whether the activity is allowed or not explicitly restricted.

Instructions: If the service or act is NOT explicitly permitted by 2 or 3 above, or explicitly restricted by 4 above, go on to Part B and/or the Decision Tree. If it is explicitly permitted, go to Part F.

Part B: Education, Credentialing, and Privileging

1. If the activity or service was *not* included in your basic DTR/RD education program, have you since completed a training program that demonstrates competence? ❑ No ❑ Yes
2. If yes, has this training been documented? ❑ No ❑ Yes
3. Is the activity or service becoming so routine across the profession that it can reasonably and prudently be assumed within scope? ❑ No ❑ Yes
4. Do the policies and procedures, your manual, or your credentialing and privileging for your employer permit the activity or service? ❑ N/A ❑ No ❑ Yes
5. Does performing the activity pass the "reasonable and prudent" test for dietetics practice? ❑ No ❑ Yes
6. Is the activity reflective of the consumer's desires and appropriately authorized? ❑ No ❑ Yes
7. Is the activity authorized by federal statute, if applicable (eg, Medicare Medical Nutrition Therapy)? ❑ N/A ❑ No ❑ Yes

Instructions: If you answered "no" to any of the above questions, the activity may not be within your scope of practice. Go to Part C for further analysis. If you answered "yes" or "N/A" to all the questions, then proceed to Part F of this tool.

Part C: Existing Documentation

1. Does information about this activity exist in nationally developed guidelines and standards of practice; or from a local, community, or national perspective? ❑ No ❑ Yes
2. Are there statements or opinions from professional groups or dietetics organizations on this activity? ❑ No ❑ Yes
3. Does the activity meet the requirements of the Dietetics Practice Act for your state, if applicable? ❑ N/A ❑ No ❑ Yes
4. Does carrying out the activity pass the "reasonable and prudent" test for dietetics practice? ❑ No ❑ Yes

Instructions: If you answer "no" to any of the above questions, go to Part D to review Advisory Opinions. If you answer "yes" or "N/A" to all these questions, your institution may want to consider including the activity in its official policies and procedures, competency, credentialing, and privileging literature. You can proceed to Part F, if you answer "yes" or "N/A" to all the questions in this section.

Figure 5. American Dietetic Association Scope of Dietetics Practice Framework Decision Analysis Tool.

---

determining their competence to provide a specific service. The ADA developed new decision aids, listed in Block Three (Figure 3), to help individual dietetics practitioners to do just that (Figure 4). By using the Decision Analysis Tool, the Decision Tree, the Definition of Terms, and other decision aids, dietetics practitioners can fully consider whether a new service is within their legitimate scope of practice and articulate their reasons for including the service based on education, credentials, licen-

sure and certification rules, recertification requirements, organizational setting, and other factors.

The Decision Analysis Tool (Figure 5) and the Decision Tree (Figure 6) are the key tools. The Decision Analysis Tool can be used alone or in conjunction with the Decision Tree. State regulations, organizational policies and procedures, and reasonability of the practice are the basics for determining whether a dietetics practitioner should perform a service. The definitions of terms are needed for consistency within the pro-

fession, and the decision analysis tool for the individual practitioner are essential tools for all dietetics practitioners.

The Decision Tree and Decision Analysis Tool are particularly helpful when state, federal, organizational, and educational guidelines have not yet expanded to address a need. However, the extent and scope of individual dietetics practice is dependent on all the resources listed in Block Three. Practitioners should apply them to seek guidance when

Part D: Advisory Opinions

1. Is there an Advisory Opinion on this activity or service?   ❏ *No*   ❏ *Yes*
2. Is the activity or service covered in the policy and procedure manual for your employer?   ❏ *No*   ❏ *Yes*
3. Is the activity or service *not* explicitly restricted by the licensure laws for your state?   ❏ *No*   ❏ *Yes*
4. Is your competence for performing this activity or service documented in your personnel file?   ❏ *No*   ❏ *Yes*
5. Does carrying out the activity or service pass the "reasonable and prudent" test for dietetics practice?   ❏ *No*   ❏ *Yes*
6. Is the activity or service reflective of the consumer's desires and appropriately authorized?   ❏ *No*   ❏ *Yes*

Instructions: If you answered "no" to any of the above questions, consider pursuing an Advisory Opinion through your organization or the ADA. To obtain an Advisory Opinion, go to Part E. If you answered "yes" to all of the above questions, go to Part F.

Part E: Obtaining an Advisory Opinion

1. Obtain and complete an Advisory Opinion Request Form from your organization or the ADA.
2. Complete the research necessary, following the guidelines for your organization[a] or the ADA[b], based on your selection in Step 1.
3. If your request is to the ADA, submit five copies of your research results to the ADA's Scope of Practice Framework Advisory Committee. The ADA's Scope of Practice Framework Advisory Committee will review the request during the first scheduled Scope of Practice Framework Advisory Committee meeting following receipt of the request. After the Scope of Practice Framework Advisory Committee review of your request, you will receive a communication indicating whether an advisory opinion will be recommended and when to expect a complete the advisory opinion. (Not all requests will result in an advisory opinion. For requests that result in an advisory opinion, the opinion may also be published in the journal or on the ADA website if appropriate). If your request is to another organization, follow that organization's guidelines for submitting your request.

Instructions: Once you have received the Advisory Opinion, proceed to Part F provided the opinion supports performance of the activity. If the Opinion does **not** support it, and you have answered "no" to any of the questions in Parts A-D, you are not authorized to perform the activity.

Part F: Performing the Service or Activity

Provided you have answered "yes" to all of the questions in any of the above sections and followed the instructions at the end of the section directing you to Part F, you may consider performing the act with valid orders when necessary and in accordance with organizational policies and procedures.

[a]Advisory Opinions are responses to questions that dietetics professionals, health care providers, and consumers have about (a) interpreting standards of practice, or (b) applying the Nutrition Care Process to their particular situation.

[b]In general, the ADA approaches Advisory Opinions by first identifying the level of credential or licensure needed. Second, the context of the clinical situation is considered: Is the question widespread and frequently asked by dietetics professionals and health care providers? Next, the degree of independence in performing the activity is considered: What level of preparation is needed to safely and competently perform the activity? Finally, questions such as the following are considered: Are there quality assessment mechanisms to evaluate the performance of the activity? What are the relevant community or national guidelines? Is there a current body of knowledge cited in the literature?

Figure 5. (continued)

making individual scope of practice decisions or when trying to effect change at the local or national level to reflect emerging trends and needs.

SUMMARY

As a whole, the Framework provides a structure for our profession by describing the full range of resources available to us all, at every stage of development. At the broadest end of the spectrum, the Framework emphasizes the dietetics practitioner's professional accountability and places decisions about boundaries of practice in the hands of the individual practitioner. It is intended to be used throughout the profession by students and educators, individual RDs and DTRs, people who have just entered the profession, people who have progressed to advanced or specialty practice, retired dietetics professionals who maintain the active RD

or DTR credential, hiring managers, certification and licensure boards, national committee members, researchers, and anyone encountering new challenges at work. It serves as a tool for everyone who engages in the profession of dietetics. And, as we individually and collectively change to respond to new developments in the health care environment, so too will our Framework evolve over time to reflect this.

Although Julie O'Sullivan Maillet, Janet Skates, and Ellen Pritchett are the authors of this article, the work reflects the entire Practice Definitions Taskforce, including Karmeen Kulkarni, MS, RD; Sandra McNeil, MA, RD, FADA; Lorna West, DTR; Beth Leonberg, MS, RD, FADA; and Sally Cohenour, MS, RD, as well as the input of the House of Delegates, the Commission on Dietetic Registration, and the Board of Directors.

References

1. American Dietetic Association. ADA Research Philosophy. Available at: http://www.eatright.org/Member/index_10895.cfm. Accessed March 2, 2005.
2. Code of Ethics for the Profession of Dietetics. *J Am Diet Assoc.* 1999;99:109-113.
3. Bruening KS, Mitchell BE, Pfeiffer MM. 2002 Accreditation Standards for Dietetics Education. *J Am Diet Assoc.* 2002;102:566-577.
4. Lacey K, Pritchett E. Nutrition care process and model: ADA adopts road map to quality care and outcomes management. *J Am Diet Assoc.* 2003;103:1061-1072.
5. Kieselhorst KJ, Skates J, Pritchett E. American Dietetic Association: Standards of Practice in Nutrition Care and updated Standards of Professional Performance. *J Am Diet Assoc.* 2005;105:641-645.

When to use the Decision Tree: Use this tool when trying to determine whether a specific activity or service (such as assuming responsibility for instructing patients with diabetes on insulin pump usage or ordering nutrition related labs) falls within your individual scope of practice.

Instructions for Use:

Start on the left side of the diagram and match numbered boxes with each "Question to Ask Yourself" on the right of the diagram. Fully consider all decision points.

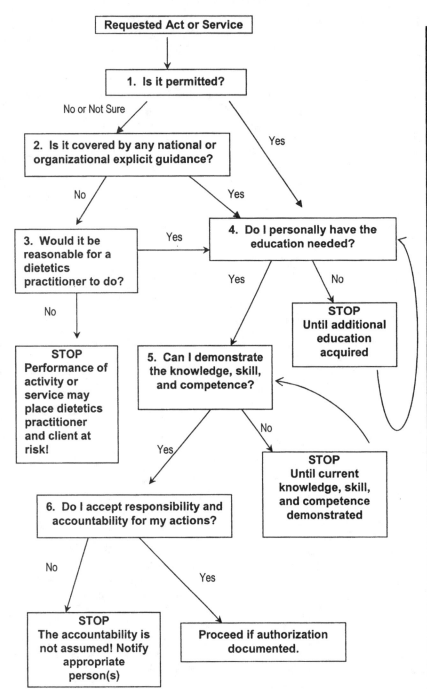

Questions to Ask Yourself

1. Does the license or credential I hold permit me to perform this activity or service?

2. Is the activity or service consistent with the following?
   - Entry level dietetics education and credentialing (CADE and CDR)
   - ADA Standards of Practice, Standards of Professional Performance, Code of Ethics
   - ADA position statements or practice papers; dietetics literature/research
   - Nutrition practice guidelines or protocols
   - National organization standards of practice
   - Institution job description or privileges
   - Accrediting Organization Standards
   - Federal Statutes and Regulations

3. Would the activity or service be within the accepted "standard of practice " that would be provided in similar circumstances by reasonable and prudent dietetics practitioners who have similar training, education, skill, competence, and experience?

4. Have I acquired the depth and breadth of knowledge needed to safely and effectively perform this activity or service through training, such as a pre-professional program, a continuing education program, or self-study?

5. Have I personally demonstrated current knowledge, skills, and competence to safely perform this activity or service?

6. Am I personally prepared to accept the consequences of my actions?

IF YOU HAVE ANSWERED YES TO EACH OF THESE QUESTIONS, perform the activity or service with valid order, when necessary, and in accordance with organizational policies and procedures.

Figure 6. American Dietetic Association Scope of Dietetics Practice Framework Decision Tree.

American Dietetic Association: Standards of Practice in Nutrition Care and Updated Standards of Professional Performance

Kessey J. Kieselhorst, MPA, RD; Janet Skates, MS, RD, FADA; Ellen Pritchett, RD

Web site exclusive!

Editor's note: The Appendix that accompanies this article is available online at www.adajournal.org.

As the most valued source of food and nutrition services, dietetics professionals are accountable and responsible for their practices and the unique services they provide. The American Dietetic Association (ADA) leads the dietetics profession by developing standards by which the quality of practice and service can be evaluated. Within the Scope of Dietetics Practice

K. Kieselhorst is the manager of Clinical Nutrition Services and director of Dietetic Internship at Geisinger Medical Center, Danville, PA; she is also the chair of the Quality Management Committee and Pennsylvania delegate to the House of Delegates. **J. Skates** is a consultant in private practice, Kingsport, TN; she is also a member of the Quality Management Committee, co-chair of the Practice Definitions Task Force, and Tennessee delegate to the House of Delegates. **E. Pritchett** is the director of Quality and Outcomes at ADA headquarters in Chicago, IL.

Questions regarding the Standards of Practice in Nutrition Care for the Registered Dietitian (RD), Standards of Practice in Nutrition Care for the Dietetic Technician, Registered (DTR), and Standards of Professional Performance for Dietetics Professionals may be addressed to Ellen Pritchett, RD, Director of Quality and Outcomes at ADA, at epritchett@eatright.org

0002-8223/05/10504-0018$30.00/0
doi: 10.1016/j.jada.2005.02.039

Framework (1), the standards, along with the Code of Ethics (2), guide and direct the practice and professional performance of dietetics in all settings (see the article by O'Sullivan Maillet and colleagues in this issue).

The standards describe a competent level of dietetics practice and professional performance. They are authoritative statements addressing four standards of practice in nutrition care, designed as two separate sets of standards—one for registered dietitians (RDs) and one for dietetic technicians, registered (DTRs)—as well as six standards of professional performance common to all registered dietetics professionals. The Standards of Practice in Nutrition Care and Standards of Professional Performance are generic standards and may evolve to include specialty and advanced practice standards for RDs in specific practice areas.

This article presents the ADA's Standards of Practice in Nutrition Care and the updated Standards of Professional Performance (see the Web site exclusive Appendix at www.adajournal.org) incorporating for the first time the ADA's Nutrition Care Process and Model (3).

STANDARDS OF PRACTICE IN NUTRITION CARE FOR THE REGISTERED DIETITIAN, STANDARDS OF PRACTICE IN NUTRITION CARE FOR THE DIETETIC TECHNICIAN, REGISTERED, AND STANDARDS OF PROFESSIONAL PERFORMANCE FOR DIETETICS PROFESSIONALS

What Are the Standards of Practice in Nutrition Care?

The Standards of Practice in Nutrition Care:

- describe in general terms a competent level of nutrition care practice as

shown by the nutrition care process, the systematic problem-solving method that dietetics professionals use to think critically and make decisions to address nutrition-related problems and provide safe, effective, high-quality nutrition care;

- are based on the Nutrition Care Process and Model, which shows that all practice is centered around relationships that are collaborative, client-focused, and individualized;
- are reflective of the Commission on Accreditation for Dietetics Education core educational competencies and research impacting the profession (4);
- reflect the evolving nature of dietetics practice as health care continues to change. The standards evolved from the need to more clearly describe a competent level of dietetics practice based on two significant developments for the profession: RDs were granted Medicare Medical Nutrition Therapy benefit provider status beginning in 2002, and the ADA adopted the Nutrition Care Process and Model in 2003, which standardized terminology for the steps of nutrition assessment, nutrition diagnosis, nutrition intervention, and nutrition monitoring and evaluation (5); and
- are designed as two separate sets of standards, one for RDs and one for DTRs. This recognizes the distinct responsibilities of the RD and DTR in providing medical nutrition therapy. It is also consistent with federal law and the action of ADA's Board of Directors in September 2003, which clarified that the DTR works under the supervision of the RD when providing medical nutrition therapy.

ADA REPORTS

What are the Standards of Professional Performance for Dietetics Professionals?

The Standards of Professional Performance:

- describe in general terms a competent level of behavior in the professional role, including activities related to quality of care and administrative practice, performance appraisal, education, professional environment, ethics, collaboration, research, and resource utilization. For clarity, the ADA's board in September 2003 changed the name of the former Standards of Professional Practice, which were last updated in 1998, to Standards of Professional Performance, to more accurately describe their content and function (6);
- include indicators and examples of outcomes reflecting enhancements from the outer rings of the ADA Nutrition Care Process and Model (3) (eg, environmental factors such as practice settings, health care systems, social systems, economics, and support system components), as well as the screening, referral, and outcomes management systems); and
- are designed as one core Standard of Professional Performance to be implemented by all dietetics professionals.

How Do the Standards of Practice in Nutrition Care Relate to the Standards of Professional Performance?

The Standards of Practice and Standards of Professional Performance are complementary documents. The Standards of Practice in Nutrition Care describe a competent level of nutrition care practice. The Standards of Professional Performance describe a competent level of behavior in the professional role. One does not replace the other; rather, both serve to describe more comprehensively the practice and professional performance of dietetics practitioners.

The Standards of Practice in Nutrition Care apply to a wide variety of public health, community, and practice settings, including clinical health care settings (ie, inpatient, ambulatory, and extended care). However, they primarily apply to dietetics practitioners who have di-

rect contact with individuals and groups.

Those dietetics practitioners who do not have direct contact with individuals and groups will find that the Standards of Professional Performance, along with the Code of Ethics, meet their needs for evaluating their professional services. This may include those professionals who primarily manage food and other material resources, market products and services, teach dietetics professionals and students, conduct research, manage human resources, or manage facilities.

Why Are They Important?

The standards are designed to promote:

- providing safe, effective, and efficient food and nutrition care and services;
- evidence-based practice;
- improving quality and health outcomes;
- continuous quality improvement;
- evaluation and research;
- leading and developing practice;
- innovation and changing practice; and
- developing the individual and others.

The standards:

- define, in general terms, desirable and achievable levels of performance;
- acknowledge the common dimensions of practice;
- provide a common base for practitioners to use in individual evaluation and the development of a high level of practice quality;
- describe responsibilities for which RDs and DTRs are accountable;
- articulate the role of dietetics and the unique services that dietetics professionals provide within the health care team;
- provide a mechanism for regulatory bodies, consumer groups, accrediting agencies, insurers, and other third-party payers to evaluate the quality of food and nutrition care and services provided;
- enable patients/clients to judge the adequacy of dietetics services;
- provide guidance for researchers to identify relationships between dietetics practice and outcomes;

- provide guidance for educators i setting objectives for educationa programs; and
- provide a blueprint for developin specialty practice and advanced RI standards.

How Are They Structured?

The standards are outcome-focusec with mainly process-based criteria because this is the most effective wa to develop and measure quality. Eac standard is equal in relevance an importance. Both the RD and DT Standards of Practice in Nutritio Care and the Standards of Profes sional Performance have the follow ing components:

- the Standards: Brief, authoritativ statement that describes a compe tent level of dietetics practice o professional performance.
- Rationales: Statements that de scribe the intent of the standard and define their purpose and impor tance in greater detail.
- Indicators: Measurable, quantifi able, concrete action statement that illustrate how each specifi standard may be applied in practic to meet the standard.
- Examples of Outcomes: Measurabl end results or changes that can b expected as a result of applying th indicators of the RD and DTR Stan dards of Practice in Nutrition Car and the Standards of Professiona Performance.

How Can I Use the Standards to Evaluate My Practice?

Standards are promoted as part of th broader professional developmen process. Standards are clearly linkec to other quality mechanisms withir the profession. To use the standards dietetics professionals do not need t apply every indicator or achieve ever outcome. The indicators and out comes are given as examples to elab orate on the standard and its indica tor. Dietetics professionals are no limited to the examples indicated o the outcomes listed in the standards and indicators may not be applicabl to all practitioners. Likewise, indica tors may not be applicable all th time.

The Figure shows a tool for reflect ing on practice in a scheduled, proac

---

Standards

The four standards of practice in nutrition care and six standards of professional performance describe a competent level of dietetics practice and professional performance.

As you read the standards and rationale statements, determine how each relates to your practice

---

Indicators

Indicators are action statements that illustrate how each standard can be applied in practice. Indicators link the standards to the outcomes.

Read each of the indicator statements. Review direct evidence of competence (eg, medical records, peer interactions, client interactions, documentation, observation, education materials)

Are you performing these activities consistently?

Examples of Outcomes

Outcomes are measurable end results or changes and are provided to help individuals set minimum goals for each standard.

Review the examples of outcomes. Review direct evidence of competence (eg, medical records, peer interactions, client interactions, documentation, observation, education materials)

Am I knowledgeable and do I consistently demonstrate it in my practice?

> If you are seeing consistent results in your practice, take a continuous improvement approach to implementing the standards, and plan to revisit and reevaluate on a regular basis.

Do I need to learn more or enhance my practice?

> Use this information to develop a Professional Development Plan. The CDR Professional Development Portfolio Process offers a framework for credentialed professionals to develop specific goals, identify learning needs, and pursue continuing education opportunities.

---

gure. Flow chart for implementing the Standards of Professional Performance. Adapted from the American Dietetic Association. Standards of 'ofessional Practice for Dietetics Professionals. *J Am Diet Assoc.* 1998;98:83-85.

ve way to self-assess knowledge, ills, and competence using the tandards of Practice and Standards f Professional Performance. This ads to identification of individual learning needs based on actual issues confronted. The practitioner can then use the results of the self-assessment and apply the Commission on Dietetic Registration Professional Develop- ment Portfolio Process to develop specific goals related to the identified needs and pursue continuing professional education to achieve those needs and goals (7).

How Do They Relate to My Everyday Practice?

Standards of Practice in Nutrition Care and Standards of Professional Performance exist to ensure that the highest quality of care and service is maintained. Standards support the learner or the novice, a more advanced beginner. For a practitioner lacking mastery, standards of practice provide a safe structure by which to practice, as they spell out what to do, in situations in which the provider has no prior experience, by breaking down the activity into smaller components and providing pertinent indicators. They act as an essential teaching guide.

It is very important to understand that while serving the essential role of guiding the novice, the standards also guide the competent level of dietetics practice and professional performance for more experienced practitioners. Standards are the conduits of the culture of care, and therefore, the very essence of that care. By serving as a teaching tool, they establish a level of expectation about food and nutrition care and service delivery (8,9).

Consistent adherence to standards also provides an added measure of safety by extending professional expertise. With the guidance of practice standards, practitioners can step into situations and perform effectively. Standards are written in general rather than specific terms to account for individual dietetics practitioners handling of new or nonroutine situations.

Standards are geared toward the typical situation and are not intended to supersede the individual, specific needs of the client at any given time. Dietetics professionals face many complex situations every day. Understanding the unique needs of each situation and the latitude in applying standards is imperative to providing effective, high-quality care and services. Strictly adhering to standards does not, in and of itself, constitute best food and nutrition care and service. It is up to the individual practitioner to recognize and interpret situations, and to know what standards apply and in what ways they apply (10).

Individual practitioners who use the standards must be aware of state and federal laws affecting their practices as well as organizational policies and guidelines. The intent of the standards is not to supersede these laws, polices, and guidelines, but to serve as a resource for the development or modification of licensure laws as well as organizational policies and guidelines.

Available on the ADA Web site is a sample Nutrition Care Policy for use in clinical health care settings (inpatient, ambulatory, and extended care) that uses the standards as the foundation of the policy. The standards are not inflexible rules and are not intended, nor should they be used, to establish a legal standard of care. Within each setting, policies and procedures may be developed to reflect site-specific conditions, to provide operational guidelines for recommended practice, and to delineate local authority, responsibility, and accountability.

It is also important to note the additional tools from the ADA Scope of Dietetics Practice Framework, the Decision Aids. Because the standards are written in a generic format, the Decision Tree, Decision Analysis Tool, and the Definitions of Terms may be helpful when state, federal, and ADA documents do not clearly delineate responsibility.

What about Standards of Practice for Specialty or Advanced-Level Practice?

The Standards of Practice in Nutrition Care and Standards of Professional Performance are designed as blueprints to accommodate the development of specialty and advanced-level practice standards for RDs.

- The generic standards, along with the definition and rationale for each, remain the same. However, the indicators for specialty level and advanced practice are expanded to reflect the unique competence expectations for specific specialty and/or advanced-level practice.
- The Standards of Practice and Standards of Professional Performance for RDs (Generalist, Specialty, and Advanced) in Diabetes Care will be the first specialty and advanced-practice standards developed by the ADA Diabetes Care and Education Dietetic Practice Group under the guidance of the Quality Management Committee. The Standards of Practice (Generalist, Specialty, and Advanced) in Diabetes Care incorporates additional indicator(s) for generalist (entry level RD or novice RD) in diabetes care, for an RD at the specialty level of practice, and for a RD in advanced diabetes practice for each standard. Work is also in progress on Oncology and Behavioral Health standards.

SUMMARY

The Standards of Practice in Nutrition Care, the Standards of Professional Performance, and Specialty and Advanced Standards, along with the Code of Ethics, compose one of the three key blocks of the new Scope of Dietetics Practice Framework. Referred to as the Evaluation Resource block, they are used collectively to gauge and guide a competent level of dietetics practice and professional performance.

These resources will continue to evolve as new trends in dietetics practice emerge. All dietetics professionals should have in their personal libraries the most recent copies of the resources that compose the Scope of Dietetics Practice Framework. To ensure that practitioners always have access to the most updated resources the latest copies will be available on the ADA Web site at www.eatright.org. Also available on the Web site will be presentation materials, case scenarios, and other application tools to support practitioners in communication about and implementation of the standards.

Although K. Kieselhorst, J. Skates and E. Pritchett are the authors of this article, the following American Dietetic Association members worked on the development of the Standards of Practice in Nutrition Care and on updating of the Standards of Professional Performance. The work also reflects the input of the American Dietetic Association House of Delegates, the Commission on Dietetic Registration, and the Board of Directors.

Quality Management Committee 2003-2004:
Karen Lacey, MS, RD, Chair
Kessey Kieselhorst, MPA, RD
Kathy Masters, MS, RD

andy McNeil, MA, RD, FADA
cene Naglik, MS, RD
arlene Russell, MS, RD, FADA
DA Staff: Ellen Pritchett, RD, Director of Quality and Outcomes
uality Management Committee 2004-2005:
essey Kieselhorst, MPA, RD, Chair
andy McNeil, MA, RD, FADA
enise L. Elmore, DTR
anet J. Skates, MS, RD, FADA
ita M. Johnson, PhD, RD, FADA
oanne B. Shearer, RD
evelopment Advisors:
tandards of Practice of Dietetic Technicians, Registered
uzanne C. Bertocchi, DTR
lichael S. Weiss, DTR
onnie L. Gerald, PhD, DTR
enise L. Elmore, DTR

eferences

1. O'Sullivan Maillet J, Skates J, Pritchett E. American Dietetic Association: Scope of Dietetics Practice Framework. *J Am Diet Assoc.* 2005;105:634-640.
2. Code of Ethics for the Profession of Dietetics. *J Am Diet Assoc.* 1999;99:109-113.
3. Lacey K, Pritchett E. Nutrition Care Process and Model: ADA adopts road map to quality care and outcomes management. *J Am Diet Assoc.* 2003;103:1061-1072.
4. Bruening KS, Mitchell BE, Pfeiffer MM. 2002 Accreditation Standards for Dietetics Education. *J Am Diet Assoc.* 2002;102:566-577.
5. Pritchett E. The impact of gaining provider status in the Medicare program: What all dietetics professionals need to know. *J Am Diet Assoc.* 2002;102:480-482.
6. American Dietetic Association. Standards of Professional Practice for Dietetic Professionals. *J Am Diet Assoc.* 1998;98:83-85.
7. Weddle DO. The professional development portfolio process: Setting goals for credentialing. *J Am Diet Assoc.* 2002;102:1439-1444.
8. Dreyfus HL, Dreyfus SE. *Mind over Machine: The Power of Human Intuitive Expertise in the Era of the Computer.* New York, NY: Free Press; 1986.
9. Batalden P, Leach D, Swing S, Dreyfus H, Dreyfus S. General competencies and accreditation in graduate medical education. *Health Affairs.* 2002;21:103-111.
10. Gates G. Ethics opinion: Dietetics professionals are ethically obligated to maintain personal competence in practice. *J Am Diet Assoc.* 2003;103:633-635.

Appendix: Standards of Practice in Nutrition Care for the Registered Dietitian, Standards of Practice in Nutrition Care for the Dietetic Technician, Registered, and Standards of Professional Performance for Dietetics Professionals

The standards describe a competent level of dietetics practice and professional performance. They are authoritative statements addressing four standards of practice in nutrition care, designed as two separate sets of standards—one for registered dietitians (RDs) and one for dietetic technicians, registered (DTRs)—as well as six standards of professional performance common to all registered dietetics professionals. The Standards of Practice in Nutrition Care and Standards of Professional Performance are generic standards and may evolve to include specialty and advanced practice standards for RDs in specific practice areas.

The Standards of Practice and Standards of Professional Performance are complementary documents. One does not replace the other; rather, both serve to more completely describe the practice and professional performance of dietetics and should be considered together. For the RD, the Standards of Practice for the RD in Nutrition Care and Standards of Professional Performance for Dietetics Professionals are to be considered together. For the DTR, the Standards of Practice for the DTR in Nutrition Care and Standards of Professional Performance for Dietetics Professionals are to be considered together. They are not inflexible rules or requirements of practice and are not intended, nor should they be used, to establish a legal standard of care.

Each standard is equal in relevance and importance and includes a definition, a rationale statement, indicators, and examples of desired outcomes. A standard is a collection of specific outcome-focused statements against which a practitioner's performance can be assessed with validity and reliability. The rationale statement describes the intent of the standard and defines its purpose and importance in greater detail. Indicators are measurable, quantifiable, concrete action statements that illustrate how each specific standard may be applied in practice. They serve to identify the level of performance of competent practitioners and to encourage and recognize professional growth.

The term client is used in this evaluation resource as a universal term. Client could also mean patient, resident, customer, participant, consumer, community, or any individual or group that receives food and nutrition services. These Standards of Practice and Standards of Professional Performance are not limited to the clinical setting. The term appropriate is used in the standards to mean selecting from a range of possibilities, one or more of which would give an acceptable result under the circumstances.

AMERICAN DIETETIC ASSOCIATION STANDARDS OF PRACTICE IN NUTRITION CARE FOR THE REGISTERED DIETITIAN

Standard 1: Nutrition Assessment

The registered dietitian obtains adequate information to identify nutrition-related problems.

Rationale: Nutrition assessment is a systematic process of obtaining, verifying, and interpreting data to make decisions about the nature and cause of nutrition-related problems. It is initiated by referral and/or screening of individuals or groups for nutritional risk factors. Nutrition assessment is an ongoing, dynamic process that involves not only initial data collection, but also continual reas- sessment and analysis of the client' or community's needs assessment. I provides the foundation for the nutri- tion diagnosis at the next step of th Nutrition Care Process.

Indicators for Standard 1: Nutrition Assess ment

1. *Each RD:*
   1.1. Evaluates dietary intake fo factors that affect health con ditions, including nutritio risk
       1.1.1. Adequacy and appro priateness of food an beverage intake (eg macronutrients an micronutrients, mea patterns)
   1.2. Evaluates health and diseas condition(s) for nutrition-re lated consequences
       1.2.1. Medical and famil history and comorbidi ties
       1.2.2. Physical findings (ie physical or clinical ex aminations)
           1.2.2.1. Anthropomet ric measurement
       1.2.3. Medication manage ment (eg, prescription over-the-counter, an herbal medications medication allergies medication/food inter action and adherence)
       1.2.4. Complications an risks
       1.2.5. Diagnostic tests, proce dures, evaluations and population-base surveys
       1.2.6. Physical activity hab its and restrictions
   1.3. Evaluates psychosocial, socio

economic, functional, and behavioral factors related to food access, selection, preparation, and understanding of health condition

   1.3.1. Uses validated developmental, cultural, ethnic, lifestyle, and functional and mental status assessments

1.4. Evaluates client(s) knowledge, readiness to learn, and potential for behavior changes

   1.4.1. History of previous nutrition care services/ medical nutrition therapy

1.5. Identifies standards by which data will be compared

1.6. Identifies possible problem areas for making nutrition diagnoses

1.7. Documents and communicates:

   1.7.1. Date and time of assessment

   1.7.2. Pertinent data collected and compared with standards

   1.7.3. Client's perceptions, values, and motivation related to presenting problems

   1.7.4. Changes in client's level of understanding, food-related behaviors, and other outcomes for appropriate follow-up

   1.7.5. Reason for discharge/ discontinuation or referral, if appropriate

Examples of Outcomes for Standard 1: Nutrition Assessment

Appropriate assessment tools and procedures (matching the assessment method to the situation) are implemented.

Assessment tools are applied in valid and reliable ways.

Appropriate data are collected.

Data are validated.

Data are organized and categorized in a meaningful framework that relates to nutrition problems.

Effective interviewing methods are utilized.

Problems that require consultation with or referral to another provider are recognized.

Documentation and communication

of assessment are complete, relevant, accurate, and timely.

Standard 2: Nutrition Diagnosis

The registered dietitian identifies and describes an actual occurrence of, risk of, or potential for developing a nutrition problem that the registered dietitian is responsible for treating independently.

Rationale: At the end of the assessment step, data are clustered, analyzed, and synthesized. This will reveal a nutrition diagnostic category from which to formulate a specific Nutrition Diagnostic Statement. A nutrition diagnosis changes as the client response changes, whereas a medical diagnosis does not change as long as the disease or condition exists. There is a firm distinction between a nutrition diagnosis and a medical diagnosis. The main difference between the two types of diagnoses is that the nutrition diagnosis does not make a final conclusion about the identity and cause of the underlying disease. A client may have the medical diagnosis of type 2 diabetes mellitus; however, after performing a nutrition assessment, the RD may determine a nutrition diagnosis using nutrition diagnostic labels such as excessive energy intake or excessive carbohydrate intake. In the community or public health setting, the nutrition diagnosis may relate to a population-based condition (eg, food safety and access) rather than a medical diagnosis. Examples of nutrition diagnostic labels might then be intake of unsafe food or limited access to food. The nutrition diagnosis shows a link to setting realistic and measurable expected outcomes, selecting appropriate interventions, and tracking progress in attaining those expected outcomes.

Indicators for Standard 2: Nutrition Diagnosis

2. *Each RD:*

  2.1. Derives the nutrition diagnosis from the assessment data

    2.1.1. Identifies and labels the problem

    2.1.2. Determines etiology (cause, contributing risk factors)

    2.1.3. Clusters signs and symptoms (defining characteristics)

  2.2. Ranks (classifies) the nutrition diagnoses

    2.2.1. Validates the nutrition diagnosis with clients/ community, family members, or other health care professionals when possible and appropriate

  2.3. Documents the nutrition diagnosis in a written statement that includes the problem, etiology, and signs and symptoms (whenever possible). This may be referred to as the PES statement, which is the format commonly used: Problem (P), Etiology (E), and Signs and Symptoms (S)

  2.4. Re-evaluates and revises nutrition diagnoses when additional assessment data become available

Examples of Outcomes for Standard 2: Nutrition Diagnosis

- A Nutrition Diagnostic Statement that is:
  - Clear and concise
  - Specific: client- or community-centered
  - Accurate: relates to the etiology
  - Based on reliable and accurate assessment data
  - Includes date (all settings) and time (acute care)
- Documentation of nutrition diagnosis(es) is relevant, accurate, and timely
- Documentation of nutrition diagnosis(es) is revised and updated as more assessment data become available

Standard 3: Nutrition Intervention

The registered dietitian identifies and implements appropriate, purposefully planned actions designed with the intent of changing a nutrition-related behavior, risk factor, environmental condition, or aspect of health status for an individual, a target group, or the community at large.

Rationale: Nutrition Intervention involves (a) selecting, (b) planning, and (c) implementing appropriate actions to meet clients' nutrition needs. The selection of nutrition interventions is driven by the nutrition diagnosis and provides the basis on which outcomes are measured and evaluated. An intervention is a specific set of activities and associated materials used to address the problem. The RD may actually perform the interventions, or may delegate or coordinate the nutrition care that others provide. All interventions must be based on scientific principles and a rationale, and when available, grounded in a high level of quality research (evidence-based interventions).

The RD works collaboratively with the client, family, caregiver, or community to create a realistic plan that has a good probability of positively influencing the nutrition diagnosis/problem. This client-driven process is a key element in the success of this step, distinguishing it from previous steps that may or may not have involved the client to this degree of participation.

Indicators for Standard 3: Nutrition Intervention

3. *In planning the nutrition intervention, each RD:*
   3.1. Prioritizes the nutrition diagnoses based on severity of problem, likelihood that nutrition intervention will impact problem, and client's perception of importance
   3.2. Consults nationally developed evidence-based practice guidelines and measures for appropriate value(s) for control or improvement of the disease or conditions as defined and supported in the literature
   3.3. Determines client-focused expected outcomes for each nutrition diagnosis
       3.3.1. Develops expected outcomes in observable and measurable terms that are clear and concise, client-centered, tailored to what is reasonable to the client's circumstances, and develops appropriate expectations for treatments and outcomes
   3.4. Consults client/community, caregivers/other health professionals, or policies and program standards as appropriate throughout planning step
   3.5. Defines intervention plan (eg,

writes a nutrition prescription, develops an education plan or community program, creates policies that influence nutrition programs and standards)
   3.6. Ensures that the intervention plan content is based on best available evidence (eg, nationally developed guidelines, published research, evidence-based libraries/databases)
       3.6.1. Selects specific intervention strategies that are focused on the etiology of the problem and that are known to be effective based on best current knowledge and evidence
   3.7. In consultation with the client/community, defines time and frequency of care, including intensity, duration, and follow-up
   3.8. Identifies resources and/or referrals needed

In implementing the nutrition intervention, each RD

   3.9. Communicates the plan of nutrition and nutrition-related care
   3.10. Carries out the plan of nutrition and nutrition-related care
   3.11. Continues data collection and modifies the plan of care as needed
   3.12. Individualizes nutrition and nutrition-related interventions to the setting and client
   3.13. Collaborates with other colleagues and health care professionals
   3.14. Follows up and verifies that implementation is occurring and needs are being met
   3.15. Revises strategies as changes in condition/response occur
   3.16. Documents:
       3.16.1. Date and time
       3.16.2. Specific treatment goals and expected outcomes
       3.16.3. Recommended interventions
       3.16.4. Any adjustments of plan and justifications
       3.16.5. Client/community receptivity
       3.16.6. Referrals made and resources used

   3.16.7. Any other informatio relevant to providin care and monitorin progress over time
   3.16.8. Plans for follow-up an frequency of care
   3.16.9. Rationale for discharg if appropriate

Examples of Outcomes for Standard 3: N trition Intervention

- Appropriate prioritizing and se ting of goals/expected outcomes done.
- An appropriate nutrition prescri tion or plan is developed.
- Interdisciplinary connections a established.
- Nutrition interventions are deli ered, and actions are carried out.
- Documentation of nutrition inte vention is relevant, accurate, an timely.
- Documentation of nutrition inte ventions is revised and updated.

Standard 4: Nutrition Monitoring and Evaluation

The registered dietitian monitors an evaluates outcome(s) directly relate to the nutrition diagnosis and t goals established in the interventio plan to determine the degree to whic progress is being made and goals desired outcomes of nutrition care a being met. Through monitoring an evaluation, the registered dietitia uses selected outcome indicato (markers) that are relevant to the cl ent-defined needs, nutrition diagn sis, nutrition goals, and disease stat condition. Progress should monitored, measured, and evaluate on a planned schedule until di charge. The registered dietitian us data from this step to create an ou comes management system.

Rationale: Progress should l monitored, measured, and evaluate on a planned schedule until di charge. Alterations in outcome ind cators such as hemoglobin A1C valu or weight are examples that trigg reactivation of the nutrition care pr cess. Monitoring specifically refers the review and measurement of th client's status at a scheduled (pr planned) follow-up point with regar to the nutrition diagnosis, interve tion plans/goals, and outcome whereas evaluation is the systemat comparison of current findings with previous status, intervention goals, or a reference standard.

Indicators for Standard 4: Nutrition Monitoring and Evaluation

4. *Each RD:*
4.1. Monitors progress
    4.1.1. Checks client understanding and adherence with plan
    4.1.2. Determines whether the intervention is being implemented as prescribed
    4.1.3. Provides evidence that the plan/intervention strategy is or is not changing client behavior or status
    4.1.4. Identifies other positive or negative outcomes
    4.1.5. Gathers information indicating reasons for lack of progress
    4.1.6. Supports conclusions with evidence
    4.1.7. Evaluates patterns, trends, and unintended variation related to problems and intervention
4.2. Measures outcomes
    4.2.1. Selects standardized, evidence-based outcome indicators that are relevant to the client and directly related to the nutrition diagnosis and the goals established in the intervention plan (eg, direct nutrition outcomes, clinical and health status outcomes, client-centered outcomes, health care utilization)
4.3. Evaluates outcomes
    4.3.1. Uses standardized indicators to compare current findings with previous status, intervention goals, and/or reference standards
4.4. Documents:
    4.4.1. Date and time
    4.4.2. Specific indicators measured and results
    4.4.3. Progress toward goals (incremental small

change can be significant; therefore, use of a Likert-type scale may be more descriptive than a goal evaluation tool that uses only met or not met categories)
    4.4.4. Factors facilitating or hampering progress
    4.4.5. Changes in client level of understanding and food-related behaviors
    4.4.6. Changes in clinical, functional, or health status outcomes assuring care/case management in the future
    4.4.7. Other positive or negative outcomes
    4.4.8. Future plans for nutrition care, monitoring, and follow-up or discharge

Examples of Outcomes for Standard 4: Nutrition Monitoring and Evaluation

- The client/community outcome(s) directly relate to the nutrition diagnosis and the goals established in the intervention plan. Examples include but are not limited to:
  ○ Direct nutrition outcomes (eg, knowledge gained, behavior change, food or nutrient intake changes, improved nutrition status);
  ○ Clinical and health status outcomes (eg, laboratory values, weight, blood pressure, risk factor profile changes, signs and symptoms, clinical status, infections, complications);
  ○ Client-centered outcomes (eg, quality of life, satisfaction, self-efficacy, self-management, functional ability); and
  ○ Health care utilization and cost outcomes (medication changes, special procedures, planned/unplanned clinic visits, preventable hospitalizations, length of hospitalization, prevention or delay of nursing home admission).
- Documentation of the monitoring and evaluation is relevant, accurate, and timely.

AMERICAN DIETETIC ASSOCIATION STANDARDS OF PRACTICE IN NUTRITION CARE FOR THE DIETETIC TECHNICIAN, REGISTERED

Standard 1: Nutrition Assessment

The dietetic technician, registered obtains adequate information to identify nutrition-related problems for uncomplicated instances of common conditions or population-based problems (eg, health promotion, disease prevention activities). The dietetic technician, registered assists with nutrition assessment of individual clients with complex medical conditions. In the nutrition assessment for medical nutrition therapy, the dietetic technician, registered works under the supervision of a registered dietitian.

Rationale: Nutrition assessment is a systematic process of obtaining, verifying, and interpreting data to make decisions about the nature and cause of nutrition-related problems. It is initiated by referral and/or screening of individuals or groups for nutritional risk factors. Nutrition assessment is an ongoing, dynamic process that involves not only initial data collection, but also continual reassessment and analysis of client or community needs. It provides the foundation for the nutrition diagnosis at the next step of the Nutrition Care Process.

Indicators for Standard 1: Nutrition Assessment

1. *Each dietetic technician, registered (DTR):*
1.1. Evaluates dietary intake for factors that affect health conditions, including nutrition risk for uncomplicated instances of common conditions or population-based problems (eg, health promotion, disease prevention activities)
    1.1.1. Adequacy and appropriateness of food and beverage intake (eg, macronutrients and micronutrients, meal patterns)
1.2. Evaluates health and disease condition(s) for nutrition-related consequences for uncomplicated instances of common conditions or population-based problems (eg, health promotion/disease prevention activities)

1.2.1. Medical and family history and comorbidities

1.2.2. Physical findings (physical or clinical examinations)

    1.2.2.1. Anthropometric measurements

1.2.3. Medication management (eg, prescription, over-the-counter, and herbal medications; medication allergies; medication/food interaction and adherence)

1.2.4. Complications and risks

1.2.5. Diagnostic tests, procedures, evaluations, and population-based surveys

1.2.6. Physical activity habits and restrictions

1.3. Evaluates psychosocial, socioeconomic, functional, and behavioral factors related to food access, selection, preparation, and understanding of health condition for uncomplicated instances of common conditions or population-based problems

    1.3.1. Uses validated developmental, cultural, ethnic, lifestyle, and functional and mental status assessments

1.4. Evaluates client(s) knowledge, readiness to learn, and potential for behavior changes for uncomplicated instances of common conditions or population-based problems

    1.4.1. History of previous nutrition care services or medical nutrition therapy

1.5. Identifies standards by which data will be compared

1.6. Identifies possible problem areas for making nutrition diagnoses for uncomplicated instances of common conditions or population-based problems

1.7. Assists the registered dietitian (RD) with nutrition assessment of individual patients/clients with complex medical conditions

1.8. Communicates findings to the RD

1.9. Documents and communicates:

    1.9.1. Date and time of assessment

    1.9.2. Pertinent data collected and comparison with standards

    1.9.3. Clients' perceptions, values, and motivation related to presenting problems

    1.9.4. Changes in client level of understanding, food-related behaviors, and other outcomes for appropriate follow-up

    1.9.5. Reason for discharge/discontinuation or referral if appropriate

Examples of Outcomes for Standard 1: Nutrition Assessment

- Appropriate assessment tools and procedures (matching the assessment method to the situation) are implemented.
- Assessment tools are applied in valid and reliable ways.
- Appropriate data are collected.
- Data are validated.
- Data are organized and categorized in a meaningful framework that relates to nutrition problems.
- Effective interviewing methods are utilized.
- Problems that require consultation with or referral to another provider are recognized.
- Documentation and communication of assessment are complete, relevant, accurate, and timely.

Standard 2: Nutrition Diagnosis

The dietetic technician, registered identifies and describes an actual occurrence of, risk of, or potential for developing a nutrition problem for uncomplicated instances of common conditions or population-based problems (eg, health promotion, disease prevention activities). The dietetic technician, registered assists the registered dietitian with nutrition diagnosis of individual clients with complex medical conditions. In the nutrition diagnosis for medical nutrition therapy, the dietetic technician, registered works under the supervision of a registered dietitian.

Rationale: At the end of the assessment step, data are clustered, analyzed, and synthesized. This will reveal a nutrition diagnostic category from which to formulate a specific nutrition diagnostic statement. A nutrition diagnosis changes as the client response changes, whereas a medical diagnosis does not change as long as the disease or condition exists. There is a firm distinction between a nutrition diagnosis and a medical diagnosis. The main difference between the two types of diagnoses is that the nutrition diagnosis does not make a final conclusion about the identity and cause of the underlying disease. A client may have the medical diagnosis of dyslipidemia, however, after performing a nutrition assessment, the DTR may determine a nutrition diagnosis using a nutrition diagnostic label such as excessive fat intake. In the community or public health setting the nutrition diagnosis may relate to a population-based condition (eg, food safety and access) rather than to a medical diagnosis. Examples of nutrition diagnosis labels may then be intake of unsafe food or limited access to food. The nutrition diagnosis demonstrates a link to setting realistic and measurable expected outcomes, selecting appropriate interventions, and tracking progress in attaining those expected outcomes.

Indicators for Standard 2: Nutrition Diagnosis

2. *Each DTR:*

2.1. Derives the nutrition diagnosis for uncomplicated instances of common conditions or population-based problems from the assessment data

    2.1.1. Identifies and labels the problem

    2.1.2. Determines etiology (cause, contributing risk factors)

    2.1.3. Clusters signs and symptoms (defining characteristics)

2.2. Ranks (classifies) the nutrition diagnoses for uncomplicated instances of common conditions or population-based problems

    2.2.1. Validates the nutrition diagnosis with clients, community, family members, or other health care professionals when possible and appropriate

2.3. Documents the nutrition diagnosis for uncomplicated instances of common or population-based conditions in a written statement(s) that includes the problem, etiology, and signs and symptoms (whenever possible). This may be referred to as the PES statement, which is the format commonly used: Problem (P), Etiology (E), and Signs and Symptoms (S)

2.4. Communicates with the RD regarding Nutrition Diagnostic Statements

2.5. Assists the RD with nutrition diagnosis of individual clients with complex medical conditions

2.6. Re-evaluates and revises nutrition diagnoses when additional assessment data become available

Examples of Outcomes for Standard 2: Nutrition Diagnosis

A Nutrition Diagnostic Statement that is:

○ Clear and concise
○ Specific: client- or community-centered
○ Accurate: relates to the etiology
○ Based on reliable and accurate assessment data
○ Includes date (all settings) and time (acute care)

Documentation of nutrition diagnosis is relevant, accurate, and timely
Documentation of nutrition diagnosis is revised and updated as more assessment data become available
Documentation of communication with the RD

Standard 3: Nutrition Intervention

The dietetic technician, registered identifies and implements appropriate, purposefully planned actions for uncomplicated instances of common conditions in individuals and populations (eg, health promotion, disease prevention activities) designed with the intent of changing a nutrition-related behavior, risk factor, environmental condition, or aspect of health status for an individual, a target group, or the community at large. The dietetic technician, registered assists the registered dietitian with the nutrition intervention of individual clients with complex medical conditions. In the nutrition intervention for medical nutrition therapy, the dietetic technician, registered works under the supervision of a registered dietitian.

Rationale: Nutrition intervention involves (a) selecting, (b) planning, and (c) implementing appropriate actions to meet clients' nutrition needs. The selection of nutrition interventions is driven by the nutrition diagnosis and provides the basis on which outcomes are measured and evaluated. An intervention is a specific set of activities and associated materials used to address the problem. The DTR may actually perform the interventions, or may delegate or coordinate the nutrition care that others provide. All interventions must be based on scientific principles and rationale, and when available, grounded in a high level of quality research (evidence-based interventions). The DTR works collaboratively with the client, family, caregiver, or community to create a realistic plan that has a good probability of positively influencing the nutrition diagnosis/problem. This client-driven process is a key element in the success of this step, distinguishing it from previous steps that may or may not have involved the client to this degree of participation.

Indicators for Standard 3: Nutrition Intervention

3. *In planning the nutrition intervention, each DTR:*

3.1. Prioritizes the nutrition diagnoses for uncomplicated instances of common conditions in individuals and populations (eg, health promotion/disease prevention activities) based on severity of problem, likelihood that nutrition intervention will impact problem, and client's perception of importance

3.2. Consults nationally developed evidence-based practice guidelines/measures for appropriate value(s) for control or improvement of the disease or conditions as defined and supported in the literature

3.3. Determines client-focused expected outcomes for each nutrition diagnosis for uncomplicated instances of common conditions in individuals and populations (eg, health promotion/disease prevention activities)

3.3.1. Develops expected outcomes for uncomplicated instances of common conditions in individuals and populations (eg, health promotion/disease prevention activities) in observable and measurable terms that are clear and concise, client-centered, tailored to what is reasonable to the client's circumstances, and develops appropriate expectations for treatments and outcomes

3.4. Confers with client/community, caregivers/other health professionals, an RD if indicated, or policies and program standards as appropriate throughout planning step

3.5. Defines intervention plan for uncomplicated instances of common conditions in individuals and populations (eg, health promotion/disease prevention activities) (eg, writes a basic nutrition prescription, participates in defining an education plan or community program, participates in creating policies that influence nutrition programs and standards)

3.6. Ensures intervention plan content for uncomplicated instances of common conditions in individuals and populations is based on best available evidence (eg, nationally developed guidelines, published research, evidence-based libraries/databases)

3.6.1. Selects specific intervention strategies for uncomplicated instances of common conditions in individuals and populations that are focused on the etiology of the problem and that are known to be effective based on best current knowledge and evidence

3.7. In consultation with the client/community, defines time and frequency of care, including intensity, duration, and follow-up for uncomplicated instances of common conditions in individuals and populations

3.8. Assists the RD with the planning of the nutrition intervention of individual clients with complex medical conditions

3.9. Identifies resources and/or referrals needed

3.10. Communicates the plan of nutrition and nutrition-related care for uncomplicated instances of common conditions in individuals and populations (eg, health promotion/ disease prevention activities)

In implementing the nutrition intervention, each DTR:

3.11. Carries out the plan of nutrition and nutrition-related care for uncomplicated instances of common conditions in individuals and populations (eg, health promotion/disease prevention activities)

3.12. Continues data collection and modifies the plan of care as needed for uncomplicated instances of common conditions in individuals and populations (eg, health promotion/disease prevention activities)

3.13. Individualizes nutrition and nutrition-related interventions to the setting and client/community for uncomplicated instances of common conditions in individuals and populations (eg, health promotion/disease prevention activities)

3.14. Collaborates and communicates with the RD, other colleagues, and health care professionals

3.15. Follows up and verifies that implementation is occurring and needs are being met

3.16. Revises strategies for uncomplicated instances of common conditions in individuals and populations (eg, health promotion/disease

prevention activities) as a change in condition/response occurs

3.17. Assists with the implementation of the nutrition intervention of individual clients with complex medical conditions

3.18. Documents:
  3.18.1. Date and time
  3.18.2. Specific treatment goals and expected outcomes
  3.18.3. Recommended interventions
  3.18.4. Any adjustments of plan and justifications
  3.18.5. Client/community receptivity
  3.18.6. Referrals made and resources used
  3.18.7. Any other information relevant to providing care and monitoring progress over time
  3.18.8. Plans for follow-up and frequency of care
  3.18.9. Rationale for discharge if appropriate
  3.18.10. Communication with RD

Examples of Outcomes for Standard 3: Nutrition Intervention

- Appropriate prioritizing and setting of goals/expected outcomes is done.
- Appropriate basic nutrition prescription or basic plan is developed.
- Interdisciplinary connections are established.
- Nutrition Interventions are delivered, and actions are carried out.
- Documentation of nutrition intervention is relevant, accurate, and timely.
- Documentation of nutrition interventions is revised and updated.
- Documentation of communication with the RD is done.

Standard 4: Nutrition Monitoring and Evaluation
The dietetic technician, registered monitors and evaluates outcome(s) directly related to the nutrition diagnosis and the goals established in the intervention plan for uncomplicated instances of common conditions in individuals and populations (eg, health promotion, disease prevention activities) to determine the degree to which progress is being made and goals or desired outcomes of nutrition care are being met. Through monitoring and evaluation, the dietetic technician registered uses selected outcome indicators (markers) that are relevant to the client's defined needs, nutrition diagnosis, nutrition goals, and disease state/condition/health status. The dietetic technician, registered uses data from this step to create an outcomes management system. The dietetic technician, registered assists the registered dietitian with the monitoring and evaluations of individual clients with complex medical conditions. In the nutrition monitoring and evaluation for medical nutrition therapy, the dietetic technician, registered works under the supervision of a registered dietitian.

Rationale: Progress should be monitored, measured, and evaluated on a planned schedule until discharge. Alterations in outcome indicators such as A1C hemoglobin value or weight are examples that trigger reactivation of the nutrition care process. Monitoring specifically refers to the review and measurement of the client's status at a scheduled (preplanned) follow-up point with regard to the nutrition diagnosis, intervention plans/goals, and outcomes whereas evaluation is the systematic comparison of current findings with previous status, intervention goals, or a reference standard.

Indicators for Standard 4: Nutrition Monitoring and Evaluation

4. *Each DTR:*
  4.1. Monitors progress for uncomplicated instances of common conditions in individuals and populations (eg, health promotion/disease prevention activities)
    4.1.1. Checks client understanding and adherence with plan
    4.1.2. Determines whether the intervention is being implemented as prescribed
    4.1.3. Provides evidence that the intervention strat-

egy is or is not changing client behavior or status

4.1.4. Identifies other positive or negative outcomes

4.1.5. Gathers information indicating reasons for lack of progress

4.1.6. Supports conclusions with evidence

4.1.7. Evaluates patterns, trends, and unintended variation related to problems and intervention

4.2. Measures outcomes for uncomplicated instances of common conditions in individuals and populations

4.2.1. Selects standardized evidence-based outcome indicators that are relevant to the client and directly related to the nutrition diagnosis and the goals established in the intervention plan (eg, direct nutrition outcomes, clinical and health status outcomes, client-centered outcomes, health care utilization)

4.3. Evaluates outcomes for uncomplicated instances of common conditions in individuals and populations

4.3.1. Uses standardized indicators to compare current findings with previous status, intervention goals, and/or reference standards

4.4. Communicates with the RD regarding monitoring and evaluation activities

4.5. Assists the RD with the monitoring, measuring, and evaluations of individual clients with complex medical conditions

4.6. Documents:

4.6.1. Date and time

4.6.2. Specific indicators measured and results

4.6.3. Progress toward goals (small, incremental changes can be significant, therefore, use of a Likert-type scale may be more descriptive

than a goal evaluation tool that uses only met or not met categories)

4.6.4. Factors facilitating or hampering progress

4.6.5. Changes in client level of understanding and food-related behaviors

4.6.6. Changes in clinical, health status, or functional outcomes assuring care/case management in the future

4.6.7. Other positive or negative outcomes

4.6.8. Future plans for nutrition care, monitoring, and follow-up or discharge

4.6.9. Communication with the RD

Examples of Outcomes for Standard 4: Nutrition Monitoring and Evaluation

- The client/community outcome(s) directly relate to the nutrition diagnosis and the goals established in the intervention plan for uncomplicated instances of common conditions in individuals and populations. Examples include, but are not limited to:
  - Direct nutrition outcomes (eg, knowledge gained, behavior change, food or nutrient intake changes, improved nutrition status)
  - Clinical and health status outcomes (eg, laboratory values, weight, blood pressure, risk factor profile changes, signs and symptoms, clinical status, infections, complications)
  - Client-centered outcomes (eg, quality of life, satisfaction, self-efficacy, self-management, functional ability)
  - Health care utilization and cost outcomes (eg, medication changes, special procedures, planned/unplanned clinic visits, preventable hospitalizations, length of hospitalization, prevention or delay of nursing home admission)
- Documentation of the monitoring and evaluation is relevant, accurate, and timely.
- Communication with the RD is documented.

AMERICAN DIETETIC ASSOCIATION STANDARDS OF PROFESSIONAL PERFORMANCE FOR DIETETICS PROFESSIONALS

Standard 1: Provision of Services

The dietetics practitioner provides quality service based on customer expectations and needs.

Rationale: Dietetics practitioners provide, facilitate, and promote quality services based on client needs and expectations, current knowledge, and professional experience.

Indicators for Standard 1: Provision of Services

1. *Each dietetics practitioner:*

1.1. Provides input on the development of appropriate screening parameters, ensuring that the right questions are asked and the screening process is effective

1.2. Contributes to the development of a referral process to ensure that the public has an identifiable method of being linked to dietetics professionals who will ultimately provide services

1.3. Collaborates with clients to assess needs, background, and resources, and to establish mutual goals

1.4. Informs clients and their families and involves them in decision making

1.5. Recognizes clients' concepts of illness and their cultural beliefs

1.6. Applies knowledge and principles of disease prevention and behavioral change appropriate for diverse populations

1.7. Collaborates and coordinates with other professionals as appropriate

1.8. Applies knowledge and skills to determine the most appropriate action plan

1.9. Implements quality practice by following an evidence-based approach for policies, procedures, legislation, licensure, credentialing, competency, regulatory requirements, and practice guidelines

1.10. Fosters excellence and shows professionalism in practice

1.11. Continuously evaluates processes and outcomes of both nutrition/health quality and service quality dimensions (ie, convenience, dignity, ease of access, privacy, comfort, client involvement in decision-making, and promptness of care)

1.12. Advocates for the provision of food and nutrition services as part of public policy

Examples of Outcomes for Standard 1: Provision of Services

- Clients actively participate in establishing goals and objectives.
- Clients' needs are met.
- Clients are satisfied with products and services provided.
- Evaluation reflects expected outcomes.
- Appropriate screening and referral systems are established.
- Public has access to food and nutrition services.

Standard 2: Application of Research

The dietetics practitioner effectively applies, participates in, or generates research to enhance practice.

Rationale: Effective application, support, and generation of dietetics research in practice encourages continuous quality improvement and provides documented support for the benefit of the client.

Indicators for Standard 2: Application of Research

2. *Each dietetics practitioner:*
2.1. Locates and reviews best available research findings for application to dietetics practice
2.2. Bases practice on sound scientific principles, best available research, and theory
2.3. Integrates best available research with clinical/managerial expertise and client values (evidence-based practice)
2.4. Promotes research through alliances and collaboration with dietetics and other professionals and organizations
2.5. Contributes to the development of new knowledge and research in dietetics
2.6. Collects measurable data and

documents outcomes within the practice setting
2.7. Shares research data and activities through various media

Examples of Outcomes for Standard 2: Application of Research

- Client receives appropriate services based on the effective application of research.
- A foundation for performance measurement and improvement is provided.
- Outcomes data support reimbursement for the services of dietetics professionals.
- Best available research findings are used for the development and revision of resources used for practice content.
- Practitioner uses benchmarking and knowledge of best practices to improve performance.

Standard 3: Communication and Application of Knowledge

The dietetics practitioner effectively applies knowledge and communicates with others.

Rationale: Dietetics practitioners work with and through others while using their unique knowledge of food, human nutrition, and management, in addition to their skills in providing services.

Indicators for Standard 3: Communication and Application of Knowledge

3. *Each dietetics practitioner:*
3.1. Has knowledge related to a specific area(s) of professional service
3.2. Communicates sound scientific principles, research, and theory
3.3. Integrates knowledge of food and human nutrition with knowledge of health, social sciences, communication, and management theory
3.4. Shares knowledge and information with clients
3.5. Helps students and clients apply knowledge and skills
3.6. Documents interpretation of relevant information and results of communication with professionals, personnel, students, or clients

3.7. Contributes to the development of new knowledge
3.8. Seeks out information to provide effective services
3.9. Communicates, manages knowledge, and supports decision making using information technology

Examples of Outcomes for Standard 3: Communication and Application of Knowledge

- Practitioner provides expertise in food, nutrition, and management information.
- Client understands the information received.
- Client receives current and appropriate information and knowledge.
- Client knows how to obtain additional guidance.

Standard 4: Utilization and Management of Resources

The dietetics practitioner uses resources effectively and efficiently in practice.

Rationale: Appropriate use of time, money, facilities, and human resources facilitates delivery of quality services.

Indicators for Standard 4: Utilization and Management of Resources

4. *Each dietetics practitioner:*
4.1. Uses a systematic approach to maintain and manage professional resources successfully
4.2. Uses measurable resources such as personnel, money, equipment, guidelines, protocols, reference materials, and time in the provision of dietetics services
4.3. Analyzes safety, effectiveness, and cost in planning and delivering products and services
4.4. Justifies use of resources by documenting consistency with plan, continuous quality improvement, and desired outcomes
4.5. Educates and helps clients and others to identify and secure appropriate and available resources and services

Examples of Outcomes for Standard 4: Utilization and Management of Resources

The dietetics practitioner documents use of resources according to plan and budget.

Resources and services are measured, and data are used to promote and validate the effectiveness of services.

Desired outcomes are achieved and documented.

Resources are managed and used cost-effectively.

Standard 5: Quality in Practice

The dietetics practitioner systematically evaluates the quality and effectiveness of practice and revises practice as needed to incorporate the results of evaluation.

Rationale: Quality practice requires regular performance evaluation and continuous improvement of services.

Indicators for Standard 5: Quality in Practice

5. *Each dietetics practitioner:*

5.1. Continually understands and measures the quality of food and nutrition services in terms of structure, process, and outcomes

5.2. Identifies performance improvement criteria to monitor effectiveness of services

5.3. Designs and tests interventions to change processes and systems of food and nutrition care and services with the objective of improving quality

5.4. Identifies errors and hazards in food and nutrition care and services

5.5. Recognizes and implements basic safety design principles, such as standardization and simplification

5.6. Identifies expected outcomes

5.7. Documents outcomes of services provided

5.8. Compares actual performance to expected outcomes

5.9. Documents action taken when discrepancies exist between active performance and expected outcomes

5.10. Continuously evaluates and refines services based on measured outcomes

5.11. Implements an outcomes management system to evaluate the effectiveness and efficiency of practice

Examples of Outcomes for Standard 5: Quality in Practice

- Performance improvement criteria are measured.
- Actual performance is evaluated.
- Aggregate of outcomes data meets established criteria (objectives/goals).
- Results of quality improvement activities direct refinement of practice.

Standard 6: Continued Competence and Professional Accountability

The dietetics practitioner engages in lifelong self-development to improve knowledge and enhance professional competence.

Rationale: Professional practice requires continuous acquisition of knowledge and skill development to maintain accountability to the public.

Indicators for Standard 6: Continued Competence and Professional Accountability

6. *Each dietetics practitioner:*

6.1. Conducts self-assessment at regular intervals to identify professional strengths and weaknesses

6.2. Identifies needs for professional development from a variety of sources

6.3. Participates in peer review and mentors others

6.4. Develops and implements a plan for professional growth

6.5. Documents professional development activities

6.6. Adheres to the Code of Ethics for the profession of dietetics and is accountable and responsible for actions and behavior

6.7. Implements the American Dietetic Association Standards of Practice and Standards of Professional Performance

6.8. Supports the application of research findings and best available evidence to professional practice

6.9. Takes active leadership roles

Examples of Outcomes for Standard 6: Continued Competence and Professional Accountability

- Self-assessments are completed.
- Development needs are identified and directed learning is demonstrated.
- Practice outcomes demonstrate adherence to the Code of Ethics, Standards of Practice, and Standards of Professional Performance.
- Practice decisions reflect best available evidence.
- Appropriate certifications are obtained.
- Commission on Dietetic Registration recertification requirements are met.

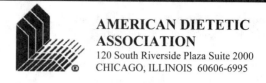

AMERICAN DIETETIC ASSOCIATION
120 South Riverside Plaza Suite 2000
CHICAGO, ILLINOIS 60606-6995

Effective Date: April 2005
Revision Date: February 2006
Review Date: February 2006

PURPOSE:

This policy establishes the process followed by the Nutrition Care Process/Standardized Language (NCP/SL) Committee to maintain a current Nutrition Care Process and list of nutrition controlled vocabulary terminology that document the Nutrition Care Process.

STRUCTURE:

The NCP/SL Committee is a joint House of Delegates and Board of Directors Committee and provides semi-annual reports to both bodies.

PROCEDURES:

The NCP/SL Committee accepts proposals for modification or additions to the Nutrition Diagnostic and Nutrition Intervention Terminology as follows:

1. Any individual ADA member or Dietetic Practice Group can submit proposals for modification or additions by completing the attached two documents:
    a. Proposed Nutrition Diagnostic or Nutrition Interventions Terminology Addition or Modification letter
    b. Reference worksheet for proposed addition or modification
2. The NCP/SL will review the submissions at their routine face-to-face meetings or teleconferences to establish the following:
    a. Is the term already represented by an existing term?
        i. If yes, the new term can be added as a synonym for the existing term or replace the existing term.
        ii. If no, then the term can be considered for addition to the list of terms as long as it meets the need for describing elements of dietetic practice in the context of the nutrition care process.
    b. Does the term overlap with an existing term, but add new elements?
        i. If yes, then the existing term can be modified to include the new elements or the proposed term can be clarified to be distinctly different from the existing term through a dialogue with the proposal submitter.
        ii. If no, then consider adding new term
    c. Is the term distinct and separate from all existing terms?
        i. If yes, then ensure that the term is in the context of dietetic practice within the Nutrition Care Process and consider adding to list of terms.
        ii. If no, then work with proposal submitter to discuss how to integrate into existing terms or create a separate term.
3. The NCP/SL will prepare a summary of comments and one representative of the NCP/SL will confer with the proposal submitter after the initial discussion to answer questions and discuss the initial input from the NCP/SL Committee. If the proposal submitter is not satisfied with the direction proposed by the NCP/SL, then they will be invited to submit

additional documentation and have time on the next teleconference/meeting agenda to personally present their concerns.

4. Changes or modifications accepted by the NCP/SL will be integrated into the Nutrition Diagnostic or Nutrition Intervention Terminology that is re-published on an annual basis.

STAFFING:
Governance and Scientific Affairs and Research provide staff support for Research Committee functions.

ATTACHMENTS:
1. Letter template for proposing a **New Term** for **Nutrition Diagnostic Terminology**
2. Letter template for proposing a **New Term** for **Nutrition Intervention Terminology**
3. Letter template for proposing **Modifications** for either Nutrition Diagnostic or Nutrition Intervention Terminology
4. Template for **Reference Sheet** to support **additions/modifications** to **Nutrition Diagnostic Terminology**
5. Completed Nutrition Diagnostic Reference Sheet
6. Template for **Reference Sheet** to support **additions/modifications** to **Nutrition Intervention Terminology**
7. Completed Nutrition Intervention Reference Sheet

SUBJECT: NUTRITION CONTROLLED VOCABULARY/TERMINOLOGY MAINTENANCE/REVIEW

Attachment 1: Letter Template for Proposing **New Term** for **Nutrition Diagnostic Terminology**

Date: _____

To: NCP/SL Committee
       Scientific Affairs and Research
       American Dietetic Association
       120 South Riverside Plaza, Suite 2000
       Chicago, IL 60606-6995
       emyers@eatright.org; lornstein@eatright.org

Subject: Proposed **Addition** to **Nutrition Diagnostic Terminology**

(I/We) would like to propose a new term, _____ (Proposed term to add to the Nutrition Diagnostic Terminology list). The reason I/we believe that this term should be added is as follows: (insert concise rationale for change and may include brief example of when the situation arose that the current term was inadequately defined)
1. (Insert first statement of rationale.)
2. (Insert second statement of rationale, if applicable.)
3. (Insert example of situation where this modification was needed.)

Other terms that are similar with explanations of why they do not exactly match our new proposed term are as follows:
1. (Insert term.) – (Insert 2-3 sentences to illustrate why the existing term does not meet your need.)
2. (Insert term.) – (Insert 2-3 sentences to illustrate why the existing term does not meet your need)
3. (Add as many as applicable.)

Attached is the a reference sheet that includes the label name, proposed domain and category, definition, examples of etiologies and signs and symptoms, references, and a case that illustrates when this term would be used and the corresponding PES statement that would be used in medical record documentation.

The point of contact for this proposal is _____ (insert name), who can be reached at _____(best contact telephone number) and _____ (e-mail address).

Thank you for considering our request.

Signature block
(Organizational unit if applicable)

Attachments: (1) Completed Reference Sheet, (2) Case

Attachment 2: Letter Template for Proposing **New Term** for **Nutrition Intervention Terminology**

Date: _____

To: NCP/SL Committee
      Scientific Affairs and Research
      American Dietetic Association
      120 South Riverside Plaza, Suite 2000
      Chicago, IL 60606-6995
      emyers@eatright.org; lornstein@eatright.org

Subject: Proposed **Addition** to **Nutrition Intervention Terminology**

(I/We) would like to propose a new term, _____ (Proposed term to add to the Nutrition Intervention Terminology list). The reason I/we believe that this term should be added is as follows: (insert concise rationale for change and may include brief example of when the situation arose that the current term was inadequately defined)
  1. (Insert first statement of rationale.)
  2. (Insert second statement of rationale, if applicable.)
  3. (Insert example of situation where this modification was needed.)

Other terms that are similar with explanations of why they do not exactly match our new proposed term are as follows:
  1. (Insert term.) – (Insert 2-3 sentences to illustrate why the existing term does not meet your need.)
  2. (Insert term.) – (Insert 2-3 sentences to illustrate why the existing term does not meet your need)
  3. (Add as many as applicable.)

Attached is the a reference sheet that includes the label name, proposed domain, definition, details of the nutrition intervention, nutrition diagnostic terminology with which it is typically used, other considerations, and references, and a case that illustrates when this term would be used.

The point of contact for this proposal is _____ (insert name), who can be reached at _____(best contact telephone number) and _____ (e-mail address).

Thank you for considering our request.

Signature block
(Organizational unit if applicable)

Attachments: (1) Completed Reference Sheet, (2) Case

Attachment 3: Letter Template for Proposing **Modifications** to Nutrition Diagnostic or
Nutrition Intervention Terminology

Date: _____

To: NCP/SL Committee
        Scientific Affairs and Research
        American Dietetic Association
        120 South Riverside Plaza, Suite 2000
        Chicago, IL 60606-6995
        emyers@eatright.org; lornstein@eatright.org

Subject: Proposed **Modification** to an existing term in **Nutrition Diagnostic or Nutrition
Intervention Terminology**

(I/We) would like to propose a modification of the term, _____ (insert
Number and Name from current Nutrition Diagnostic or Nutrition Intervention Terminology
lists). The reason I/we believe that this term should be modified is as follows (insert concise
rationale for change and may include brief example of when the situation arose that the
current term was inadequately defined):
    1. (Insert first statement of rationale.)
    2. (Insert second statement of rationale, if applicable.)
    3. (Insert example of situation where this modification was needed.)

Attached is the revised Nutrition Diagnostic or Nutrition Intervention reference sheet that
shows the changes highlighted or bolded for your consideration.

The point of contact for this proposal is _____ (insert
name), who can be reached at _____ (best contact telephone number) and
_____ (e-mail address).

Thank you for considering our request.

Signature block
(Organizational unit if applicable)

Attachments: (1) Modified Reference Sheet, (2) Case, if needed

Attachment 4: Template for **Reference Sheet** to support **additions/modifications** to **Nutrition Diagnostic Terminology**

DOMAIN
(Intake, Clinical or Behavioral-Environmental)

Category
(e.g., Functional Balance)

Nutrition Diagnostic Label (Leave number blank)
(Insert 1- to 4-word label)

Definition
(Insert 1 sentence that describes the intent of the label)

Etiology (Cause/Contributing Risk Factors)
Factors gathered during the nutrition assessment process that contribute to the existence of or the maintenance of pathophysiological, psychosocial, situational, developmental, cultural, and/or environmental problems.

- (Insert common etiologies for Nutrition Diagnostic Label)

Signs/Symptoms (Defining Characteristics)
A typical cluster of subjective and objective signs and symptoms gathered during the nutrition assessment process that provide evidence that a problem exists; quantify the problem and describe its severity.

Nutrition Assessment Category	Potential Indicators of this Nutrition Diagnosis (one or more must be present)
Biochemical Data, Medical Tests and Procedures	• (Insert as appropriate)
Anthropometric Measurements	• (Insert as appropriate)
Physical Exam Findings	• (Insert as appropriate)
Food/Nutrition History	• (Insert as appropriate)
Client History	• (Insert as appropriate)

References:

Cite references

Attachment 5: Completed Nutrition Diagnosis Reference Sheet

DOMAIN: CLINICAL

Category: Functional Balance

Nutrition Diagnostic Label NC-1.1
Swallowing difficulty

Definition
Impaired movement of food and liquid from the mouth to the stomach

Etiology (Cause/Contributing Risk Factors)
Factors gathered during the nutrition assessment process that contribute to the existence of or the maintenance of pathophysiological, psychosocial, situational, developmental, cultural, and/or environmental problems.

- Mechanical causes, e.g., inflammation; surgery; stricture; or oral, pharyngeal, and esophageal tumors
- Motor causes, e.g., neurological or muscular disorders, such as cerebral palsy, stroke, multiple sclerosis, scleroderma, or prematurity

Signs/Symptoms (Defining Characteristics)
A typical cluster of subjective and objective signs and symptoms gathered during the nutrition assessment process that provide evidence that a problem exists; quantify the problem and describe its severity.

Nutrition Assessment Category	Potential Indicators of this Nutrition Diagnosis (one or more must be present)
Biochemical Data, Medical Tests and Procedures	• Radiological findings, e.g., abnormal swallowing studies
Anthropometric Measurements	
Physical Exam Findings	• Evidence of dehydration, e.g., dry mucous membranes, poor skin turgor
Food/Nutrition History	Reports or observations of: • Coughing, choking, prolonged chewing, pouching of food, regurgitation, facial expression changes during eating, prolonged feeding time, drooling, noisy wet upper airway sounds, feeling of "food getting stuck," pain while swallowing • Decreased food intake • Avoidance of foods • Mealtime resistance
Client History	• Conditions associated with a diagnosis or treatment of dysphagia, achalasia • Repeated upper respiratory infections and or pneumonia

References:
1. Braunwald E, Fauci AS, Kasper DL, Hauser SL, Longo DL, Jameson JL, ed. *Harrison's Principles of Internal Medicine. 15th Edition.* New York, NY: McGraw-Hill,.2001.

Attachment 6: Template for **Reference Sheet** to support **additions/modifications** to **Nutrition Intervention Terminology**

Nutrition Intervention Label (Leave number blank)
(Insert 1- to 4-word label)

DOMAIN
(Food and/ or Nutrient Delivery, Nutrition Education, Nutrition Counseling, or Coordination of Nutrition Care)

Definition
(Insert 1 sentence that describes the intent of the label)

Details of Intervention
A typical intervention might be further described related the following details.
- Insert as appropriate

Typically used with the following

Nutrition Diagnostic Terminology Used in PES Statements	Common Examples (Not intended to be inclusive)
Nutrition Diagnoses	• (Insert as appropriate)
Etiology	• (Insert as appropriate)
Signs and Symptoms	• (Insert as appropriate)

Other considerations *(e.g., patient/client negotiation, patient/client needs and desires, readiness to change)*
List other considerations

References

Cite references

Attachment 7: Completed Nutrition Intervention Reference Sheet

Initial/Brief Nutrition Education (E-1)

DOMAIN: Education

Definition: Instruction or training intended to build or reinforce basic nutrition-related knowledge, or to provide essential nutrition-related information until patient/client returns

Details of Intervention:

A typical intervention might be further described related to the following details:
- Discuss the purpose of the nutrition education intervention
- Communicate relationship between nutrition and specific disease/health issue
- Begin instruction of nutrition issue of most concern to patient/client's health and well being
- Provide basic nutrition-related educational information until client is able to return for comprehensive education

Typically used with the following:

Nutrition Diagnostic Terminology Used in PES Statements	Common Examples (Not intended to be inclusive)
Nutrition Diagnoses	• Food–medication interaction (NC-2.3) • Food- and nutrition-related knowledge deficit (NB-1.1) • Harmful beliefs/attitudes about food- or nutrition-related topics (NB-1.2) • Self-monitoring deficit (NB-1.4) • Other: Any diagnoses related to inadequate, excessive, inappropriate, or inconsistent intake
Etiology	• Capacity for learning • Knowledge deficit related to newly diagnosed medical condition • Interest and/or motivation • Medical or surgical procedure requiring modified diet • Unable to distinguish legitimate from false information
Signs and Symptoms	• Unable to explain purpose of the nutrition prescription or rationale for nutrition prescription in relationship to disease/health • Expresses need for additional information or clarification of education or additional time to learn information • Unable to select appropriate foods or supplements • Unable to choose appropriate timing, volume, or preparation/handling of foods

Other considerations *(e.g., patient/client negotiation, patient/client needs and desires, readiness to change)*
- Met with several providers in one day and is unable or unwilling to receive more nutrition education at this time
- Profile reflects complicated situation warranting additional education/instruction
- Being discharged from the hospital
- Caregiver unavailable at time of nutrition education
- Baseline knowledge
- Learning style
- Other education and learning needs, e.g., new medication or other treatment administration

SUBJECT: NUTRITION CONTROLLED VOCABULARY/TERMINOLOGY MAINTENANCE/REVIEW

References:
1. Position of the American Dietetic Association: Total diet approach to communicating food and nutrition information. *J Am Diet Assoc.* 2002;102:100-108.
2. Holli BB, Calabrese RJ, O'Sullivan-Maillet J. *Communication and Education Skills for Dietetics Professionals. 4th ed.* New York, NY: Lipincott Williams and Wilkins. 2003.
3. Sahyoun NR, Pratt CA, Anderson A. Evaluation of nutrition education interventions for older adults: A proposed framework. *J Am Diet Assoc.* 2004;104:58-69.
4. Contento I. The effectiveness of nutrition education and implications for nutrition education policy, programs, and research: a review of research. *J Nutr Educ.* 1995;27: 279-283.
5. Medeiros LC, Butkus SN, Chipman H, Cox RH, Jones L, Little D. A logic model framework for community nutrition education. *J Nutr Educ Behav.* 2002;37: 197-202.

Standardized Language Task Force and Terminology Expert Reviewers

Standardized Language Task Force

Chair
Patricia Splett, PhD, MPH, RD
Splett & Associates
3219 Midland Ave
St. Paul, MN 55110
Task Force Member 2003-2006

Vice Chair
Annalynn Skipper, PhD, RD, FADA
PO Box 45
Oak Park, IL 60303-0045
Task Force Member 2005-2006

Sylvia Escott-Stump, MA, RD, LDN
Dietetic Programs Director
East Carolina University
155 Rivers Building, Dept. NUHM
Greenville, NC 27858
Task Force Past Chair and Member 2003-2006

Peter Beyer, MS, RD, LD
Associate Professor
University of Kansas Medical Center
Dietetics & Nutrition
3900 Rainbow, Mail stop 4013
Kansas City, KS 66160
Task Force Member 2003-2006

Pam Charney, PhD, RD, CNSD
2460 64th Ave SE
Mercer Island, WA 98040
Task Force Member 2003-2006

Mary Jane Oakland, PhD, RD, LD, FADA
Associate Professor
Food Science and Human Nutrition
1612 Truman Dr
Ames, IA 50010-4344
Task Force Member 2003-2006

Nancy Lewis, PhD, RD, FADA
Professor
Nutrition and Health Sciences
University of Nebraska
4507 E Eden Dr
Lincoln, NE 68506
Task Force Member 2005-2006

Mary Russell, MS, RD, LDN, CNSD
1101 S State St #807
Chicago IL 60605
Task Force Member 2005-2006

Trisha Fuhrman, MS, RD, LD, FADA, CNSD
1932 Prospector Ridge Dr
Ballwin, MO 63011-4808
Task Force Member 2005-2006

Donna A Israel, PhD, RD, LD, LPC, FADA
The Fitness Formula Inc.
Professional Nutrition Therapist
3611 Dartmouth Ave
Dallas, TX 75205-3238
Task Force Member 2005-2006

Joanne Shearer, MS, RD, CDE, LN
Team Leader, Food & Nutrition Services
Avera Heart Hospital of South Dakota
4500 West 69th St
Ex-Officio Task Force Member 2005-2006

Kristy Hendricks, DSc, RD
Tufts University, Jaharis 262
150 Harrison Ave
Boston, MA 02111-1817
Ex-Officio/Research Committee
Task Force Member 2005-2006

Standardized Language Task Force Past Members and Contributors

Christina Biesemeier MS, RD, LDN, FADA
313 Logans Circle
Franklin, TN 37067-1363
Task Force Member 2003-2005

Marion Franz, MS, RD, CDE
6635 Limerick Dr
Minneapolis, MN 55439-1260
Task Force Member 2003-2005

Karen Lacey, MS, RD, CD
500 Saint Mary's Blvd
Green Bay, WI 54301-2610
Task Force Member 2003-2005

Kathleen Niedert, MBA, RD, LD, FADA
PO Box 843
110 Ardis St
Hudson, IA 50643-0843
Task Force Member 2003-2005

Frances Tyus, MS, RD, LD
19412 Mayfair Ln
Cleveland, OH 44128-2727
Task Force Member 2003-2005

Standardized Language Task Force and Terminology Expert Reviewers

Naomi Trostler, PhD, RD
Institute of Biochemistry, Food Science, and
Nutrition
Faculty of Agriculture, Food and Environmental
Quality Sciences
The Hebrew University of Jerusalem
PO Box 12
Rehovot 76100, Israel
Task Force Member 2004-2005

Robin Leonhardt, RD
1905 North 24th St
Sheboygan, WI 53081-2124
*Attended Face-to-Face Meeting in Summer
2003*

Staff Liaisons
Esther Myers, PhD, RD, FADA
Director of Scientific Affairs and Research
American Dietetic Association
120 South Riverside Plaza, Suite 2000
Chicago, IL 60606
Work (312) 899-4860
Fax (312) 899-4757
E-mail: emyers@eatright.org

Pam Michael, MBA, RD
Director, Nutrition Services Coverage Team
American Dietetic Association
120 South Riverside Plaza, Suite 2000
Chicago, IL 60606
Work (312) 899-4747
E-Mail: pmichael@eatright.org

Major Kim Thomsen, MA, MHA, RD, LD, CHE
US Army Training with Industry Program
American Dietetic Association
120 South Riverside Plaza, Suite 2000
Chicago, IL 60606
Work (312) 899-4797
Fax (312) 899-4812
E-Mail: kthomsen@eatright.org

Ellen Pritchett, RD, CPHQ
Staff Liaison 2003-2005

Lt Col Vivian Hutson, MA, MHA, RD, LD,
FACHE
Staff Liaison 2003-2004

Consultants
Donna G. Pertel, MEd, RD
5 Bonny Ln
Clinton, CT 06413

Patricia Splett, PhD, MPH, RD
Splett & Associates
3219 Midland Ave
St. Paul, MN 55110

Melinda L. Jenkins, PhD, FNP
Assistant Professor of Clinical Nursing
Columbia University School of Nursing
630 W 168 St, mail code 6
New York, NY 10032

Annalynn Skipper, PhD, RD, FADA
P.O. Box 45
Oak Park, IL 60303-0045

Expert Reviewers
Nutrition Diagnosis Terminology

Nutrition Diagnostic Label	Label #	Reviewers
CLINICAL DOMAIN – Functional Balance		
Swallowing difficulty	NC-1.1	Moshe Shike, MD (Memorial Sloan Kettering)
Chewing (masticatory) difficulty	NC-1.2	Helen Smiciklas-Wright, PhD, RD (Penn State) Riva Touger-Decker, PhD, RD (UMDNJ)
Breastfeeding difficulty	NC-1.3	Maureen A. Murtaugh, PhD, RD (University of Utah)
Altered GI function	NC-1.4	Larry Cheskin, MD (Johns Hopkins)
CLINICAL DOMAIN – Biochemical Balance		
Impaired nutrient utilization	NC-2.1	Laura Matarese, MS, RD, CNSD (Cleveland Clinic)
Altered nutrition-related laboratory values	NC-2.2	Denise Baird Schwartz, MS, RD, CNSD (Clinical practice)
Food medication interaction	NC-2.3	Andrea Hutchins, PhD, RD (Arizona State University East, Mesa, AZ)
CLINICAL DOMAIN – Weight Balance		
Underweight	NC-3.1	Bonnie Spear, PhD, RD (University of Alabama, Birmingham
Involuntary weight loss	NC-3.2	Jody Vogelzang, MS, RD, LD, CD, FADA (Texas Women's University)
Overweight/obesity	NC-3.3	Rebecca Mullis, PhD, RD (Georgia)
Involuntary weight gain	NC-3.4	Celia Hayes, MS, RD (HRSA)
BEHAVIORAL-ENVIRONMENTAL DOMAIN – Knowledge and Beliefs		
Food- and nutrition-related knowledge deficit	NB-1.1	Penny Kris-Etherton, PhD, RD (Penn State)
Harmful beliefs/attitudes about food, nutrition, and nutrition-related topics	NB-1.2	Keith-Thomas Ayoob, PhD, RD (Albert Einstein)
Not ready for diet/lifestyle change	NB-1.3	Geoffrey Greene, PhD, RD (University of Rhode Island)
Self-monitoring deficit	NB-1.4	Linda Delahanty, MS, RD (Harvard)
Disordered eating pattern	NB-1.5	Eileen Stellefson Myers, PhD, RD (Private practice) Leah Graves, MS, RD (Saint Francis Hospital, Tulsa, OK)
Limited adherence to nutrition-related recommendations	NB-1.6	Ellen Parham, PhD, RD (Northern Illinois University)
Undesirable food choices	NB-1.7	Kathy Cobb, MS, RD (Centers for Disease Control)
BEHAVIORAL-ENVIRONMENTAL DOMAIN – Physical Activity Balance and Function		
Physical inactivity	NB-2.1	Melinda Manore, PhD, RD (Oregon State)
Excessive exercise	NB-2.2	Katherine Beals, PhD, RD (Industry, formerly Ball State)
Inability to manage self-care	NB-2.3	Emily Gier, MS, RD (Cornell)
Impaired ability to prepare foods/meals	NB-2.4	Marla Reicks, PhD, RD (U of MN)
Poor nutrition quality of life	NB-2.5	Elvira Johnson, MS, RD (Private practice)
Self-feeding difficulty	NB-2.6	Mary Cluskey, PhD, RD (Oregon State)
BEHAVIORAL-ENVIRONMENTAL DOMAIN – Food Safety and Access		
Intake of unsafe food	NB-3.1	Johanna Dwyer, DSc, RD (Tufts)
Limited access to food	NB-3.2	Sondra King, PhD, RD (Northern Illinois University)

Nutrition Diagnostic Label	Label #	Reviewers
INTAKE DOMAIN – Caloric Energy Balance		
Hypermetabolism	NI-1.1	Jonathan Waitman, MD for Louis Arrone, MD (Cornell)
Increased energy expenditure (when part of hypermetabolism)	NI-1.2	Jonathan Waitman, MD for Louis Arrone, MD (Cornell)
Hypometabolism	NI-1.3	Edith Lerner, PhD (Case Western Reserve University)
Inadequate energy intake	NI-1.4	Joel Mason, MD (Tufts)
Excessive energy intake	NI-1.5	Jim Hill, MD (University of Colorado)
INTAKE DOMAIN – Oral or Nutrition Support Intake		
Inadequate oral food/beverage intake	NI-2.1	Anne Voss, PhD, RD (Ross Labs)
Excessive oral food/beverage intake	NI-2.2	Jessica Krenkel, MS, RD (University of Nevada)
Inadequate intake from enteral/parenteral nutrition	NI-2.3	Kenneth Kudsk, MD (University of Wisconsin)
Excessive intake from enteral/parenteral nutrition	NI-2.4	Annalynn Skipper, PhD, RD, FADA (Oak Park, IL)
Inappropriate infusion of enteral/parenteral nutrition	NI-2.5	Annalynn Skipper, PhD, RD, FADA (Oak Park, IL)
INTAKE DOMAIN – Fluid Intake Balance		
Inadequate fluid intake	NI-3.1	Ann Grandjean, EdD, RD (International Center for Sports Nutrition)
Excessive fluid intake	NI-3.2	Joel Kopple, MD (UCLA)
INTAKE DOMAIN – Bioactive Substances Balance		
Inadequate bioactive substance intake	NI-4.1	Johanna Lappe, PhD, RN (Creighton University)
Excess bioactive substance	NI-4.2	Elizabeth Jeffery, PhD (University of Illinois, Champaign)
Excessive alcohol intake	NI-4.3	Janice Harris, PhD, RD (University of Kansas)
INTAKE DOMAIN – Nutrient Balance		
Increased nutrient (specify) needs	NI-5.1	Carol Braunschweig, PhD, RD (University of Illinois, Chicago)
Evident protein-energy malnutrition	NI-5.2	Charlette R. Gallagher Allred, PhD, RD (Retired-Ross Labs)
Inadequate protein energy intake	NI-5.3	Trisha Fuhrman, MS, RD (Coram Healthcare)
Decreased nutrient (specify) needs	NI-5.4	Jeannmarie Beiseigel, PhD, RD (USDA)
Imbalance of nutrients	NI-5.5	Molly Kretsch, PhD, RD (USDA)
INTAKE DOMAIN – Nutrient Balance – Fat and Cholesterol Balance		
Inadequate fat intake	NI-51.1	Alice Lichtenstein, DSc (Tufts)
Excessive fat intake	NI-51.2	Wendy Mueller Cunnigham, PhD, RD (Cal State)
Inappropriate intake of food fats	NI-51.3	Nancy Lewis, PhD, RD (University of Nebraska-Lincoln)
INTAKE DOMAIN – Nutrient Balance – Protein Balance		
Inadequate protein intake	NI-52.1	Don Layman, PhD (University of Illinois-Champaign)
Excessive or unbalanced protein intake	NI-52.2	Linda A. Vaughan, PhD, RD (Arizona State University)
Inappropriate intake of amino acids	NI-52.3	Allison Yates, PhD, RD (Industry, formerly Director of the IOM Food and Nutrition Board)
INTAKE DOMAIN – Nutrient Balance – Carbohydrate Balance		
Inadequate carbohydrate intake	NI-53.1	Robert Wolfe, PhD (University of Texas)
Excessive carbohydrate intake	NI-53.2	Anne Daly, MS, RD, BC-ADM, CDE (Springfield, IL)
Inappropriate intake of types of carbohydrate	NI-53.3	Lyn Wheeler, MS, RD, CD, FADA, CDE (Indiana University School of Medicine)
Inconsistent intake of carbohydrate	NI-53.4	Maggie Powers, MS, RD, CDE (International Diabetes Center)
Inadequate fiber intake	NI-53.5	Joanne Slavin, PhD, RD (University of Minnesota)
Excess fiber intake	NI-53.6	Judith Marlett, PhD, RD (University of Wisconsin)

Nutrition Diagnostic Label	Label #	Reviewers
INTAKE DOMAIN – Nutrient Balance – Vitamin Balance		
Inadequate vitamin intake (specify)	NI-54.1	Laurie A. Kruzich, MS, RD (Iowa State)
		Kristina Penniston, PhD, RD (University of Wisconsin)
Excess vitamin intake	NI-54.2	Kristina Penniston, PhD, RD (University of Wisconsin)
INTAKE DOMAIN – Nutrient Balance – Mineral Balance		
Inadequate mineral intake (specify)	NI-55.1	Bob Heaney, MD (Creighton University)
Excessive mineral intake	NI-55.2	Joan Fischer, PhD, RD (University of Georgia)

Expert Reviewers
Nutrition Intervention Terminology

Nutrition Intervention	Label #	Reviewers
Food and/or Nutrient Delivery		
Meals and Snacks	ND-1	Marion J Franz, MS, RD, CDE
		Rene Brand, RD, LN
Enteral and Parenteral Nutrition	ND-2	Carol Ireton-Jones, PhD, RD, LD, CNSD
		Mary Hise, PhD, RD
Medical Food Supplement	ND-3.1	Marion J. Franz, MS, RD, CDE
		Rene Brand, RD, LN
		Mary Hise, PhD, RD
Vitamin and Mineral Supplement	ND-3.2	Marion J. Franz, MS, RD, CDE
		Rene Brand, RD, LN
		Mary Hise, PhD, RD
Bioactive Substance Supplement	ND-3.3	Marion J. Franz, MS, RD, CDE
		Rene Brand, RD, LN
		Mary Hise, PhD, RD
Feeding Assistance	ND-4	Mary Ellen E. Posthauer, RD, CD, LD
		Kathleen Niedert, MBA, RD, LD, FADA
Feeding Environment	ND-5	Mary Ellen E. Posthauer, RD, CD, LD
		Kathleen Niedert, MBA, RD, LD, FADA
Nutrition-Related Medication Management	ND-6	Marion J Franz, MS, RD, CDE
		Kathleen Niedert, MBA, RD, LD, FADA
Nutrition Education		
Initial/Brief Education	E-1	Laura Graney, MS, RD, CD
		Shirley Gerrior, PhD, RD, LD
Comprehensive Education	E-2	Laura Graney, MS, RD, CD
		Shirley Gerrior, PhD, RD, LD
Nutrition Counseling		
Nutrition Counseling	C-1	Linda G. Snetselaar, RD, PhD
		Tay Kennedy, PhD, RD
Coordination of Nutrition Care		
Coordination of Other Care During Nutrition Care	RC-1	Joanne Guthrie, PhD, RD
		Carol Ireton-Jones, PhD, RD, LD, CNSD
Discharge and Transfer of Nutrition Care to New Setting or Provider	RC-2	Joanne Guthrie, PhD, RD
		Carol Ireton-Jones, PhD, RD, LD, CNSD

FEEDBACK FORM

Please provide us with feedback on revisions you would suggest to the next version of this reference related to Nutrition Diagnosis and Intervention. Please indicate whether each section should still be included and also identify what questions you would like answered in the next version as well as additional materials that you would find helpful.

Please Check

The following items should be included in the next version:

	YES	NO

Nutrition Diagnosis and Intervention Introduction
Nutrition Care Process and Model Article

	YES	NO

Step 1: Nutrition Assessment Introduction
Nutrition Assessment Matrix

Step 2: Nutrition Diagnosis Introduction
Nutrition Diagnosis Terminology
Nutrition Diagnosis Terms and Definitions
Nutrition Diagnosis Reference Sheets

Step 3: Nutrition Intervention Introduction
Nutrition Intervention Terminology
Nutrition Intervention Terms and Definitions
Nutrition Intervention Reference Sheets

Case Study A and Examples of Charting in Various Formats
Case Study B and Examples of Charting in Various Formats
Implementing Nutrition Diagnosis, Step Two in the Nutrition Care Process Article
Scope of Dietetics Practice Framework Article
Standards of Practice in Nutrition Care Article

What questions would you like answered in the 2008 version?

What additional materials would be helpful in the 2008 version?

Please remove from packet and mail form or e-mail information to:
Scientific Affairs and Research
American Dietetic Association
Standardized Language/Nutrition Care Process Committee
120 South Riverside Plaza, Suite 2000
Chicago, IL 60606-6995
emyers@eatright.org; lornstein@eatright.org

INTAKE   NI

Defined as "actual problems related to intake of energy, nutrients, fluids, bioactive substances through oral diet or nutrition support"

Energy Balance (1)

Defined as "actual or estimated changes in energy (kcal)"

❑ Hypermetabolism (Increased energy needs)	NI-1.1
❑ Increased energy expenditure	NI-1.2
❑ Hypometabolism (Decreased energy needs)	NI-1.3
❑ Inadequate energy intake	NI-1.4
❑ Excessive energy intake	NI-1.5

Oral or Nutrition Support Intake (2)

Defined as "actual or estimated food and beverage intake from oral diet or nutrition support compared with patient goal"

❑ Inadequate oral food/beverage intake	NI-2.1
❑ Excessive oral food/beverage intake	NI-2.2
❑ Inadequate intake from enteral/parenteral nutrition infusion	NI-2.3
❑ Excessive intake from enteral/parenteral nutrition	NI-2.4
❑ Inappropriate infusion of enteral/parenteral nutrition (use with caution)	NI-2.5

Fluid Intake (3)

Defined as "actual or estimated fluid intake compared with patient goal"

❑ Inadequate fluid intake	NI-3.1
❑ Excessive fluid intake	NI-3.2

Bioactive Substances (4)

Defined as "actual or observed intake of bioactive substances, including single or multiple functional food components, ingredients, dietary supplements, alcohol"

❑ Inadequate bioactive substance intake	NI-4.1
❑ Excessive bioactive substance intake	NI-4.2
❑ Excessive alcohol intake	NI-4.3

Nutrient (5)

Defined as "actual or estimated intake of specific nutrient groups or single nutrients as compared with desired levels"

❑ Increased nutrient needs (specify) _____	NI-5.1
❑ Evident protein-energy malnutrition	NI-5.2
❑ Inadequate protein-energy intake	NI-5.3
❑ Decreased nutrient needs (specify) _____	NI-5.4
❑ Imbalance of nutrients	NI-5.5

Fat and Cholesterol (51)

❑ Inadequate fat intake	NI-51.1
❑ Excessive fat intake	NI-51.2
❑ Inappropriate intake of food fats (specify) _____	NI-51.3

Protein (52)

❑ Inadequate protein intake	NI-52.1
❑ Excessive protein intake	NI-52.2
❑ Inappropriate intake of amino acids (specify) _____	NI-52.3

Carbohydrate and Fiber (53)

❑ Inadequate carbohydrate intake	NI-53.1
❑ Excessive carbohydrate intake	NI-53.2
❑ Inappropriate intake of types of carbohydrate (specify) _____	NI-53.3
❑ Inconsistent carbohydrate intake	NI-53.4
❑ Inadequate fiber intake	NI-53.5
❑ Excessive fiber intake	NI-53.6

Vitamin (54)

❑ Inadequate vitamin intake (specify)	NI-54.1
❑ Excessive vitamin intake (specify)	NI-54.2

❑ A	❑ C
❑ Thiamin	❑ D
❑ Riboflavin	❑ E
❑ Niacin	❑ K
❑ Folate	❑ Other

Mineral (55)

❑ Inadequate mineral intake (specify)	NI-55.1

❑ Calcium	❑ Iron
❑ Potassium	❑ Zinc
❑ Other	

❑ Excessive mineral intake (specify)	NI-55.2

❑ Calcium	❑ Iron
❑ Potassium	❑ Zinc
❑ Other	

CLINICAL   NC

Defined as "nutritional findings/problems identified as related to medical or physical conditions"

Functional (1)

Defined as "change in physical or mechanical functioning that interferes with or prevents desired nutritional consequences"

❑ Swallowing difficulty	NC-1.1
❑ Chewing (masticatory) difficulty	NC-1.2
❑ Breastfeeding difficulty	NC-1.3
❑ Altered GI function	NC-1.4

Biochemical (2)

Defined as "change in capacity to metabolize nutrients as a result of medications, or surgery, or as indicated by altered lab values"

❑ Impaired nutrient utilization	NC-2.1
❑ Altered nutrition-related laboratory values	NC-2.2
❑ Food-medication interaction	NC-2.3

Weight (3)

Defined as "chronic weight or changed weight status when compared with usual or desired body weight"

❑ Underweight	NC-3.1
❑ Involuntary weight loss	NC-3.2
❑ Overweight/obesity	NC-3.3
❑ Involuntary weight gain	NC-3.4

BEHAVIORAL-ENVIRONMENTAL   NB

Defined as "nutritional findings/problems identified that relate to knowledge, attitudes/beliefs, physical environment, access to food, or food safety"

Knowledge and Beliefs (1)

Defined as "actual knowledge and beliefs as observed or documented"

❑ Food- and nutrition-related knowledge deficit	NB-1.1
❑ Harmful beliefs/attitudes about food- or nutrition-related topics (use with caution)	NB-1.2
❑ Not ready for diet/lifestyle change	NB-1.3
❑ Self-monitoring deficit	NB-1.4
❑ Disordered eating pattern	NB-1.5
❑ Limited adherence to nutrition-related recommendations	NB-1.6
❑ Undesirable food choices	NB-1.7

Physical Activity and Function (2)

Defined as "actual physical activity, self-care, and quality-of-life problems as reported, observed, or documented"

❑ Physical inactivity	NB-2.1
❑ Excessive exercise	NB-2.2
❑ Inability or lack of desire to manage self-care	NB-2.3
❑ Impaired ability to prepare foods/meals	NB-2.4
❑ Poor nutrition quality of life	NB-2.5
❑ Self-feeding difficulty	NB-2.6

Food Safety and Access (3)

Defined as "actual problems with food access or food safety"

❑ Intake of unsafe food	NB-3.1
❑ Limited access to food	NB-3.2

NUTRITION COUNSELING — C

Nutrition Counseling — C-1
A supportive process to set priorities, establish goals, and create individualized action plans that acknowledge and foster responsibility for self-care.

□ Theory or approach
□ Cognitive-behavioral theory
□ Behavior modification
□ Social learning theory
□ Transtheoretical
□ Other (*specify*)

□ Strategies
□ Cognitive restructuring
□ Goal setting
□ Motivational interviewing
□ Problem solving
□ Rewards/reinforcement
□ Self-monitoring
□ Social support
□ Stimulus control/contingency mgmt
□ Stress management
□ Other (*specify*)

□ Phase
□ Involving
□ Exploring
□ Resolving
□ Closing

COORDINATION OF NUTRITION CARE — RC

Coordination of Other Care During Nutrition Care — RC-1
Facilitating services with other professionals, institutions, or agencies during nutrition care.

□ Team meeting
□ Referral to RD with different expertise
□ Collaboration/referral to other providers
□ Referral to community agencies/programs
(*specify*)

Discharge and Transfer of Nutrition Care to New Setting or Provider — RC-2
Discharge planning and transfer of nutrition care from one level or location of care to another.

□ Collaboration/referral to other providers
□ Referral to community agencies/programs
(*specify*)

Feeding Environment — ND-5
Adjustment of the factors where food is served that impact food consumption.

□ Lighting
□ Odors
□ Distractions
□ Table height
□ Table service/set up
□ Room temperature
□ Other (*specify*)

Nutrition-Related Medication Management — ND-6
Modification of a drug or herbal to optimize patient/client nutritional or health status.

□ Initiate
□ Dose change
□ Form change
□ Route change
□ Administration schedule
□ Discontinue
(*specify*)

NUTRITION EDUCATION — E

Initial/Brief Nutrition Education — E-1
Build or reinforce basic or essential nutrition-related knowledge.

□ Purpose of the nutrition education
□ Priority modifications
□ Survival information
□ Other (*specify*)

Comprehensive Nutrition Education — E-2
Instruction or training leading to in-depth nutrition-related knowledge or skills.

□ Purpose of the nutrition education
□ Recommended modifications
□ Advanced or related topics
□ Result interpretation
□ Other (*specify*)

FOOD AND/OR NUTRIENT DELIVERY — ND

Meal and Snacks — ND-1
Regular eating event (meal); food served between regular meals (snack).

□ General/healthful diet
□ Modify distribution, type, or amount of food and nutrients within meals or at specified time
□ Specific foods/beverages or groups
□ Other (*specify*)

Enteral and Parenteral Nutrition — ND-2
Nutrition provided through the GI tract via tube, catheter, or stoma (enteral) or intravenously (centrally, or peripherally) (parenteral).

□ Initiate enteral or parenteral nutrition
□ Modify rate, concentration, composition or schedule
□ Discontinue enteral or parenteral nutrition
□ Insert enteral feeding tube
□ Site care
□ Other (*specify*)

SUPPLEMENTS — ND

Medical Food Supplements — ND-3.1
Commercial or prepared foods or beverages that supplement energy, protein, carbohydrate, fiber, fat intake.

Type
□ Commercial beverage
□ Commercial food
□ Modified beverage
□ Modified food

Purpose
(*specify*)

Vitamin and Mineral Supplements — ND-3.2
Supplemental vitamins or minerals.

□ Multivitamin/mineral
□ Vitamin

□ A	□ C
□ Thiamin	□ D
□ Riboflavin	□ E
□ Niacin	□ K
□ Folate	□ Multivitamin
□ Other (*specify*)	

□ Mineral

□ Calcium	□ Iron
□ Potassium	□ Zinc
□ Phosphorus	□ Magnesium
□ Multi-trace elements	
□ Other (*specify*)	

Bioactive Substance Supplement — ND-3.3
Supplemental bioactive substances.

□ Initiate
□ Dose change
□ Form change
□ Route change
□ Administration schedule
□ Discontinue
(*specify*)

Feeding Assistance — ND-4
Accommodation or assistance in eating.

□ Adaptive equipment
□ Feeding position
□ Meal set-up
□ Mouth care
□ Other (*specify*)